HYGIENE AND ITS ROLE IN HEALTH

HYGIENE AND ITS ROLE IN HEALTH

PATRICK L. ANDERSON AND JEROME P. LACHAN
EDITORS

Nova Science Publishers, Inc.
New York

For permission to use material from this book please contact us:
Telephone 631-231-7269; Fax 631-231-8175
Web Site: http://www.novapublishers.com

NOTICE TO THE READER

The Publisher has taken reasonable care in the preparation of this book, but makes no expressed or implied warranty of any kind and assumes no responsibility for any errors or omissions. No liability is assumed for incidental or consequential damages in connection with or arising out of information contained in this book. The Publisher shall not be liable for any special, consequential, or exemplary damages resulting, in whole or in part, from the readers' use of, or reliance upon, this material. Any parts of this book based on government reports are so indicated and copyright is claimed for those parts to the extent applicable to compilations of such works.

Independent verification should be sought for any data, advice or recommendations contained in this book. In addition, no responsibility is assumed by the publisher for any injury and/or damage to persons or property arising from any methods, products, instructions, ideas or otherwise contained in this publication.

This publication is designed to provide accurate and authoritative information with regard to the subject matter covered herein. It is sold with the clear understanding that the Publisher is not engaged in rendering legal or any other professional services. If legal or any other expert assistance is required, the services of a competent person should be sought. FROM A DECLARATION OF PARTICIPANTS JOINTLY ADOPTED BY A COMMITTEE OF THE AMERICAN BAR ASSOCIATION AND A COMMITTEE OF PUBLISHERS.

Library of Congress Cataloging-in-Publication Data

Hygiene and its role in health / Patrick L. Anderson and Jerome P. Lachan (editors).
      p. ; cm.
Includes bibliographical reference and index.
ISBN 978-1-60456-195-1 (hardcover)
1. Hygiene. 2. Public health. 3. Medicine, Preventive. 4. Health promotion. I. Anderson, Patrick L. II. Lachan, Jerome P.
[DNLM: 1. Hygiene. 2. Communicable Disease Control. 3. Health Promotion. QT 180 H996 2007]
RA425.H94 2007
613--dc22   2007046680

Published by Nova Science Publishers, Inc. ≃ New York

Hygiene and its Role in Health Errata   (ISBN: 978-1-60456-195-1)
Editors: Patrick L. Anderson and Jerome P. Lachan

Is Hand Hygiene Linked to Health Benefits in the Community in Developed Countries? (Thea F. van de Mortel) should be Chapter 6

Contents

Preface

Hygiene refers to practices associated with ensuring good health and cleanliness. The scientific term "hygiene" refers to the maintenance of health and healthy living. The term appears in phrases such as personal hygiene, domestic hygiene, dental hygiene, and occupational hygiene and is frequently used in connection with public health. The term "hygiene" is derived from Hygieia, the Greek goddess of health, cleanliness and sanitation. Hygiene is also a science that deals with the promotion and preservation of health. This new book presents recent and important research in this field.

Expert Commentary - In several studies, primarily from developed countries, an association between hepatitis A virus (HAV) and atopic diseases, including asthma, allergic rhinitis, and atopic dermatitis has been found. Whereas such an association has not been found in other studies, but thise studies primary came from underdeveloped countries. The finding that being seropositive to HAV is associated with a lower prevalence of atopy and respiratory allergies has been interpreted as HAV infection protecting against atopy. But this assumption can only be true if the HAV infection precedes the establishment of the atopic phenotype. If the atopic phenotype precedes the HAV infection, then the opposite assumption must be true i.e., it is the atopic phenotype that protects against HAV infections. An HAV infection is of short duration, and the virus is permanently cleared from the body. The finding of an association between atopy and HAV was taken as an indirect evidence for "the hygiene hypothesis". Recently, by studying different polymorphisms in the TIM-1 allele and their interactions with HAV it was argued that a special insertion variant in combination with HAV infection protects against atopy and that this was the first genetic evidence for the hygiene hypothesis. In this study, the authors discuss these findings and show that the interaction with HAV and the TIM-1 alleles cannot be taken as a genetic evidence for the hygiene hypothesis. Because atopy and the TIM-1 alleles are not independent variables, the argument, that the insertion variant in combination with HAV infection protecting against atopy, is not valid. Additionally, despite epidemiological findings of an interaction between HAV infections and atopy there is not necessarily a causal relationship to the development of atopy. Indeed, the opposite assumption could be true, that the atopic condition protects or is associated with mechanisms that protect against HAV infections.

Chapter 1 - Oral health is known to be associated with general health. Much oral significance is closely related to systemic diseases. There are several categories of systemic patients for whom specific needs of dental care and counseling are needed. In some instances, so as to reach the optimal total health care, a combination of medical and dental care is necessary. Furthermore, poor oral hygiene itself is a risk factor for systemic diseases such as periodontal status which can increase the severity of heart disease and diabetes.

Oral hygiene assessments are important so as to eliminate predisposing factors for oral complications such as nasopharynx cancer, immune-compromised disease, diabetes and valvular heart diseases in patients. Since early assessment can reduce both the incidence and severity of oral complications, some early appropriate interventions can be engaged according to the individual's treatment needs. It is necessary to carry out consistency in the treatment by including periodically follow up and appropriate counseling to the patients, so they may be able to take care of themselves up to the desired outcome. This review focuses on the oral health care for specific groups of the systemic patients *i.e.* diabetes, head and neck cancers, cardiovascular disease, and AIDS.

Chapter 2 – Nowadays hygiene and asepsis took an important place in all the medical fields and particularly in Dentistry, because the "hand of the dentist" can constitute a important source of infection. So, one basic measure of infection control, supposes a careful hand washing and the use of gloves which form a physical barrier and protect the Health Care Workers from occupational exposure to blood and saliva.

The authors' study carried out with the University Dental Clinic of Monastir (Tunisia) aims to evaluate knowledge in dental practice and to investigate their attitudes and practices toward the use of the gloves. It consists of a survey by auto-administrated questionnaire managed to a sample of 106 dental practitioners including 16 teachers, 26 trainees and 64 dental students.

Findings revealed that about 78.3% of dentists wore gloves, 21.7% wore masks and 2% wore protective eyeglasses. The students have a minimum necessary knowledge about gloves use but do not have a correct practice while the other practitioners have the good knowledge and the good practical attitudes.

The authors' study shows an important need to improve the students' behaviour with respect of occupational hygiene and safety conditions in order to reduce occupational blood exposure hazards.

Chapter 3 - Norovirus disease, a highly infectious gastroenteritis, traditionally known as winter vomiting disease, is spreading rapidly across many countries and continents. Schools, hospitals, hotels, cruise ships and facilities for the elderly are particularly prone to outbreaks of infection. Although few persons die from the infection, the burden of illness is high since many people can be afflicted in outbreaks. Norovirus is known to occur after eating contaminated food however the majority of cases have resulted from person to person transmission and via environmental contamination. This can occur when persons or health care workers have poor personal hygiene or where there is failure to clean common areas properly.

A protracted outbreak of Norovirus occurred in a hotel in Malta between March and October 2006 with four identified outbreaks affecting a total of 337 persons. The recurrent waves of infection in successive cohorts of tourists indicated a source of environmental contamination. Traditional cleaning agents were not sufficient to eliminate the source of infection. The outbreaks were only successfully curtailed with isolation of ill patients;

environmental cleaning with appropriate agents; specific prevention strategies including the early identification of patients; contact precautions with patients; enhanced patient and staff hygiene and training and discipline during food preparation and serving.

Environmental contamination has been shown to be implicated in Norovirus outbreaks. Hygiene measures are not a luxury but a necessity to help reduce the burden of this highly contagious infectious disease.

Chapter 4 - Street-vended food raises concerns with respect to their potential for serious foodborne bacterial and viral illnesses. Food associated viruses such as gastroenteritis Human calicivirus (HuCV) Norovirus (NLV), Rotavirus (RV), Hepatitis A Virus (HAV), Poliovirus (PV) are responsible for a high number of infectious diseases in human. In addition to foodborne viruses via faecal contamination in the food chain, there are emerging zoonotic viral agents such as Avian Influenza Virus (AIV) H_5N_1 and Severe Acute Respiratory Syndrome Coronavirus: SARS-CoV. Food my be a vetor for this agent asociated to raw foodstuffs in primary production level. Epidemiological data on foodborne viruses analysis shown that one of the most prominent emerging food safety problems stem from viruses because they are not well-known and classical food safety measures are not alsways efficient on them. International concepts such as *Food Safety Objectives* (FSO), *Hazards Analysis and Critical Control Points* (HACCP) and *Behavioral Risk Factors Surveillance System* (BRFS), used for risk assessment were applied to street food process, for indentification of factors playing an important role for contamination by viruses and bacteria during the food processing. These principles were allowed to well-know epidemiology of foodborne pathogens. Epidemiology of foodborne viral diseases is changing, and reemerging viral diseases take place through a complex interaction of social, economic, evolutionary, and ecological factors. They included changes in the pathogens; development, urbanization and new lifestyles; cuts in health systems; unknowledge on viruses, demographic changes, farming system, food handling behaviors, food processing system, environmental conditions, poverty and pollution. As recommends by the Advisory Committee on Microbial Safety of Food to use Kaplan criteria which can give strong circumstantial evidence that an outbreak is attribuable to pathogen agent; these criteria were took into account to give more accurate reflection of the involvement of viruses in incidence of foodborne diseases. Understanding the factors associated with safe street food handling will assist in development of effective safe-street-vended food instruction programs.

Chapter 5 - *Escherichia coli* O157:H7 is an important foodborne pathogen. It was recognized as a cause of severe human illness only in the early 1980's. Since then it has been implicated in foodborne disease outbreaks in many countries throughout the world. Cattle are the main reservoir of this microrganism, and transmission of the infection to humans occurs primarily through the consumption of contaminated food. The pathogenicity of *E. coli* O157:H7 is associated to genes encoding for a number of virulence factors, especially the verotoxin-encoding genes. The infective dose is extremely low - in the order of a few bacterial units. *E. coli* O157:H7 is acid-tolerant and survives in acidic environments such as the gastric barrier and acidic foods. The most severe illnesses induced by *E. coli* O157:H7 are Hemorrhagic Colitis and Hemolytic Uremic Syndrome. Both these clinical forms are characterized by severe morbidity and might sometimes be lethal. Children are the most commonly affected age group and they are affected by the highest death rate. *E. coli*

O157:H7 is one of the main food safety hazards having important implications for human health worldwide, since outbreaks lead sometimes to cases of mortality. This review examines the etiological and epidemiological aspects of *E. coli* O157:H7 infection and focuses on the food safety concerns raised by *E. coli* O157:H7 and on control methods for the prevention of food poisoning.

Chapter 6 - Mortality rates from infectious diseases have declined dramatically in developed countries over the last century, largely due to improvements in nutrition, sanitation, and vaccination, and to the development of effective antimicrobials. Research has demonstrated that hands can be contaminated by pathogens, and that washing hands or using a waterless hand sanitizer can reduce that microbial contamination. Increased frequency of hand hygiene in homes, child care facilities, schools, and workplaces is therefore hypothesized to reduce infectious illness in the community, thus reducing morbidity and mortality and improving productivity as well as providing both a health and a cost benefit to the community. There is some evidence to support this hypothesis in the developing world, where infectious illnesses are very common and a major source of morbidity and mortality for the population, particularly for children. However, in a modern society that has proper sanitation, clean water, plentiful food and access to good health care, does increased hand hygiene frequency or the use of antimicrobial hand hygiene solutions significantly improve health and reduce costs in the community outside of the hospital setting? Various studies have examined infectious illness and/or illness absenteeism outcomes in response to hand hygiene programs in first world homes, child care facilities, elementary schools, colleges and some workplaces, with effects ranging from a lack of significant improvement to reductions in illness and illness absenteeism of up to 50%. However, the studies are often confounded by poor research design, including lack of randomisation and blinding, failure to calculate sample sizes and power, failure to analyse on the basis of intention to treat, and failure to take clustering into account when calculating sample sizes and analysing data, most of which have a tendency to increase the chance of spurious positive findings. Reductions in mild infectious illnesses, such as colds, must also be offset against possible adverse effects of frequent hand hygiene such as skin damage and the increased risk of atopy in children exposed to a very hygienic environment in early life. This chapter will discuss the relative benefits and costs of hand hygiene programs in developed countries in the community setting and make some suggestions on the design and analysis of future programs.

Chapter 7 - The purpose of this study was to improve the understanding of sexuality and sexual behaviors of adolescents and to identify factors that are relevant for sexual health promotion and HIV/AIDS prevention in adolescents. In order to achieve these goals, two studies, one quantitative, and one qualitative were undertaken. The quantitative study described knowledge, attitudes and sexual behaviors that are important to AIDS prevention and examined the relationship between adolescent sexual behavior and demographic factors, personal characteristics, and social context of young people (family, peers, school and community). Data were collected from the Portuguese sample of Health Behaviour in School-aged Children/WHO study, 2002. The qualitative study was used to identify and understand the dynamics of protective and risk factors relevant to AIDS prevention at individual and contextual level. In this study, 12 focus groups were conducted in six secondary schools from different geographic areas of Portugal. In the quantitative study the percent of adolescents reporting ever had sexual intercourse was 23.7%. With respect to use of condoms, 29.9% of the adolescents reported that they or their partner didn't use a condom last time they had engage in sexual intercourse. The findings put forward differences in gender and age in knowledge, attitudes and sexual behaviors. The logistic regression analysis showed that the variables "have sexual intercourse" and "didn't used condom last time they engage in sexual intercourse" are associated with socio-demographic characteristics, individual, family, peers, school and community variables. The qualitative study results underline that issues related to sexuality are complex and knowledge, attitudes and sexual behaviors are influenced by multiple determinants at different levels: individual, family, peers, school and community. The findings suggest that protective and risk factors interact with each other within a network of possible relations that either reduce or increase the probability of involvement in risk behaviors. The results of the two studies suggest that adolescents can't be seen like a homogeneous group concerning knowledge, attitudes and sexual behaviors and HIV/AIDS. They highlight the significance of early interventions that involve young people, but also agents of socialization in the reduction of risk factors and the promotion of protecting factors. This study confirms that complementary use of different methodologies is an appropriate strategy to increase knowledge and understanding about complex meanings in which sexuality is submersed. This work can be useful to design and implement a comprehensive programme on sexual health promotion and AIDS prevention in young people.

Chapter 8 - School Health Program (SHP) is defined with respect to environment, services, and education. It should be a plan with a good vision so that it will be fruitful. School Health Program is to be conducted to ensure a healthy environment in schools and to promote the health of the school children. It helps to prevent the different diseases and make the children conscious about their health. SHP makes easy for early diagnosis, treatment, follow-up, and check regularly to the diseased and non-diseased students. A new concept of SHP, which is an emerging need for developing countries, is also included in this study. It is one of the cost effective program if implemented at a national and international level and make aware all the nongovernmental organizations/international non-governmental organizations/donors to spend their money in this type of program.

Chapter 9 - This study describes potential personal, household and community hygiene motivators and de-motivators among 494 villagers in the Eastern Cape. Over 50% were 26-50 years, male, married, employed and had secondary education. Individual interviews were conducted using an interview schedule with open ended questions. More than 50% viewed access to regular water supply as a hygiene motivator and the lack thereof as a de-motivator. Personal hygiene (30%), refuse/solid waste disposal (14.2%), safe human excreta disposal (28.5%) and safe liquid waste disposal (12.0%) facilities were viewed as hygiene motivators and the lack of these as de-motivators. Hygiene education was identified as a motivator for personal (7.5%), household (7.6%) and community (7.8%) hygiene and the lack of it as a de-motivator. Protected household water storage facilities (10.2%), money to purchase both personal hygiene items (10.5%) and domestic hygiene detergents (8.4%) were seen as hygiene motivators and the lack of these as de-motivators.

Chapter 10 - *Introduction:* According to the opinion of gerontologists, it is possible to prevent or delay the negative influence of aging on mental and physical health status by healthy behaviors. "Active aging" people bring a lot for their societies and that's why activity is the value not only for the elderly but also for the societies.

Aim: The purpose of the research was to assess the impact of various forms of the activity (physical, pro-social and intellectual) on the health condition people who are 65 years old and older.

Material and Methods: The research was conducted by anonymous questionnaire forms. A nation-wide research had been preceded by a pilot study. After a preliminary qualification and selection of 2,072 questionnaires, a further analysis of 1,910 questionnaires (92.6%) have been finally classified. The condition of health has been evaluated on the basis of information: illness and health problems, self-evaluation of health condition, body weight, use of medical assistance, and other aids, hospitalization and reasons for it and presence of at least one group of disabled persons whose mobility is limited and reasons for these limitations. The extent of psycho-social health has been evaluated on the basis of moods such as sadness, depression, limited life enthusiasm, assessment of satisfaction resulting from contacts with relatives and other persons, and identification of problems connected with aging.

Results: Active persons determine their health condition more positively, they suffer from fewer CVDs and their health is more stable, they have a better psychological condition (loneliness, depression), and they are less often use medical services in hospitals.

Disability recognized in legal terms and formal disability, except 1st disability category (the hardest cases) and persons who are immobile does not constitute any barrier in becoming active. Similarly, diseases don't exclude activity, except pathologies that limit or prevent elderly people from partaking in any activities. Activity has a positive impact on keeping a proper body weight. Active persons stay independent, are satisfied with life more often, feel that they are needed, and their self-esteem is high. It seems that a barrier in the psychological sense in becoming active by elderly people is the fact that they are less willing to become active. The majority of respondents have admitted that their health condition has deteriorated drastically at the age of 63 to 64.

Conclusion: Analysis of results has confirmed the existence of a relation between activity and health condition. Activity (different kinds) is deciding about healthy aging and it is simultaneously a positive indicator.

In: Hygiene and Its Role in Health
Editors: P. L. Anderson and J. P. Lachan

ISBN 978-1-60456-195-1
© 2008 Nova Science Publishers, Inc.

Expert Commentary

Does Hepatitis A Offer Protection against Asthma or Does Asthma Offer Protection Against Hepatitis A?

Lars-Georg Hersoug[*a] and *José Arnau*[b]

[a]Research Centre for Prevention and Health,
Copenhagen County, Denmark
[b]Unizyme Laboratories A/S, Dr. Neergaardsvej 17,
DK-2970 Hoersholm, Denmark

Abstract

In several studies, primarily from developed countries, an association between hepatitis A virus (HAV) and atopic diseases, including asthma, allergic rhinitis, and atopic dermatitis has been found. Whereas such an association has not been found in other studies, but thise studies primary came from underdeveloped countries. The finding that being seropositive to HAV is associated with a lower prevalence of atopy and respiratory allergies has been interpreted as HAV infection protecting against atopy. But this assumption can only be true if the HAV infection precedes the establishment of the atopic phenotype. If the atopic phenotype precedes the HAV infection, then the opposite assumption must be true i.e., it is the atopic phenotype that protects against HAV infections. An HAV infection is of short duration, and the virus is permanently cleared from the body. The finding of an association between atopy and HAV was taken as an indirect evidence for "the hygiene hypothesis". Recently, by studying different polymorphisms in the TIM-1 allele and their interactions with HAV it was argued that a special insertion variant in combination with HAV infection protects against atopy and

---

[*] Corresponding author: Lars-Georg Hersoug, M.Sc., Research Centre for Prevention and Health, Glostrup University Hospital, 57 Nrd Ringvej, building 84/85, DK-2600 Glostrup, Denmark. Phone +45 43233260 Fax +45 43233977 E-mail: hersoug@vip.cybercity.dk or lagehe01@glo.regionh.dk

that this was the first genetic evidence for the hygiene hypothesis. In this study, we discuss these findings and show that the interaction with HAV and the TIM-1 alleles cannot be taken as a genetic evidence for the hygiene hypothesis. Because atopy and the TIM-1 alleles are not independent variables, the argument, that the insertion variant in combination with HAV infection protecting against atopy, is not valid. Additionally, despite epidemiological findings of an interaction between HAV infections and atopy there is not necessarily a causal relationship to the development of atopy. Indeed, the opposite assumption could be true, that the atopic condition protects or is associated with mechanisms that protect against HAV infections.

Keywords: *Hepatitis A, atopy, asthma, hygiene hypothesis, TIM-1.*

Abbreviations: *HAV = hepatitis A virus.*

Introduction

Atopic diseases, including asthma, allergic rhinitis, and atopic dermatitis have increased dramatically over the past three decades [1;2]. Strachan (1989) observed an inverse relation between the number of older siblings and allergic diseases. He formulated "the hygiene hypothesis", proposing that protection from these diseases might be exerted by infections acquired early, often during childhood, as the result of unhygienic contact with older siblings [3-6]. A number of studies had shown a dose-related protection of atopy and respiratory allergy with orofecal-foodborne microbial load including exposure to hepatitis A (HAV) [7-9]. Another study [10] found a protective effect on atopy from orofecal-foodborne infections on the basis of *helicobacter pylori* infections, but infections with HAV had the opposite trend. A recent study carried out in Iceland, Estonia, and Sweden did not find a protective effect on atopy from HAV [11]. However, in this study the prevalence of HAV infection was low (14%) and more than half of the positive subjects came from Estonia. This may have decreased the power of the study to detect a significant relationship between HAV infections and atopy. The studies that have shown a protective effect associated with HAV infections have predominantly been from developed countries [7-9;12] whereas, others not showing a protective effect have been mostly from underdeveloped countries [13-18]. Why HAV infections have such an inconsistent effect on atopy in different populations is difficult to determine. It is necessary to be very careful in the interpretation of scientific results. Otherwise, as we shall see below, we may easily come to the wrong conclusions.

Is There A Link between HAV and Atopic Diseases?

A study among Italian military students showed an association between seropositivity to HAV and atopy. Atopy was less common among HAV seropositive than seronegative subjects. This finding was taken as indirect evidence for "the hygiene hypothesis" where common infections acquired early in life was assumed to reduce the risk of developing atopy [8].

HAV is one of the most reliable markers of being exposed to unhygienical conditions. The presence of HAV antibodies is considered as the result of exposure to an infectious environment is considered in Southern Europe to [19]. Having many older siblings is also assumed to be a marker for an infectious environment. They conclude that because of the presence of many older siblings (among seronegative subjects) or because of unhygienic living conditions (among seropositive subjects) that the finding of the association between HAV and atopy added evidence to the working hypothesis that common infections acquired early in life (i.e., HAV) may have reduced the risk of developing atopy. For this conclusion to hold, they must assume that the infection with HAV should be acquired before the development of the atopic phenotype. If the development of the atopic phenotype precedes the HAV infection then the opposite assumption must be true i.e., it is the atopic phenotype that protects against HAV infections. It is well established that atopy most often develops early in life. The working hypothesis postulates that pregnancy causes a natural deviation against a Th2 phenotype in the mother and child. This is an evolutionary adaptation designed to protect against rejection of the maternal unit. After birth, the normal child will gradually change phenotype towards Th1. In the atopic child, a failure of the immune deviation will result in a continuing expression of the Th2 phenotype and this will favour an allergen-driven immune response [20]. In developed populations there will be a low probability of being infected with HAV early in life. In the Italian study [8] it is likely that the atopic condition has developed before HAV infection occurs. The study was a prospective study and the data about the time of HAV infection was not available. If the infection with HAV had occurred after the development of atopy, then the correct assumption would be that the atopic condition protects or is associated with mechanisms that protects against HAV (figure 1).

Recently McIntyre et al. [21] discovered a genetic interaction between HAV and a TIM-1 allele and claimed that this was the first genetic evidence for the hygiene hypothesis.

These results have also been published elsewhere [22-24]. By positional cloning, a special gene, TIM-1, was identified as a strong candidate for atopy and asthma. TIM-1 (also known as HAVcr-1) is the only known cell-surface receptor used by HAV to infect human cells [24]. TIM-1 is expressed in CD4$^+$ T cells, which play a critical role in the regulation of airway hyper reactivity (AHR) and in the pathogenesis of asthma. TIM-1 transcription occurs during primary antigen stimulation, a period crucial in influencing T-cell differentiation and commitment to Th2 cytokine production [25]. Several variants of TIM-1 were identified e.g., a six-amino-acid insertion (ins) at residue 157, termed 157insMTTTVP and two single-amino-acid changes, 195delT (where "del" refers to a deletion) and A206T.

The 157insMTTTVP variant results in efficient HAV un-coating and it are suggested that this variation may affect the efficiency of viral entry [26].

To determine the effect of the insertion 157insMTTTVP on the occurrence of atopy, a cross-sectional study was carried out on 375 individuals who were evaluated by history and tested serologically for atopy and prior HAV infections. Among them, 185 individuals carried the 157insMTTTVP variant of TIM-1 and 136 had the wild type allele. Data is shown in table 1. Based on this data it was concluded that HAV seropositivity protects against atopy, but only in individuals with the 157insMTTTVP variant of TIM-1.

The relationship between HAV and atopy.

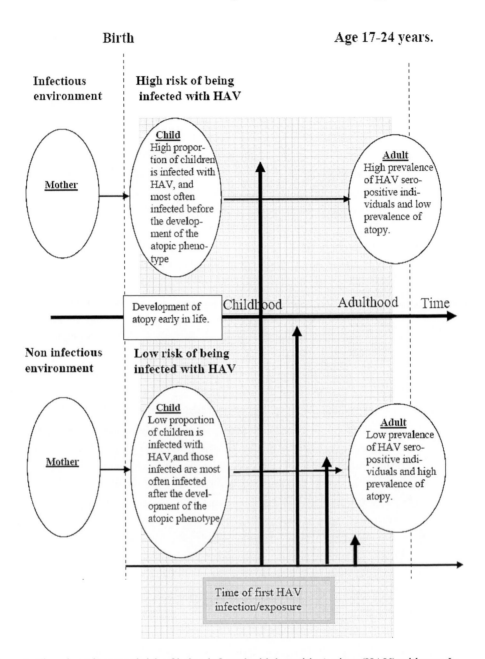

Figure 1. There is an increased risk of being infected with hepatitis A virus (HAV) with age. In infectious environments (in underdeveloped countries) most of the children are infected before the atopic phenotype is established. In non-infectious environments (developed countries) children are normally infected after the atopic phenotype is established.

These data are indeed interesting but there is a serious problem with the data the authors presented to support the postulate (table 1). Because TIM-1 is proposed as an asthma-susceptible gene and, therefore, we must assume that the insertion 157insMTTTVP must influence the prevalence of asthma and atopy. In addition, TIM-1 is the surface receptor for HAV entry. It is clear that none of these factors are independent. Nevertheless, the authors stratify the data by dividing them in groups of seropositive and seronegative HAV individuals. This is equivalent to solving an equation with more than one unknown factor.

Table 1. TIM-1 insertion 157insMTTTVP and protection against atopy subdivided in hepatitis A status

(n=321) HAV status	157insMTTTVP genotype	Total	Atopic	Non-atopic	χ^2 (P)
Seronegative (n=198)	Insertion	120	83 (69%)	37 (31%)	0.463
	No insertion	78	50 (64%)	28 (36%)	(0.496)
Seropositive (n=123)	Insertion	65	31 (48%)	34 (52%)	11.978
	No insertion	58	46 (79%)	12 (21%)	(0.0005)

Data from table 1: McIntyre et al. *Nature* 425;576 (2003). Printed with permission from the authors and NPG (Nature's Publishing Group).

Table 2. TIM-1 insertion 157insMTTTVP and protection against atopy with no subdivision in hepatitis A status

(n=321)	157insMTTTVP genotype	Total	Atopic	Non-atopic	χ^2 (P)
	Insertion	185	114 (62%)	71 (38%)	10.376
	No insertion	136	96 (71%)	40 (29%)	(<0.01)

Data from table 1 is used to create data in this table. The χ^2-test shows that there are significant differences between the two groups with and without the insertion.

Table 3. TIM-1 insertion 157insMTTTVP and hepatitis A (HAV) status

(n=321)	HAV status	Total	157insMTTTVP genotype	χ^2 (P)
	seronegative	198	120 (61%)	1.8713
	seropositive	123	65 (53%)	(<0.20)

Data from table 1 is used to create data in this table. The χ^2-test shows that there is no significant difference between the two groups with and without the insertion.

This might explain the inadequate interpretation of the data from table 1. In table 2 it is illustrated why the proposed mechanisms might be misleading. Taken away the stratification on HAV status it is possible to establish the effect of 157insMTTTVP on the prevalence of atopy. The atopic prevalence for subjects with 157insMTTTVP is 62% while it is 71% for individuals with wild type TIM-1. Therefore it may be concluded that there is only a slightly higher protection against atopy for 157insMTTTVP allele. Additionally, it was proposed that the 157insMTTTVP should be more effective in un-coating HAV and, therefore, we must assume that having the 157insMTTTVP allele should increase the risk of being infected with HAV. In table 3, it is shown that there is not a significant difference between the prevalence of being seronegative or seropositive with the 157insMTTTVP allele. If any thing, there seems to be a trend in the opposite direction, the prevalence of being seronegative with the 157insMTTTVP was 61% and being seropositive with the 157insMTTTVP allele was 53%. Therefore, it is not possible to conclude that having the 157insMTTTVP allele should increase the risk of being infected with HAV. On the contrary, the assumption that the atopic condition protects or is associated with mechanisms that protect against HAV infections may be more correct because it is in better accordance with the assumption that the development of the atopic phenotype most often precedes the HVA infection. If the observed protective effect of HAV on atopy should be interpreted as a protective effect of atopy on the HAV infection, then we also get the answers to why there are differences between developed and underdeveloped countries. The protective effect of HAV infections on atopy has predominantly been observed in epidemiological studies from developed countries where the probability of getting a HAV infection is more likely to occur after the atopic phenotype is acquired and therefore potentially could inhibit HAV infection. Whereas, in underdeveloped countries where it is more likely to be infected before the atopic phenotype is established there would be no effect on HAV infection. The immune system has two phenotypes the normal (dominated by Th1-helper cells) and the atopic (dominated by Th2- helper cells). It may be reasonable to assume, because an HAV infection is of short duration, that the actual immunological phenotype, at the time of infection, is more likely to influence the susceptibility to HAV than the HAV infection and could be responsible to the immune deviation towards the atopic phenotype, even for a long time after it has been eliminated by the immune system.

It has been assumed, because HAV is not a respiratory pathogen, and because HAV is transmitted through fecal-oral routes, that infections with HAV are not necessarily causally related to the development of atopy but could only be a marker for living in an unhygienic environment. This argument may only hold in underdeveloped countries.

Conclusion

A number of studies have found that being seropositive to HAV is associated with a lower prevalence of atopy and respiratory allergies. This has been interpreted as if HAV infection protects against atopy. But this assumption can only be true if the HAV infection precedes the establishment of the atopic phenotype. If the atopic phenotype precedes the HAV infection then the opposite assumption that it is the atopic phenotype that protects against HAV infections must be true. Additionally, the proposed interaction between TIM-1 insertion 157insMTTTVP and HAV as a genetic evidence for the hygiene hypothesis is indeed not convincing. At the moment there is no proof for the hypothesis that the TIM-1 gene is involved in the protective effect of HAV against the development of atopy. On the contrary, the assumption that the atopic condition protects or is associated with mechanisms that protect against HAV infections may be more correct. The differentiated effect of the immunological phenotypes (Th1 or Th2) on susceptibility to infections is not investigated and it is clear that much more research in this field is needed.

References

[1]   Woolcock AJ, Peat JK. Evidence for the increase in asthma worldwide. *Ciba Found.Symp.* 1997;206:122-34.

[2]   Bjorksten B. Environmental factors and respiratory hypersensitivity: experiences from studies in Eastern and Western Europe. *Toxicol Lett.* 1996;86:93-8.

[3]   Strachan DP. Hay fever, hygiene, and household size. *BMJ* 1989;299:1259-60.

[4]   Strachan DP, Griffith JM, Anderson HR, Johnston IDA. Allergic sensitization and position in the sibship: anational study of yong British adults. *Thorax* 1994;49:1053P.

[5]   Strachan DP. Epidemiology of hay fever: towards a community diagnosis. *Clin. Exp. Allergy* 1995;25:296-303.

[6]   Williams HC, Strachan DP, Hay RJ. Childhood eczema: disease of the advantaged? *BMJ* 1994;308:1132-5.

[7]   Linneberg A, Ostergaard C, Tvede M et al. IgG antibodies against microorganisms and atopic disease in Danish adults: the Copenhagen Allergy Study. *J. Allergy Clin. Immunol.* 2003;111:847-53.

[8]   Matricardi PM, Rosmini F, Ferrigno L et al. Cross sectional retrospective study of prevalence of atopy among Italian military students with antibodies against hepatitis A virus. *BMJ* 1997;314:999-1003.

[9]   Matricardi PM, Rosmini F, Panetta V, Ferrigno L, Bonini S. Hay fever and asthma in relation to markers of infection in the United States. *J. Allergy Clin. Immunol.* 2002;110:381-7.

[10]   von Hertzen LC, Laatikainen T, Makela MJ et al. Infectious burden as a determinant of atopy-- a comparison between adults in Finnish and Russian Karelia. *Int. Arch. Allergy Immunol.* 2006;140:89-95.

[11]   Janson C, Asbjornsdottir H, Birgisdottir A et al. The effect of infectious burden on the prevalence of atopy and respiratory allergies in Iceland, Estonia, and Sweden. *J. Allergy Clin. Immunol.* 2007.

[12]   Kosunen TU, Hook-Nikanne J, Salomaa A, Sarna S, Aromaa A, Haahtela T. Increase of allergen-specific immunoglobulin E antibodies from 1973 to 1994 in a Finnish population and a possible relationship to Helicobacter pylori infections. *Clin. Exp. Allergy* 2002;32:373-8.

[13]   Law M, Morris JK, Wald N, Luczynska C, Burney P. Changes in atopy over a quarter of a century, based on cross sectional data at three time periods. *BMJ* 2005;330:1187-8.

[14]   Gonzalez-Quintela A, Gude F, Boquete O et al. Association of hepatitis A virus infection with allergic sensitization in a population with high prevalence of hepatitis A virus exposure. *Allergy* 2005;60:98-103.

[15] Uter W, Stock C, Pfahlberg A et al. Association between infections and signs and symptoms of 'atopic' hypersensitivity--results of a cross-sectional survey among first-year university students in Germany and Spain. *Allergy* 2003;58:580-4.

[16] Bodner C, Anderson WJ, Reid TS, Godden DJ. Childhood exposure to infection and risk of adult onset wheeze and atopy. *Thorax* 2000;55:383-7.

[17] Scrivener S, Yemaneberhan H, Zebenigus M et al. Independent effects of intestinal parasite infection and domestic allergen exposure on risk of wheeze in Ethiopia: a nested case-control study. *Lancet* 2001;358:1493-9.

[18] Jarvis D, Luczynska C, Chinn S, Burney P. The association of hepatitis A and Helicobacter pylori with sensitization to common allergens, asthma and hay fever in a population of young British adults. *Allergy* 2004;59:1063-7.

[19] Papaevangelou G. Epidemiology of hepatitis A in Mediteranean countries. *Vaccine* 1992;10(suppl):63-6.

[20] Holt PG. Programming for Responsiveness to Environmental Antigens That Trigger Allergic Respiratory Disease in Adulthood Is Initiated during the Perinatal Period. *Environ. Health Perspect.* 1998;106:795-800.

[21] McIntire JJ, Umetsu SE, Macaubas C et al. Immunology: hepatitis A virus link to atopic disease. *Nature* 2003;425:576.

[22] Umetsu DT, McIntire JJ, DeKruyff RH. TIM-1, hepatitis A virus and the hygiene theory of atopy: association of TIM-1 with atopy. *J. Pediatr. Gastroenterol. Nutr.* 2005;40 Suppl 1:S43.

[23] Umetsu DT, DeKruyff RH. Regulation of tolerance in the respiratory tract: TIM-1, hygiene, and the environment. *Ann. NY Acad. Sci.* 2004;1029:88-93.

[24] McIntire JJ, Umetsu DT, DeKruyff RH. TIM-1, a novel allergy and asthma susceptibility gene. *Springer Semin. Immunopathol.* 2004;25:335-48.

[25] McIntire JJ, Umetsu SE, Akbari O et al. Identification of Tapr (an airway hyperreactivity regulatory locus) and the linked Tim gene family. *Nat. Immunol.* 2001;2:1109-16.

[26] Silberstein E, Xing L, van de BW, Lu J, Cheng H, Kaplan GG. Alteration of hepatitis A virus (HAV) particles by a soluble form of HAV cellular receptor 1 containing the immunoglobin-and mucin-like regions. *J. Virol.* 2003;77:8765-74.

In: Hygiene and Its Role in Health   ISBN 978-1-60456-195-1
Editors: P. L. Anderson and J. P. Lachan   © 2008 Nova Science Publishers, Inc.

Chapter 1

Oral Health Care in Systemic Diseases

Sirikarn Sutthavong*, Pornchai Jansisyanont** and Atik Sangasapaviriya***

*Dental Department, Phramongkutklao Hospital,
Bangkok 10400 Thailand
**Department of Oral and Maxillofacial Surgery,
Faculty of Dentistry, Chulalongkorn University,
Bangkok 10300 Thailand
***Department of Medicine, Phramongkutklao Hospital,
Bangkok 10400 Thailand*

Abstract

Oral health is known to be associated with general health. Much oral significance is closely related to systemic diseases. There are several categories of systemic patients for whom specific needs of dental care and counseling are needed. In some instances, so as to reach the optimal total health care, a combination of medical and dental care is necessary. Furthermore, poor oral hygiene itself is a risk factor for systemic diseases such as periodontal status which can increase the severity of heart disease and diabetes.

Oral hygiene assessments are important so as to eliminate predisposing factors for oral complications such as nasopharynx cancer, immune-compromised disease, diabetes and valvular heart diseases in patients. Since early assessment can reduce both the incidence and severity of oral complications, some early appropriate interventions can be engaged according to the individual's treatment needs. It is necessary to carry out consistency in the treatment by including periodically follow up and appropriate counseling to the patients, so they may be able to take care of themselves up to the desired outcome. This review focuses on the oral health care for specific groups of the systemic patients *i.e.* diabetes, head and neck cancers, cardiovascular disease, and AIDS.

* Correspondance to: Sutthavong S, Dental Department, Phramongkutklao Hospital, Bangkok 10400, Thailand.
E-mail address: oisiri@yahoo.com

Introduction

General health and oral health cannot be parted. The relations between oral and systemic health are complex and reciprocal, associating many pathophysiological and psychosomatic systems. In several occurrences, oral problems commence in favor of a systemic condition, by which the discrepancy of systemic diseases may result in an impairment of organic functions, exacerbate oral diseases and oral health behavior; vice-versa, the oral conditions can be the premises of systemic deterioration resembling the forming of a vicious cycle. The correlations between oral and systemic health can usually be observed as of the oral manifestations of the systemic conditions per se, oral complications from systemic treatments and drug therapies, localized oropharyngeal infections as the reservoir of pathogens or foci of infections which may exacerbate inflammation and the spread of oral pathogens and their toxins to other organs and tissues. In addition, in the sense of patients' total well being, oral conditions were significantly associated to psycho-physiological health such as pain, discomfort, anxiety, functions and aesthetics which affect the quality of life, and economic efficiency. Health care providers cannot deny that patients are unable to be healthy without good oral health thus, so as to achieve the optimal total health care, the integration of medical and dental care is essential. In addition to that, many patients with systemic diseases have significant needs of oral care in order to maintain the oral health per se or to maintain the recovery of the systemic compromised [1, 2].

Oral hygiene becomes the key role as a risk factor of systemic diseases since meticulous oral hygiene control and regularly maintaining the highest level of oral health is required to prevent the sequel complications. The presenting of dental plaque on the surfaces of the teeth demonstrates an inadequate oral health care. Despite, dental plaque harbors specific bacteria that are the causes of oral diseases such as periodontitis and dental caries. Bacterial levels in dental plaque can reach more than 10^{11} microorganisms/mg and the most common isolated microorganisms were anaerobic and gram negative rods organisms [3-7].

The importance of oral microorganisms: there are definite microorganisms that originate in the oral cavity as the foci of infections and the origin for dissemination of pathogenic organisms to the systemic especially in those who are immunocompromised such as diabetes, and under chemotherapy for treatment of cancer. The increasing levels of the periodontal bacteria including *Actinobacillus actinomycetem comitans*, *Porphyromonas gingivali*, *Tannerella forsythensis* and *Treponima denticola* were observed related to carotid atherosclerosis and coronary heart disease [8-10]. The probable routes of oral infections to the systemic are metastatic infections from oral cavity via transient bacteremia, metastatic injury from circulation of oral microbial toxins and metastatic inflammation caused by immunological injury from oral microorganisms. Trauma to oral mucosal surface is one of the common causes of dissemination of oral microorganisms into the blood circulation particularly at the gingival crevice around the teeth in patients with impaired defense mechanism of the body. The episode of dissemination of pathogens is less than 1 minute after an oral treatment procedure [11, 12]. The occurences of bacteremia following dental procedures and routine daily activities have been observed; in the invasive operations cases such as tooth extractions, endodontic treatment, periodontal surgery, root scaling, and other oral surgery like surgical removal of impacted teeth. In addition, several of oral hygiene care such as tooth brushing, flossing, the use of wooden toothpicks, water irrigation and chewing food has been observed causing bacteremia [13, 14]. Thus, poor oral health particularly in children with chronic illness and in the immunocompromised patients can be a major cause of morbidity and risk factor for severe complications, some of which can even be life threatening. Dental caries is one of the major oral diseases which can lead to pain and infection if left untreated [5, 7, 13-18].

There are several categories of systemic patients, for whom specific needs of dental care and counseling are needed especially those who were admitted in the hospital for a long period of time. They had been observed of having several significant dental needs and about 80% of them required treatments for specific oral conditions and their majority were ignorant of such problems [2]. The main objective of this review is to discuss the oral health care for specific groups of the systemic patients. The diseases selected for discussion are at the top most from the survey of the systemic patients who seek treatment for dental services at our hospital; they are: cardiovascular diseases, diabetes mellitus, allergic diseases, nasopharynx cancer and others respectively. There were a number of patients with HIV infection who required dental services, but did not divulge to their patrician during the inquiry about their health history. The cases recorded were obtained only from those with some specific oral or systemic manifestations and the referred known cases of AIDS. It has not been known exactly how many patients disclosed their HIV status. The disease draws attention to health team due to accumulative number of HIV patients in Thailand. The discussion will focus on the necessary to dental care rather than the details about the drug and treatment modalities of certain systemic diseases.

Cardiovascular Diseases

Cardiovascular diseases (CVD) are the most common causes of death and disability in industrialized countries. The major risk factors associated with CVD were dyslipidemia, low level of high density lipoprotein, smoking, hypertension, and diabetes as well as periodontal disease [19]. There are 6 common groups of patients with CVD can be identified which are ischemic heart disease (IHD) insufficient blood supply to the heart muscle, myocardial infarction (MI) previous ischemic heart muscle, hypertension blood pressure greater than 140/90 mmHg, vulvular and congenital heart disease, arrhythmias and congestive heart failure (CHF) incompetent heart muscle [2, 20].

The relationship between oral health and CVD has been a topic of increasing researches recently, and is supported by data of possible transient bacteremia and elevated inflammatory markers. Since oral mucosa is populated with a dense endogenous microflora, trauma to oral mucosal surface, particularly at gingival crevice around teeth, and oropharynx, many different microbial species can be released transiently into bloodstream. Periodontal disease principally may cause infective endocarditis (IE) which is the net result of the complex interaction between the bloodstream pathogens with matrix molecules and platelets at the sites of endocardial cell damage [14, 21, 22]. Transient bacteremia were observed commonly caused by viridians group streptococci and some other oral microflora associated with invasive procedures such as dental extractions, periodontal surgery, scaling and root planing, tooth cleaning and endodontic procedures or other dental procedures.

Some studies have shown a link between infections of the mouth such as periodontitis and coronary artery disease. Both CVD and periodontal disease are more likely to occur in old people, male, as well as those with low level of education and socioeconomic status. Bacteria from periodontal disease may enter the blood circulation and contribute directly to the atheromatous or thrombotic processes [23]. Systemic factors alter the immuno-inflammatory process involved in both periodontal and cardiovascular disease. Infection is now recognized as a risk factor for atherogenesis and thromboembolic events and may cause direct injury to the epithelium and partially activate the inflammatory response seen with atherosclerosis. *Chlamydia pneumoniae, Helicobacter pylori*, cytomegalovirus and other periodontal bacteria are observed associated with heart disease [24].

With daily routine activities as tooth brushing and flossing, the use of wooden toothpicks and chewing food were found to cause transient bacteremia and are much more likely to cause IE than a dental procedure [13, 14], as it is presumed that the frequency and cumulative duration of exposure to bacteremia are much higher from daily activities than those that result from dental procedures [2, 25, 26].

Poor oral hygiene and dental diseases were proposed to be more significant as a cause of IE than the dental procedures and unfortunately, poor dental health was significantly observed in patients with CVD compare to the controls [14, 19]. In addition, there were available evidence that supported an importance on maintaining good oral hygiene and eradicating dental diseases to decrease the frequency of bacteremia from routine activities [14, 27].

Comprehensive Considerations for Dental Care in CVD

There are some of the preliminary precautions for the dentists to consider from the first contact with patients. Since the symptoms of CVD vary from patient to patient; and that many are asymptomatic, they make the disease difficult to detect, while others have advanced symptoms and require intensive management such as patients with coronary heart disease. Thus, all dental practices should be prepared for an emergency event possibly lead to critical and fatal of the patient that may occur during dental procedures including the followings.

Prior to dental appointment: the patient's complete and current medical history including prescription and non prescription medications, allergies, special diets and a list of medical diagnoses with specific reference to respiratory and cardiac problems, a record of vital signs, stress tolerance of the patient as well as dental history should be reviewed. Communication with the patient's cardiologist in the questionable or uncontrolled cases, sometimes the written document of improved management of the patients is required [28].

The readiness for an office emergency: it is recommended that all dental offices maintain at least basic emergency equipment and drugs. Emergencies usually found in dental clinic include seizures, cardiovascular and respiratory distress, altered consciousness, chest pain. Cabinets stocked with current necessary non-expired drugs such as adrenaline 1:1000 (injectable), hydrocortisone, antihistamine (Chlorpheniramine, Hydroxyzine), atropine, nitroglycerine (sublingual tablet), bronchodilator are necessary. Emergency resuscitation equipment including oxygen should be available at all times. The content and design of these kits should be based upon each practitioner's training and individual requirements. For offices in which emergency medical services, or EMS, personnel with defibrillation skill and equipment are not available within a reasonable time frame, the dentist may wish to consider automated external defibrillator (AED), consistent with AED training acquired in the BLS section of the health care provider courses. Emergency procedures should be written and regularly reviewed. All dental staffs should be certified in basic cardiopulmonary resuscitation training and updated periodically [28-30].

The first dental visit: all patients should have their blood pressure checked, especially those who are hypertensive or have a history of hypertension, since it is the most frequent medical problem which is a major risk factor for cardiovascular morbidity and mortality. The routine check of blood pressure should be done at all dental visits. After complete oral examination and a treatment plan is designed. For patients presented with severe elevated blood pressure (180/110 or greater), elective dental procedures should be postponed until adequate control is achieved. If an emergency treatment is needed, such as a tooth extraction, consultation with the cardiologist is recommended. Blood pressure control during dental procedures may require the intravenous use of medications such as nitroglycerin. Sublingual nitroglycerin or calcium channel blockers also produce a transient reduction in blood pressure. Management of these patients should be made in conjunction with an anesthesiologist in a hospital setting [28, 31].

Reduction of the patient's stress and anxiety, medications taken on the day of dental procedures; The dentist should encourage the patients to take all their prescribed cardiac medications such as anti-hypertensive medications on the day of dental procedures. It is suggested that let the patients bring their medications with them to confirm prescriptions and doses before dental procedure, thus the appointment should be in the morning when the patient is well rested and has a greater physical reserve. Shorter appointments are preferred [23, 28]. Preoperative or intraoperative conscious sedation or both is suggested for stress reduction since with physical activity or emotional stress in dental atmosphere and during dental treatment has the potential to significantly alter hemodynamic stability [32-34].

For example; some patients with CVD may develop angina pectoris during dental procedures. They may complain of chest discomfort and very short breath, palpitation, sweating and syncope. The symptoms usually last about 1-5 minutes and may subsides when the stress is stopped usually with comfortable positioning, reassuring statements as well as the use of preoperative sedation. The symptoms typically respond to sublingual nitrates. The patients should have their own supply of nitroglycerin available at the time of dental procedure. Pre-treatment with sublingual nitroglycerin may be indicated in some patients [28]. The patient's physician should be notified for further treatment which usually consists of bed-rest, analgesic (morphine), anti-platelet agents (Aspirin), thrombolytic therapy (for selected patients presenting within 12 hours of chest pain onset) [28].

Patients who have had a myocardial infarction *within the last 6 months* are at risk for another infarction. Accordingly, dental procedures should be performed with caution, and only in consultation with the patient's physician [28].

Minimize discomfort with the use of profound local anesthesia is recommended since stress may be induced by pain during dental treatment. Excellent postoperative analgesia is preferred [33, 34]. The uses of local anesthetic agents with vasoconstrictors in patients with cardiovascular disease remains controversial for fearing of precipitating ischemic heart disease and develop myocardial infarction. However, patients receiving local anesthetic without vasoconstrictor often have significantly impaired pain control compared with those receiving local anesthetic with epinephrine. For this reason, patients with cardiovascular disease may be at greater risk of experiencing massive endogenous epinephrine release secondary to poor local anesthesia, than they are from the small amount of vasoconstrictor used in local anesthesics [35]. It is recommended that patients with mild or moderate cardiovascular disease receive the smallest amount of local anesthetic needed to provide profound anesthesia, with aspiration performed to prevent intravascular injection.

Although small amounts of vasoconstrictors produce little risk for the average patient with cardiovascular disease, in the patients with severely compromised cardiovascular condition, exogenous vasoconstrictors is contraindicated [34, 36-39].

Patients who recently had myocardial infarction attack are commonly recommended to postpone routine dental care for at least six months. This suggestion is due to the fact that the mortality rate following myocardial infarction commonly occurs during the first year and the patients are high risk of developing another attack [28, 40]. During this period, dental treatment is recommended only to managing acute dental needs, and consultation with the patient's physician is needed [41]. However, acute dental needs are indicated, since consistent pain may aggravate hemodynamic alterations leading to dangerous cardiac arrhythmias [33, 39].

Patients taking antiarrhythmic drugs may have oral side effects such as gingival overgrowth or xerostomia and may have an impact on the dentition or periodontium. In addition the use of local anesthetics with vasoconstrictors may be contraindicated in the patients with refractory arrhythmias [36]. Dental treatment should be performed with medications and cardiac monitoring [39].

Management in patients with pacemaker monitoring and automatic defibrillators usually does not require prophylactic antibiotic coverage before dental therapy because of considering a low risk of infective endocarditis [42]. The use of equipment in an oral surgery procedure that generates an electromagnetic field, such as electrocautery units could interfere with older pacemaker models which were unipolar [45].

Position of the patient during dental procedure: The dental chair should be comfortable, a lumbar and back support are suggested, which can be adjusted for each patient. Especially patients with congestive heart failure should be kept in the upright position as much as possible [28]. Intra-operative oxygen at low flow (2 L/min) via nasal canula is useful for patient with frequent attack of angina or symptomatic heart failure [30].

Antibiotic Prophylaxis: The main purpose of antibiotic coverage with dental procedures is to get the antibiotics into the blood stream to eliminate the microorganisms before they reach the target organs and invading organisms at/in the target organs [2]. However, with the broad use of antibiotics, bacterial resistance to antibiotics is a serious concern. There is the basis for a debate whether prophylactic antibiotic coverage should be administered to at risk patients with certain cardiovascular manifestations. According to The American Heart

Association 2007 [14] "Cardiac conditions associated with highest risk of adverse outcome from endocarditis for which prophylaxis with dental procedures is recommended."

The need of prophylaxis is included in all dental procedures involved with manipulation of gingival tissues or the periapical region of teeth or perforations of the oral mucosa.

The exemptions of prophylaxis can be done in the following procedures and events: routine anesthetic injections through non-infected tissues, taking dental radiograph, placement of removable prosthodontics or orthodontic appliances, adjustment of orthodontic appliances and brackets, exfoliation of deciduous teeth, and bleeding from trauma to the lips or oral mucosa.

Endocarditis prophylaxis before dental procedures is recommended for the patients with one of the following conditions: *prosthetic cardiac valve, previous IE, and cardiac transplantation recipients who develop cardiac valvulopathy.*

Antibiotic prophylaxis is recommended for the following conditions of the congenital heart disease (CHD):

Unrepaired cyanotic CHD, including palliative shunts and conduits, *Complete repaired congenital heart defect with prosthetic material or device,* whether placed by surgery or by catheter intervention, during the first 6 months after the procedure. Prophylaxis is recommended because endothelialization of prosthetic material occurs within 6 months after the procedure.

Repaired CHD with residual defects at the site or adjacent to the site of prosthetic patch or prosthetic device (with inhibited endothelialization).

Antibiotic prophylaxis is no longer recommended for any other forms of CHD other than the exceptional conditions which previous mentioned [14].

In dental procedures Amoxicillin is the preferred choice of antibiotics because of its good absorbance in the GI tract, providing high and sustained serum concentration. In the cases of allergies to Amoxicillin, the use of Cephalexin or another first generation oral cephalosporin, Clindamycin, Azithromycin and Clarithromycin is recommended. Cephalosporins should not used in the patients with history of anaphylaxis, angioedema, or urticaria with Penicillins or Ampicillin and Amoxicillin [43]. The doses and route of drug administration recommended by AHA 2007 is shown in Table 1.

Patients at risk for bleeding from medications; There are increasing numbers of dental patients who take drugs interfering with hemostasis. The major concern is that an invasive dental procedure may create many difficulties particularly postsurgical hemorrhage. There are medications used that may interfere with hemostasis which the dentists should aware of such Aspirin and Aspirin-containing compounds, non-steroidal anti-inflammatory drugs (NSAIDS), antibiotics/antifungals and some other medications including anticoagulant drugs, cancer chemotherapy as well as alcohol [44].

Anticoagulants therapy is commonly used to decrease the incidence of thromboembolic in at risk patients. When patients on anticoagulant drugs show up for an invasive dental procedures one question comes up for the clinicians who perform the dental surgery what to be done: whether to withdraw, reduce or alter anticoagulation therapy before dental treatment, since management of patients receiving anticoagulation therapy remains controversial for dental procedures [45].

Recommended management of the patients on anticoagulants therapy should include full medical history-taking, consideration of specific laboratory tests and the consultation with the patients' physician.

Table 1. The recommended prophylactic management before dental procedures

Drugs	Route	Single dose 30 to 60 min before procedure	Other comments
Amoxicillin	oral	50 mg/kg in children 2 gm single dose in adult	
Amoxicillin Cefazolin Ceftriaxone	Intravenous	50 mg/kg max 2 gm 50 mg/kg max 1 gm 50 mg/kg max 1 gm	Unable to take oral medication
Allergic to penicillins or ampicillin Cephalexin Clindamycin Azithromycin Clarithromycin	oral	50 mg/kg max 2 gm 20 mg/kg max 600 mg 15 mg/kg max 500 mg 15 mg/kg max 500 mg	Equivalent adult or pediatric dosage
Allergic to penicillins or ampicillin Cefazolin Ceftriaxone Clindamycin	Intravenous	50 mg/kg max 1 gm 50 mg/kg max 1 gm 20 mg/kg max 600 mg	Unable to take oral medication

Full medical history-taking to identify at risk patients, standard medical history questionnaires with more detailed questioning about specific medications which may interfere with hemostasis, the reason of the patient receiving anticoagulant therapy, previous problematic bleeding as well as the history of thromboembolitic events should be performed [44, 46].

Specific laboratory tests usually include several laboratory tests used to evaluate coagulapathies from drugs prior to invasive dental procedures.

Bleeding Time (BT) is for testing platelet function (normal range:2-7 min).

International Normalized Ratio (INR) for patients taking Warfarin measures of extrinsic clotting cascade (normal range around 1.0).

Partial thromboplastin time (PTT) for patients on heparin measure of intrinsic clotting cascade normal range is 25-35 seconds. Platelet count (full complete blood count) is for patients on cancer chemotherapy (normal range 150-450,000/µl) [44].

The consultation with the patients' physician: carefully discuss the type of dental care and risk assessment of hemorrhage from dental procedures against the risks of emboli from stopping the anticoagulant therapy. In addition, the evaluation whether the need to alter the anticoagulant regimen or to determine the patients' international normalized ratio (INR) and discuss whether dental treatment should be delayed until the INR value is within therapeutic levels (INR=2.0-3.0) [44, 45, 47].

There are two types of oral anticoagulant agents that are commonly prescribed for outpatients to decrease the risk for thromboembolism; prothombin blockers such as Warfarin, and antiplatelets agents such as Aspirin and Dipyridamole.

Platelet inhibition or antiplatelet; Aspirin has been found to be effective in the prophylaxis of angina, acute myocardial infarction, transient ischemic attack and stroke. It has weak antiplatelet activity through acetylating and irreversibly inactivating the enzyme cyclo-oxygenase which prevents the conversion of arachidonic acid to thromboxane A, the prostaglandin required to stimulate platelet activation and aggregation [48-51]. Platelet inhibition usually begins about 1 hour after Aspirin ingestion, the effect is irreversible and last for the lifetime of the affected platelet which is around 7-10 days [48-50]. The patients who have taken any Aspirin containing medications are recommended to halt the antiplatelet and delay invasive dental procedures for one week. The bleeding time should be performed before the dental procedures [47].

Prothombin blockers; Warfarin is one of the worldwide commonly used oral anticoagulants, for prevention of embolic phenomenon from atrial fibrillation and clots around prosthetic heart valves. It is a vitamin K antagonist which is necessary for thrombin formation and the synthesis of the vitamin K-dependent coagulant protein factor II (prothrombin), VII, IX, and X, and the other vitamin K dependent protein C and S [52, 53]. After ingestion Warfarin is rapidly and completely absorbed, and peak plasma concentration can be observed within 1 hour; its half life being approximately 36 hours, it may take up to 4 days for INR to reach 1.5 after Warfarin has been stopped and depending upon the original INR value of the patients [44, 52, 54]. It is often recommended to stop Warfarin 2-4 days prior to an invasive dental procedure so as to decrease INR value to less than 2.0-3.0 [44] . If Warfarin is withdrawn, it usually takes about 4-6 days for the coagulation process to return to normal [54, 55]. When restarted it takes about 3 days to reach an INR of 2.0, such that patients may have at least 2-3 days of subtherapeutic anticoagulant around the time of surgery. This is an especially worrisome practice in patients that have had a thromboembolic event within the past month. Since recurrent embolic event are more frequent, and some will be fatal, elective oral surgery should be delayed in these circumstances [44]. In addition there were reported of embolic complications cases in patients whose Warfarin therapy was discontinued for dental treatment [56, 57].

The patients that have more than one anticoagulant therapy are at greater risk of intra-and post-operative bleeding from dental procedures, such as the use of Aspirin with patients taking Warfarin as well as non Aspirin NSAIDs such as Ibuprofen [44]. There are drugs that can interact adversely with Warfarin such as common analgesics e.g. Acetaminophen, Aspirin, nonsteroids anti-inflammatory drugs and cyclooxygenase-2 inhibitors, broad spectrum antibiotics e. g. Amoxicillin, macrolides (Erythromycin), Cotrimoxazole as well as alcohol [44, 59]. Some anticonvulsant; Carbamazepine, Phenytoin, antituberculosis drug; Rifampicin, antiarrhythmic drugs; Amiodarone are also a high risk of generating pharmacokinetic interactions with Warfarin [60]. Medications prescribed for post dental procedures such as analgesics for postoperative pain and the antibiotics should be carefully considered in the patients taking anticoagulant drugs.

When there is a high risk of thromboembolism for patients to discontinue Warfarin and required oral surgery, alteration of the anticoagulant therapy is necessary. Unfractionated Heparin is used as a substitute of oral anticoagulant, the patients should be administered four days before surgical procedure to stop Warfarin and set up for intravenous heparin. On the fifth day approximate 4-6 hours before the procedure heparin is stopped for the surgery, and shortly after the procedure Warfarin is restarted. The patients remain in the hospital until adequate therapeutic levels of Warfarin are reestablished [45, 46, 59]. Low molecular weight heparins (LMWHs) are now being used in the out patients. It is suggested to be effective to the dental patients since it has high predictive bioactivity and can be self administered, and save cost and time of hospitalization (5-7 days). Patients will discontinue Warfarin and self-administer start LMWHs according to the prescription and then undergo outpatient surgery and reinitiate Warfarin under the guidance of their physician [45, 46].

If emergency dental procedure has to be done in patients taking anticoagulant drugs, the dentist should be prepared for bleeding that might go beyond the normal circumstances and be ready to provide haemostatic measures. It was observed that there were no significantly different types of bleeding complications in both group of patient with or without coagulative therapy [61], and if there were the incidence of postoperative bleeding the percentage was low and all of which were effectively controlled with local hemostatic measures [62, 63]. The local effective haemostatic measures that are commonly used include the use of gelatin sponges, placed oxidized cellulose in the surgical site and stabilize it with silk sutures; the use of mouth rinse forms of tranexamic acid or placing gauze square saturated with tranexamic acid on the surgical site for 30-60 min; vasoconstrictors in local anesthesia; and atraumatic surgical technique [46].

The maintenance of good oral health: According to AHA in regard to the prevention of bacterial endocarditis, the recommendations emphasize the importance of establishing and maintaining the best possible oral health to reduce potential sources of bacterial seeding [14].

The *professional therapy* to reduce of all carious teeth and periodontal inflammation, as well as *oral hygiene instruction* is highly recommended.

Dentists and physicians should work aggressively to educate CVD patients about poor oral hygiene as the cause of developing oral diseases; and that most cases of infective endocarditis are involving oral microorganisms probably are caused by dental diseases (dental caries, periodontal disease), mastication and oral hygiene procedures [14] in an effort to improve the quality of health and contribute to their long-term survival. The dental health care provider should counsel the patient about the importance of meticulous oral hygiene. Modify oral hygiene instruments to ease individuals use may be needed, perhaps in consultation with an occupational therapist.

Topical antiseptic rinses such as Chlorhexidine and Povidone-iodine are highly recommended for prevention or halt the growth or action of oral microorganisms. A long term regimen of Chlorhexidine rinses to aid in plaque control can be done [14, 64].

Dental treatment in patients with cardiovascular disease the more aggressive interventional therapy such as tooth extraction is recommended in the teeth with uncertain prognosis, recurrence of disease or uncontrollable of disease progression although they are functional and asymptomatic. Retention of questionable teeth may be an inappropriate treatment for those with cardiovascular disease since adverse affected by periodontal diseases may be occurred even with those who have regularly effective supportive periodontal therapy [65].

Diabetes Mellitus

Diabetes Mellitus is somewhat a group of metabolic disorder not only being a single disease which characterized by common principal feature of hyperglycemia resulting from defects in insulin secretion, insulin action or both. The etiologies or pathogenic processes involved in the development of hyperglycemia vary widely however, the vast majority of cases of diabetes fall into one of two major classes: type 1 diabetes or type 2 diabetes, and somehow, there are some of other specific types of diabetes and gestational diabetes.

Type 1 diabetes represents approximately 10-20% of all cases of diabetes mellitus characterised by an absolute deficiency lack of insulin caused by pancreatic β-cell destruction and labeled as insulin-dependent diabetes mellitus (IDDM). The incidence of type 1 diabetes has been reported to increase by about 3% annually. The diagnosed usually is before 21 of age and the peak incidence is among age 10-14 years. There are genetically and environmental influences on the development of type 1 diabetes. There is a possibility of environmental activates in genetics prone individuals including viruses and toxins or destruction of the pancreases beta cells as the result of an autoimmune early in life.

Type 2 diabetes is the most common diabetes; the average of cases is between 85% and 95% depending on the ethnic groups of the patients. The prevalence of type 2 diabetes is rising steadily in many regions worldwide and often is associated with obesity and is rather relative to inactive individuals. It is characterized by slow onset of symptoms, usually in the patients older than 40 years however, it was now observed in younger people, including children and adolescents. In developing countries, the average ages of the patients at diagnosis are lower at age 40-45 years, compared with those age > 60 years in developed countries, and many delayed in attendance and often with serious infections or diabetic complications [66, 67].

The chronic diabetic hyperglycemia and attendant metabolic dysregulation may associate with long term damage, dysfunction and failure of various organs, especially the eyes, kidney, nerves, heart and blood vessels. Criteria for diagnosis of symptoms of diabetes plus either random blood glucose concentration ≥ 200 mg/dL or fasting plasma glucose ≥ 126 mg/dL, or two hour plasma glucose ≥ 200 mg/dL during an oral glucose tolerance test [68].

There are multiple immunity defects which may cause the susceptibility to infections. Diabetic host are prone to have infection more frequently which some predominantly occur in diabetic subjects, such as urinary tract infection (UTI), respiratory tract infection, deep soft tissues infection with bacterial and fungus, and etc. The course of infection may be different and more aggressive in diabetes. Moreover, frequent hospitalization, delayed wound healing and chronic renal failure can be anticipated in diabetes [69].

The Significance Oral Conditions Associate to Diabetes

There are several oral manifestations of diabetes mellitus which the progression of symptoms depend on the ages of the patients, and duration of disease. They are likely to be more severe, and faster in those with poor glycemic control [70]. Oral infection is the common oral manifestations of diabetes mellitus.

Oral infections: there are two major oral diseases involving bacterial infection which associate to the patients with diabetes; dental caries and periodontal diseases. Other oral soft tissue pathologies including lesion associated with delayed healing, recurrent intraoral abscess. Oropharyngeal candidiasis; the fungal infection is also a specific complication of uncontrolled diabetes mellitus as well as viral infections such as herpes simplex, recurrent herpes stomatosis [69]. Xerostomia of diabetes may act as a precipitating factor of oral infections [70].

Periodontal disease is the most common oral condition in poorly controlled diabetes, usually periodontal disease consist of two elements, gingivitis and periodontitis. Gingivitis is an inflammatory response of the gingival to dental plaque characterized by redness, swelling and easily bleeding. Gingivitis is observed in younger population with poor glycemic control and is reversible with effective plaque control through good dental hygiene. Gingivitis may develop more rapidly in older people than in young individuals [65]. Gingivitis may be a precursor of chronic periodontitis which becomes irreversible along with destruction of the periodontium and leads to loss of the teeth in adults.

There are important factors to consider in assessing the periodontal status of diabetic patients including the followings: degree of metabolic control, duration of diseases, presence of other long term complications such as retinopathy, angiopathy, nephropathy, neuropathy, and delayed wound healing. In addition, coexisting risk factors such as present of dental plaque, smoking, stress, and medications taken, as well as hormonal variations in adolescence, pregnancy, and menopause are also essential to consider [71] In general, the severity of periodontal diseases is associated with age, and duration of the diseases; nevertheless, there is a controversy about the disease development as a result of increase of periodontal breakdown with time. Besides, those who take good care of their oral hygiene do not have periodontitis except if age-related [72-74]. Severe periodontal disease often coexists with severe diabetes. It seems to be a risk factor for severe periodontal disease and vice versa, periodontal disease can either predispose or exacerbate the diabetic conditions [75]. A significant effect of infections may be the development of diabetic ketoacidosis (DKA) and hyperglycemic hyperosmolar state (HHS) which are caused by alter the endocrinologic-metabolic control of blood glucose and increased insulin requirement [68].

Periodontitis progression observed is more rapidly and results in more tooth loss in poorly controlled, insulin-dependent diabetes [65] However, those with good glycemic control who have received regularly supportive periodontal therapy and who achieve good plaque control are not prone to develop severe periodontitis and respond well with treatment [76].

Dental caries: There were some important factors that observed to be associated with caries in diabetes including poor metabolic control of diabetes, poor oral hygiene, previous caries experience and a high level of cariogenic bacteria, and also higher glucose in the resting saliva [77, 88]. Diabetic patients are known with tendency to develop caries in inaccessible areas particularly in the root or dental neck regions. Saliva has been identified as a factor related to the manifestation of dental neck caries [79-81]. In children caries is worsen with malocclusions and crowding of teeth. There were also reports of dental caries relate to age of the patients, the increased gingival recession, and the presence of concomitant kidney disease [81]. Specific diet based on carbohydrates, with an incorrect provision of calcium and phosphorus has also been related to caries of diabetes [79]. However, with the fact that patients with good diabetes control have reduced sugar intakes and have good oral self care with an effective plaque removal have lower decay, missing and filling tooth surfaces (DMFS) and lower count of cariogenic metabolism [2, 83].

Oral mucosa diseases: diabetes is associated with a greater possibility of developing certain oral mucosal disorders with high prevalence of lichen planus and recurrent aphthous stomatitis, as well as oral fungal infections. Other oral soft tissue condition including lesion associated with delayed healing, recurrent intraoral abscess were also reported [69].

Oropharyngeal candidiasis: a fungal infection is a specific complication associated with diabetes which may be as a result of high concentration of salivary glucose combined with dysregulation salivary secretion as well as xerostomia. *Candida albicans* species is the most isolated form. In addition, the higher rate of colonization is observed in uncontrolled diabetic patients [84]. The manifestations of oral candidiasis include median rhomboid glossitis, angular cheilitis and denture stomatitis. Candidiasis is also higher among diabetics wearing dentures either full or partial. The symptoms are dry mouth and erythomatous mucosa underneath dentures [84-87]. Erythematous candidiasis is also present as central papillary atrophy of the dorsal tongue papillae and is up to 30% due to diabetes. Since *C. albicans* can adhere to acrylic dentures material, dentures turn into a reservoir for this typical yeast. In addition candidiasis associated to dentures is reported to relate to poor hygienic condition of the prostheses, the long time of usage and the modifications of the hard supporting tissues [88, 89]. Oral candidiasis occasionally can be invasive, resistant to treatment, and potentially lethal. Diabetes is considered as an important risk factor for candidaemia or systemic candidiasis which can become a medical emergency with high mortality rate and long stay in the hospital [90]. Mucormycosis is rare but serious systemic fungal infections that may found in uncontrolled diabetes, higher incidence were also observed in IDDM. Oral manifestations usually demonstrate as palatal ulceration or necrosis with systemic involvement as facial cellulitis and numbness, nasal discharge, fever, headache and lethargy [70, 94].

Oral lichen planus (OLP) is an inflammatory keratotic disease of the mucosa which has been observed in association to diabetes [92-94]. OLP may predispose to the development of squamous cell carcinoma within lesions [95]. However, there were some reports that the side effect of wide range using of drugs such as oral hypoglycemic agents or antihypertensive would probably induce lichenoid reactions, clinically identical to lichen planus [93, 96, 97].

Topical corticosteroids for localized OLP, systemic corticosteroids are used to treat patients with systemic lichen planus and should be carefully prescribed to patients with systemic diseases.

Viral Infection in Diabetes: Herpes simplex viruses (HSV) have recently been reported to be associated with diabetes mellitus; they usually are associated with gingivostomatitis lesions.

Other oral soft tissue pathologies including lesions associated with delayed healing: Traumatic ulcers and irritation fibromas were reported with higher prevalence in type 1 diabetes than in non-diabetic control subjects which may be related to altered wound healing patterns in diabetic patients [97].

Xerostomia and Salivary Gland Dysfunction

Diabetic patients have been reported with the complaint of dry mouth, or xerostomia, and experience salivary gland dysfunction [98-100]. There was reported of impaired salivary uptake and excretion by salivary scintigraphy in adults with type 2 diabetes [101]. The causes is unknown, nevertheless, this may be related to polyuria, the greater amounts of fluids are eliminated via the urine and the less is available for the saliva or to alterations in the basement membranes of salivary glands [102]. In contrast xerostomia in diabetes may actually refer to dry mouth sensation to peripheral neuropathy, rather than to actually diminished saliva output [103]. There were reported no differences in basal and stimulated saliva flow between diabetes patients and healthy controls [103]. The appropriate therapy for xerostemia of diabetes origin is to restore insulin balance [102].

Dysgeusia or Taste dysfunction: the taste impairment is adverse effect in diabetes. It is reported that more than one-third of diabetic adults had hypogeusia or diminished taste perception. This sensory dysfunction can inhibit the ability to maintain a proper diet and can lead to poor glycemic regulation [104].

Neurosensory disorder: burning mouth syndrome or glossodynia or oral dysesthesias were reported as related to diabetes and increased with patient complaints. Long lasting oral dysesthesias could affect oral hygiene maintenance. The burning and painful sensation can impair daily oral hygiene procedures [105].

Another indirect effect of diabetes to the oral cavity such as in diabetic retinopathy which causes visual disturbances could impair daily oral and prostheses hygiene [106]. Dysphagia also is a sequel of diabetes [107].

The Comprehensive Considerations during Dental Care in Diabetic Patients

Routine history taken of the past and present illness followed by a complete oral examination is a priority to the other managements. There are several effective measures in controlling the oral conditions of the diabetes which many treatments are similar to those recommended to the non-diabetes. However, oral managements in diabetic patients do have more comprehensive considerations as of the followings;

Check the level of blood glucose before dental work.: in the patients with diabetes hypoglycemia can do more harm than hyperglycemia, especially in juvenile diabetes: blood glucose levels may be difficult to control however; hypoglycemia is more likely to happen according to inadequate ingested carbohydrate or did not have meal after having taken morning insulin. In addition, increasing carbohydrate utilization causes lower blood glucose concentration due to exercise and stress. The dentist must be familiar with the diabetic status of the patients such as lethargy, change of the mood, sweating, palpitation and syncope. Regular communication and consultation with the physicians to monitor glycemic control before dental appointment is recommended.

Intensive follow up, for those with poor glycemic control, a frequent follow up is recommended as well as careful surveillance to acute oral infections [104].

Consideration of more aggressive interventional therapy rather than observation, similar to the patients with cardiovascular disease the more aggressive interventional therapy such as tooth extraction is recommended in the teeth with questionable prognosis, and has the history of recurrence or uncontrollable of disease progression although they are functional and asymptomatic [65]. Since retention of those teeth may be a risk of infection and is considered an inappropriate treatment for diabetes patients. An undesirable effect of acute infections may occur, and aggravate the glycemic controlled in diabetes.

Maintenance of good oral hygiene is one of the principle measures which many professionals have highly recommended for diabetic patients. The improvement of personal oral hygiene by mechanical plaque removal is a favorable prevention and treatment of oral infections such as dental caries and periodontitis. Controlling oral infections could lead to the improvement of metabolic control in diabetes [75, 108].

Antibiotic coverage: The antibiotic prophylaxis is not recommended in well controlled diabetic (HbA$_{1c}$ < 8%) because there is no greater risk of postoperative infection than in the non-diabetic. [109]. However, when dental surgery is required in poorly controlled diabetes, the antibiotic prophylaxis is highly recommended. If a significant decrease in blood sugar level and subsequent insulin requirement are observed, antibiotic coverage may help prevent impaired and delayed wound healing in invasive treatment [75, 103, 104].

Management of oropharyngeal candidiasis usually includes:

Carefully examine of the soft and hard palate, as well as the buccal mucosa is recommended especially in those wearing dentures. Good oral hygiene and topical antifungals are usually adequate for uncomplicated candidiasis. Oral hygiene measures are not only cleaning the teeth, the oral mucosa surfaces on the tongue, palate and buccal cavity should also be gently cleaned with a soft brush and the dentures as well. Removal of dentures overnight is recommended and they should be left out at least 6 hours since continuous worn denture is a predisposing factor of candidiasis. Daily cleaning and disinfecting denture is recommended when not wearing it. Clean denture with long soft bristles brush is recommended but just brushing might not be effective for removal of fungus, since acrylic denture has irregular and porous surfaces which harbor Candida easily. Soaking denture in a denture cleaning solution, such as antiseptic solution and Chlorhexidine can be done. After disinfection, dentures should be left to air dry, as it is good to eradicate the fungus. Discoloration of dentures and natural teeth can be observed using Chlorhexidine if not adequately removed after disinfection. Topical antifungal mouth rinses can be used by rinsing and held in the mouth for a few minutes to ensure that the whole mucosa is coated. Dentures should be removed to allow contact between mucosa underneath and the antifungal rinses. The integration of an antifungal with a denture liner is recommended to those who have problems holding the antifungal in their mouth for a few minutes. New denture might be necessary in long time wearing, poorly fitted and with frequent repeated infection [110].

Topical antifungal agents; Chlorhexidine digluconate and Nystatin mouth rinses are the first recommended treatment for uncomplicated oral candidiasis. When systemic treatment is needed, the continued use of topical antifungal agents helps reducing the requirement of dose and duration of systemic antifungal therapy; Fluconazole 200 mg/ml/day, or Itraconazole 200 mg/ml/day. Glycemic control has been shown to reduce mortality and morbidity [110].

Chronic Renal Failure

Chronic renal failure (CRF) is a progressive decline in renal function associated with a reduced glomerular infiltration rate, gradually destroying the nephrons, and eventually causing irreversible loss of endogenous renal function that leads to end-stage renal disease (ESRD). There are multiple etiologies such as diabetes mellitus, hypertension, and glomerulonephritis, uropathy, and autoimmune diseases [111]. Hypertension is considered a significant risk factor for the development ESRD and is also the concern of dentists. The triangular relation between chronic heart failure, chronic renal insufficiency and anemia was suggested as a vicious circle since each of the three can either be the cause or be caused by the others. The incidence of CRF continues to rise worldwide, and increases with age. The prognosis in patients with diabetics and/or hypertension is worse than those with glomerulonephritis alone [68, 111].

Without specific interventions, approximately 80% of type 1 diabetics and 20% to 40% of type 2 diabetics will develop overt nephropathy with microalbuminuria and macroalbuminuria (>300 mg of urinary albumin per day) over 10 to 15 years, usually accompanied by the appearance of hypertension. The progression from overt nephropathy to end-stage renal disease can be highly variable. By 20 years, more than 75% of type 1 diabetics and approximately 20% of type 2 diabetics with overt nephropathy will develop ERSD, requiring dialysis or renal transplantation [68].

Oral manifestations related CRF and those who require dialysis are a wide range affecting the hard and soft tissues of the mouth either from the systemic conditions per se, or as the result from the treatments which include the followings; fluid restriction and dietary changes, correction of systemic complications, dialysis and kidney transplantation. Despite these treatments, most patients progress to end stage renal disease (ESRD) and need dialysis or transplantation. The factors possibly related to oral conditions of the patients with CRF and those who require dialysis including; immunosuppressed, medications taken, renal osteodystrophy and bone loss as well as malnutrition and the result of limit amount of oral fluid ingestion. Oral common complications among those dialysis patients are periodontitis, premature tooth loss, xerostomia and local infections [111].

Anemia is a systemic condition in hemodialysis patients. Anemia is considered a multifactorials including; a decreased erythropoietin production due to loss of functional renal glomerular, malnutritional, and chronic illness. Anemia can lead to bleeding tendency from platelet dysfunction and uremia causes easily bleeding. The pallor of the oral mucous membrane, with ecchymosis and petechia can be noticed from the cause of anemia as well as gingival bleeding [112]. Hemostasis problems are usually observed in chronic renal failure due to abnormal platelet adhesion and aggregation (Von Willebrand factor defect), decrease of platelet factor III and alteration in prothrombin [113]. Thus, the dental treatment usually is recommended on the following day after hemodialysis in order to minimize the patient's stress and the risk of prolonged bleeding which probably resulted from the residual presence of heparin used in dialysis. In addition, after dialysis the patient is in better health condition as azothemia had been eliminated.

Uremia is a toxic condition resulting from renal failure (high blood levels of urea). There are many systemic dysfunctions caused by uremia such as uremic encephalopathy, metabolic acidosis, platelets dysfunction. The high concentration of urea in saliva causes some of oral manifestations in ESRD patients such as taste changes. The patients may complain of having change of taste sensation such as unpleasant and/or metallic taste as well as the sense of an enlarged tongue. Bad odor (halitosis) usually has ammonia–like smell due to break down of urea to ammonia as well as high saliva pH and buffering capacity [114, 115]. Patients with uremia are also at risk of infection such as candida infections, uremic stomatitis, and periodontal diseases [113]. The ESRD patients had some form of periodontal diseases, severe gingivitis was observed as well as early periodontitis. This may be the result of poor oral hygiene and the increased deposits of calculus. However, there were reports of premature tooth loss and localized supperative osteomyelitis, as a result of periodontitis in hemodialysis patients [2, 115, 116].

Osteodystrophy; orofacial features of renal osteodystrophy are due to the stage of hyperparathyroidism which results from a high phosphorus serum level and low serum calcium and calcitriol levels due to decreased renal clearance and hydroxylation of 25–hydroxyvitamin D_3 in kidneys [113]. Bone dystrophies can be noticed in dental radiography such as loss of lamina dura surrounding the root of the teeth and abnormal bone trabeculae. The effect of bone demineralization can lead to rapid bone destruction and periodontitis. Decreased trabeculation and thickness of cortical bone at mandible angle and surrounding of maxillary sinuses, and ground-glass appearance of bone can be noticed in radiography. The patient may have abnormal bone healing after tooth extraction and possibility of jaw fracture during dental surgery [113, 115, 117, 118].

Xerostomia in hemodialysis patients is possibly due to the excess loss of fluid through the diseased kidney, the limit amount of oral fluid ingestion and side effect of drug therapy. Long term xerostomia may cause common sequels similar to the dry mouth from other systemic causes in previous discussion such as predispose to oral infections such as dental caries, gingivitis, other fungal and viral infections. In addition, speech difficulties and dentures retention are also a burden; ill-fitting dentures particularly induce trauma to oral mucosa and may be a major risk of septicemia in those who underwent hemodialysis [2, 111, 115].

In children if the onset of renal failure develops during the growth phase, the patients might have delayed growth or rickets (renal osteodystrophy) before the completion of tooth development. There is a possibility of having enamel hypoplasia of both the primary and permanent teeth as well as intrinsic stain or the brown discoloration of the teeth due to the high blood level of urea and calcium deficiency. In addition the intrinsic stain of the teeth is completely infused all through the enamel and cannot be removed by scaling and prophylaxis. A delayed eruption of permanent teeth has been reported. In addition micronagthia and malocclusion can be anticipated [113, 115].

Antibiotic prophylaxis consideration prior to any invasive dental procedures that can cause bleeding may be done for hemodialysis patients, to avoid bacteremia and possibly infection to the shunt; a consultation with the nephrologist is recommended. According to the AHA recommendation; the standard single dose of 2 g Amoxycillin orally or 600 mg Clindamycin (if allergy to penicillin) orally 1 hour preoperatively [118].

Nephrotoxic drugs must be avoided, *i.e.* aminoglycosides, sulfonamides, and opiates. Dosage modification may be necessary to adjust, otherwise it may cause undesirably enhanced or prolonged activity. The dosage modification depends on the degree of residual renal function or the patient's dialysis schedule [119].

Candidate for Kidney Transplantation

When the kidney transplant is determined to normalize kidney function for ESRD the oral hygiene and healthy dentition becomes very important. Infections become the major complication of renal transplantation patients which can be a potential of life-threatening condition, the dental and periodontal infections are included as well. During the waiting period, the consultation with the dentist should be done for the complete oral assessment and treatment procedures. All the dental treatment should be done before the transplant. The extraction must be done in the tooth with root furcation involved lesions, periodontal abscesses, or those required more invasive surgical procedures [113]. Consistency maintenance of healthy oral condition and compliance with regularity periodically recall is necessary.

Once the successful kidney transplantation is done, the patients need lifelong daily immunosuppressive drug therapy for anti-graft rejection. Immunosuppressive drugs commonly used are Prednisolone, Azathioprine, Cyclosporine and Tacrolimus. Each has been associated with potentially serious side effects, which can give rise to oral side effects such as infections.

Oral infections become the major causes of morbidity and mortality of those who become immunosuppressive due to the drug prescribed. Angular cheilitis has been reported up to 4% prevalence in hemodialysis and transplantation followed by other oral candidal lesions erythematous 3.8%, chronic atrophic 3.8% and pseudomembranous candidiasis 1.9% respectively [115]. Prophylactic systemic antifungal are commonly prescribed hence, the figures susceptibility of immunosuppressed kidney transplanted patients to fungal disease has been declined [120]. Besides, viral infection has been significantly decreased because the use of antiviral drugs; Acyclovir, Gancyclovir, Valacyclovir. Previously it had been reported up to 50% of kidney transplanted patients shown seropositive for herpes simplex and experienced recurrent, severe and prolonged HSV infection [115].

Antibiotic prophylaxis is recommended for all dental procedures involving perforation of the oral mucosa or that can cause bleeding in the patients with kidney transplantation [118].

Gingival hypertrophy or gingival enlargement may be the side effect of drug therapy of those who take immunosuppressive drug such as Cyclosporine, calcium channel blockers and/or the combination of both. It usually affects labial inter-dental papillae gingiva. It can become more severe involving the gingival margins of the lingual and palatal surfaces which gradually may require the treatment of gingivectomy or oral flap surgery. Recurrence is common especially with the poor oral hygiene. Meticulous oral hygiene can reduce this side effect; however, long term effective plaque control is needed and as well as the use of additional anti-plaque agents such as topical Chlorhexidine gluconate or Tricosan preparations [115].

Other mucosal lesions including white patches and/or ulceration, *lichen planus-like* have been observed in individuals receiving dialysis and kidney transplantation. They may be the result of the associated drug therapy. *Oral hairy leukoplakia* can occur from drug related immunosuppression, and during uremia which the lesion may resolve with treatment of the uremia [115].

Narrowing or calcification of the pulp chamber of the teeth (resulting in difficult root canal treatment for the exposed pulp) can be observed in adult with CRF for which the cause of change is unknown. However, a significantly higher prevalence in patients with kidney transplantation than those receiving hemodialysis was observed [121].

Head and Neck Cancer

Head and neck cancer remains one of the most challenging diseases since the incidence of new cases is rising and mortality rate is high. The development of recurrence of the diseases is high particular in the oropharyngeal region. The most common risk factors are smoking and the use of smokeless tobacco, excessive alcohol consumption, and some viral infections such as papillomavirus. Unfortunately most of head and neck cancer patients usually are late diagnosed with the advanced lesions which cause poor survival and functional outcome despite with the aggressive treatments [2, 122].

Managements of head and neck cancers need several modalities treatments, usually are the conventional treatment modalities which consist of surgery, radiation, chemotherapy or a combination of those. Each treatment has specific effects depend on the tumor sites, treatment doses and host susceptibility. The oral complications are the most common of the head and neck cancer treatment which needed the special attention to the dental professionals. The consequences may have an effect on the competence of cancer therapy and may disrupt and halt the course of treatment. The quality of life of the patients is significantly changed from the toxic, pain and discomfort. Some of oral complications occur early as soon as the treatments begin and some may not showed until many years later and some lasted for life long. Chemotherapy causes myelosuppresion, immunosuppression or direct cytotoxic effects of chemical agents which may manifest in the oral cavity as mucositis, soft tissue ulceration, increase infections and bleeding. Radiotherapy can damage the surrounding tissues, not only the cancer cell itself since the radiation fields usually cover a large area of head and neck to ensure that tumor bed and regional lymph nodes receive an adequate dose. Many side effects develop shortly after radiation (mucositis, dermatitis, loss of taste and xerostomia) whereas some effects will not appear until many years later (osteoradionecrosis, trismus and extensive dental caries or rampant caries) [123, 124]. For example, the standard of care for locally advanced oropharyngeal tumor is radiation, followed by surgeries which include surgical resection of the large amount of the normal tissue to achieve tumor-free margins. Definitely the surgery of the oropharynx bears significant morbidity such as severe speech dysfunction, and dysphagia (swallowing dysfunction), such severity depending on the extension of tongue and soft palate resection. If these conditions are compounded with the postoperative radiation xerostomia and scarring of the pharyngeal muscles, the anxiety and depression were frequently observed [125-130].

Oral Assessment and Dental Care Services

After the diagnosis of head and neck cancer and treatment modalities has been desired the patients have to undergo a series of examinations and tests which associate with the treatment of cancer as well as dental services. Oral assessment and care are important before cancer therapies in order to eradicate all the potential sources of infection and trauma which may lead to severe complications during and after cancer treatment [131]. There are reported that the majority of head and neck patients need oral care before cancer therapy because of poor oral hygiene and noncompliant of routine dental care [123, 132-135].

In order to reach the desired prevention and compliance of the treatment plan, a high cooperation of the patients in particular the continuous self-meticulous oral hygiene is required. Thus the patients must be informed and understand the rationale of the oral hygiene program as well as the potential effects of cancer therapy: radiation therapy and chemotherapy. If radiation is the therapeutic modality, the knowledge of radiation dose, modality of treatment, field of radiation and tumor prognosis are necessary for the dental treatment plan [136, 137].

Ideally, the oral assessment should be performed at least one month before the beginning of cancer treatment so as to provide enough time for the adequate healing, especially when invasive dental procedures such as root canal treatment, tooth extraction and alveolectomy are performed [137].

The oral examination must include the radiographic examination for both dentate and edentate patients, panoramic, selected periapicals and bitewings [138]. A careful assessment of existing dental and periodontal diseases, complete dental and periodontal charting should be done to set up the baseline information. Carefully evaluate the condition of oral soft tissues which including hard and soft palate, labial and buccal mucosa as well as the tongue [136]. Assess the conditions of dental prostheses, not only the removable, fixed prostheses such as implants, crown and bridge.

Saliva flow of the patients should also be assessed as the base line evaluation. An average person produces at least 500 ml of saliva per day, salivary flow rates vary depending on the demand or the current physiologic status of patients, the non-stimulated or resting flow rate is 0.3 ml/min, and flow rate during sleep is 0.1 ml/min, during eating or chewing increases to 4.0 to 5.0 ml/min [139, 140].

Measurement of maximum mouth opening should be evaluated for base line measurement before radiotherapy, and frequent measurement should be performed to ensure the maintenance of maximum mouth opening [141].

Oral Preventive Counseling Prior to Cancer Treatment

Primary preventive measures, such as appropriate nutritional intake, effective oral hygiene practices, the use of topical chemotherapeutic agents and early detection of oral lesions are important prior cancer treatment since the severity of oral complications from cancer treatment can be reduced significantly when an aggressive approach to stabilizing oral health is initiated [137, 142]. The patients must achieve to the desire oral hygiene before the beginning of cancer treatment.

Dietary control, although, an adequate intake of diet is recommended, the diet intake should be seriously considered particularly as it can lead to dental caries (refined carbohydrates and sugar). Multiple extractions may be needed in patients with poor oral hygiene and non compliance with treatments, thus pain and chewing difficulty can be anticipated. The counseling of diet modification is necessary for prevention of weight loss. Patients's weight and nutritional input should be assessed at the beginning and regularly weekly throughout cancer treatment [143].

Effective oral hygiene practices include mechanical plaque removal, interproximal cleaning and the use of other cleaning devices. The assessment of the patients self awareness of dental health, their motivation and their ability to perform oral hygiene procedures is important for the preventive measures [136].

The use of topical chemotherapeutic agents such as topical fluoride and prophylactic rinses are essential since fluoride can reduce dental caries, and Chlorhexidine reduce oral microorganisms in the mouth such as mutans streptococci, and lactobacilli [144, 145]. The potential benefit of prophylactic rinsing with Chlorhexidine is to control plaque levels, gingivitis, reduced caries risk, and oropharyngeal candidiasis [137, 138, 146].

Dental Managements before Cancer Treatment

Since infections of dental or periodontal origin are considered as a severe risk to head and neck cancer, serious consequences can be anticipated when the patients become immunocompromised from cancer treatments. Furthermore, with radiotherapy, the more serious complication such as osteoradionecrosis can be predictable. Tooth extraction and dental diseases in irradiated area have been known as major risks factors for the development of osteoradionecrosis. Thus, the more aggressive dental managements were considered in patients with poor oral hygiene, and evidence of past periodontal diseases as well as those who have neglected, non-compliance or limited previous dental care. Several dental procedures should already be done before the time of cancer treatment as the followings [123, 130].

All teeth should be cleaned including dental prophylaxis, full mouth scaling and polishing. All the oral diseases should be treated such as dental caries and periodontal diseases.

Tooth restorations/fillings should be up to an acceptable level. All irritating factors which may traumatize the oral mucosa such as sharp edge teeth, rough filling, and overhang filling should be smoothed and polished. All broken or leakage fillings should be repaired and replaced as well.

Dental prostheses; ill-fitting or broken of both full and removable dentures should be adjusted and repaired, for prevention of trauma to the ridges. All fixed prostheses including implants, crown and bridges should be in good retained and hygienic [134, 148, 149].

Prophylactic tooth extraction may be required in the patient receiving radiotherapy. The criteria used for extractions before radiotherapy are not universally accepted and are subject to clinical experiences and judgment of the dental team [138, 148]. However, tooth extractions are recommended in the following circumstances: all teeth in direct association with an intra oral tumor, teeth in the high-dose radiation field with a questionable prognosis, retained root, non-opposed tooth and compromised hygiene, partial impaction or partially eruption tooth, periodontitis with the furcation involvement, non-restorable caries, tooth with extensive periapical lesions [149-151]. Dental implants with poor maintenance of peri-implants health should be removed [152]. Antibiotics coverage before and after is recommended if the tooth extraction is unavoidable although, there are evidences that the incidence of osteoradionecrosis (ORN) is not different with or without antibiotics prophylaxis. However, many clinicians recommend antibiotics coverage for the prevention of preradiation or postradiation induced ORN [153]. A non-traumatic approach and good surgical technique are suggested for the extraction. The bone at the wound margin and sharpen bone spicules should be trimmed evenly. Alveolectomy should be done to ensure smooth alveolar ridge and prepare for construction of denture after treatment. Optimal post surgical time prior radiotherapy is suggested within 2 to 3 weeks [149, 151, 154].

However, there are some exemptions, if the patient demonstrates a history of good oral hygiene care and compliancy with routine and ongoing professional dental visit; asymptomatic teeth such as chronically involved root furcation without mobility or any acute infection are not subjected to extraction [151]. Complete bony impaction can be left [155].

Usually proper endodontic treatment is recommended for pulpal involved teeth. Periodontal surgery should be avoided because of prolonged healing and the meticulous oral hygiene necessary for the good end result [152]. Metallic crown and bridges or implants should be replaced with plastic temporary crowns or removed during radiation. Orthodontic appliances should be removed and the treatment suspended for 1 year after the completion of cancer therapy [133, 137].

In children all primary teeth in children with any risk of pulpal involvement and those that will exfoliate within 3 months should be removed, the use of sealants is recommended on all exposed tooth surfaces. The parents should be informed that cancer therapy may also result in long term complications including enamel hypoplasia, microdontia, delay or failure of tooth development and eruption, altered root formation, as well as mal-development in the craniofacial skeleton that may affect the facial esthetics such as micrognathia. The effect of high dose of radiation to condylar cartilage of temporomandibular joints (TMJ) may cause TMJ ankylosis and the consequences effect the growth and movement of jaw. In children orofacial complications are three times more severe than adults who having similar treatment [133, 137].

Oral Health Managements during Cancer Therapy

There are several oral complications that can occur during treatment of cancer from both chemotherapy and radiotherapy. Acute toxicity such as mucositis and infections was significant. The hematological toxicity was also significant with neutropenia and anemia and could lead to sepsis and death. Besides, the combinations of treatment modalities induce long term damage to the digestive tract. Stases of the bolus and in severe cases, aspiration were observed after chemoradiation [125-130].

Mucositis is common, approximately 95-100% of the patients develop mucositis after radiation and 75% of chemotherapy patients. Mucositis from chemotherapy usually begins 3 to 5 days after initiation of chemotherapy and peaks at 7-14 days. Without infections, mucositis will spontaneously heal within 2 to 4 weeks [134, 139, 142]. Mucositis caused by radiotherapy is a function of cumulative tissue dose usually begins at dose about 15 Gy to 20 Gy of standard or conventional fractioned radiation therapy which has the average dosage of 200 rads or 2 Gy per fraction, one fraction daily for 5 days a week. [151, 156] Around the second weeks of radiation or at doses of 30 Gy ulcerative mucositis appears and will last for 6 to 8 weeks depends on the duration of treatment [146]. Spontaneous healing can be anticipated within 3 weeks of the treatment, delay healing of mucositis is caused by high dose radiotherapy and smoking tobacco [157].

Oral mucositis is characterized by mucosal erythematous, erosive and ulcerative lesions which may be covered by a white pseudomembrane. Mucositis is usually painful, causes discomfort and may lead to compromised nutritional intake, communication and sleep. The serious concern is increasing the risk of infections when the patients are immuno-compromised. The risk of septicemia was observed four times higher in the patients with oral mucositis and neutropenia [133, 134, 140, 142, 158].

The main objectives for prevention and treatment of oral mucositis usually are palliative and conservative treatments which consist of maintenance of good oral hygiene, eliminating all the mucosal-irritating factors, and symptomatic treatments of infections, oral mucosal dryness, pain and inflammation [134, 142,146, 148].

Maintenance of oral hygiene is the most important measure for the prevention of oral mucositis, since good oral hygiene can decrease mucosa breakdown and promote mucosa healing [142]. Daily mechanical plaque removal is encouraged as long as oral self care remains atraumatic. Toothbrushing and flossing can be done and continued unless contraindicated by neutropenia and thrombocytopenia. It is suggested the patients discontinue flossing if they have fewer than 20,000 to 50,000 platelets/mm^3 or fewer than 500 to1,000 neutrophils/mm^3. The use of ultra soft toothbrush or sponge on stick (toothettes®) is recommended, the oral soft tissues such as alveolar ridge palate and tongue may be cleaned by using toothettes® [134, 137].

Mild flavoring toothpastes with fluoride are recommended since strongly flavored toothpastes may irritate the mucosa of the mouth. If toothpaste irritation occurs, patients should be encouraged to brush with salt water, using 1 teaspoon of salt in 4 cups of water [144]. Discontinuation of routine oral hygiene can increase local and systemic infection risk due to bacterial plaque accumulation leading to gingival bleeding, gingivitis and periodontitis. Thus, if the mouth is too painful for brushing, wipe mouth and teeth gently with a wet gauze soaked salted water to remove particles, or use cotton bud or gauze soaked aqueous base Chlorhexidine. Swab the oral tissues 3 to 4 times daily. Sponges on stick are softer than cotton buds and cause less bleeding and pain when applied to the inflammatic mucosa However, the use of foam brush, cotton buds or toothettes® cannot adequately remove dental plaque, routine care of oral hygiene by brushing and flossing should be resumed when the pain is subsided. Encourage the patients to rinse their mouths frequently, as rinsing helps remove particles and bacteria from the mouth and prevents crusting of sores in the mouth [134, 136]. Oral rinses such as isotonic saline or sodium bicarbonate solution are often suggested. Use 8 to 12 oz of rinse, hold and expectorate; repeat every 2 to 4 hours as needed for pain. Avoid the use of mouthwash containing alcohol, hydrogen peroxide and some acidic non prescription oral preparations for preventive oral hygiene since they can cause erosion and tooth sensitivity or damage the mucosa and delay wound healing [140]. The use of topical fluoride is essential and must be continued; during mucositis period in some patients fluoride gel may be irritating.

During mucositis the patient should be advised to feed on a certain diet, such as a soft, bland diet, and non acidic fruits such as banana, melon, ripe sweet mango, peach and pear. Frozen yogurt, or ice cream may be especially soothing. It is recommended to drink water in high volume to maintain the moistness of tissue and the body fluid balance [161], and to avoid certain foods that may cause mucosal irritation or damage fragile mucosa, especially in patients with existing mucosa ulcer including hard, rough, salty, spices and acidic. Alcohol drinks, tobacco, acidic fruit and hot temperature drinks may irritate the oral mucosa. Acidic juices, fruit flavored ice cubed and soda or carbonated fizzy drinks should be avoided since the low pH usually between 2.5 to 3.8 may contribute to tooth sensitivity and irritating the oral mucosa [146].

Mucositis is typically painful, prevents the patient from oral feeding and leads to long term gastrostomy tube feeding. Patients's weight and nutritional input should be assessed regularly weekly throughout the course of cancer treatment. Adequate nutrition intake during and after treatment is essential when the patients lose more than 5 kg weight or 5% to 10% of their body weight or consume less than 50% of daily nutritional requirements; in these cases, enteral feeding (nasogastric feeding tube, gastrostomy tube feeding) should be initiated [143]. Nutrition has an impact on host's immune response and the integrity of the hard and soft tissues of the oral tissues [162]. Malnutrition may lead to a rising number of oral health problems [162-164]. Even during the tube feeding, the patients should be encouraged to maintain good oral hygiene.

For patients wearing removable dentures, their use should be limited to meal times only. Discontinue use if the denture causes trauma to the mucosa, and during ulcerative mucositis. The appliances should be left out of the mouth when sleeping. Encourage the patients to brush their natural teeth first then clean their dentures with soft brushes and rinse well whenever after eating before reinserted dentures back to the mouth. Disinfect the denture when is not worn; soak it in antimicrobial solution such as denture cleansing tablet, denture bath [136].

Pain managements during mucositis include topical and systemic analgesics and anti-inflammations such as: Benzydamine (Benzydamine HCl topical rinse) has been used for the prophylaxis and to reduce the severity of mucositis in head and neck radiated patients. Opioid drugs may be used in control of pain. NSAIDS, Aspirin-type analgesics should be avoided because of bleeding risk in chemotherapy induced mucositis. Topical anesthetic agents may give symptomatic relief of pain such as Diclonine hydrochloride 0.5-1% or Xylocaine 2-5%, Lidocaine, Benzocaine viscous sprays or gels [147].

The recommended use of mucosal coating agents for covering localized ulcerative lesions and protecting against trauma such as kaolin with pectin suspension, a mixture of aluminum or magnesia hydroxide suspensions and many antacids or cellulose film-forming agents as well as lanolin-based cream and ointments were observed to be effective. Hydroxypropyl methylcellulose combined with topical anesthesia was reported as an effective relief of pain. Lip care products containing petroleum-based oils and waxed can be used for preventing dryness of the lips and reducing risk of tissue injury in chemotherapy patients. However, during radiotherapy a non petroleum lip balm against dryness of the lips is suggested; oral hydration and lubrication is recommended by using a water spray or saliva substitute [133, 137, 161].

Many agents and protocols have been promoted for management or prevention of mucositis. There are reports on the use of combination of drugs and supportive treatments with some degrees of success with mild and moderate mucositis pain, but with little relief for severe mucositis. The prevention and management of oral mucositis remains unsatisfactory and basically unpreventable which because of having inadequately supported by randomized controlled clinical trials [137, 165].

Oral Infections

Infections can occur during mucositis and are more common and more severe in patients with chemotherapy than those with radiotherapy alone [152]. The common infections are *Candida* spp. and *Herpes simplex* virus infections [152, 166, 167]. Systemic dissemination may occur from the ulceration and inflammation of mucosal. One of the important factors that increase the risk of oral infections is the reduction of salivary flow due to radiation damage of salivary glands. There are many consequences of decrease salivary flow which are the loss of mechanical oral flushing, decrease production of electrolyte, immunoglobulin, saliva enzymes such as lysozymes and peroxidases, loss of saliva buffering capacity and lower of saliva pH which cause oral level of cariogenic microflora and fungal to increase [133, 145,168].

Fungal infection; candidiasis commonly manifests itself as pseudomembranous, hyperplastic, or atrophic, erythematous oral lesions and angular cheilitis. Oral candidiasis occasionally can be invasive, show resistance to drug treatment, and is potentially lethal. In children with chemotherapy, systemic candidiasis can become a medical emergency [152]. Antifungals should be used following the detection of oral candida. Systemic azole antifungals are effective in reducing overall oral fungal colonization levels and the frequency of fungal infections. Azoles may be used as prophylactic antifungals in the radiotherapy patients. Fluconazole is recommended as the drug of choice for antifungal especially in resistant fungal infections. Administration of Fluconazole: Once daily 50 or 100 mg tablets or 50 mg/5 ml of suspension 4 times daily has been suggested [166, 167]. Nystatin has been used as antifungal for a long period of time. Two-minute swishing and swallowing of 2-5 ml of Nystatin suspension (100,000 units/ml) have been used 4 times a day. Alternatively, 1 tablet of Nystatin pastilles or lozenges (200,000 units) to dissolve in the mouth 5 times daily. However, several studies indicated that the use of Nystatin suspension ineffectively reduce the incidence of oropharyngeal candidiasis in the patients receiving chemotherapy or radiation [168, 170, 171]. Using Nystatin concurrent with Chlorhexidine is not recommended because of their antagonistic effects. A self-administration of one drug should be at least one hour apart from the other [170]. Topical antifungal can be used such as Miconazole varnish or gel (25 mg/ml) by applying thin coat to the affected areas for 4 to 5 times daily. If patients wear denture, the drugs should be applied to the inner surface of denture. However, these drugs should be avoided for the patients on Warfarin because the increased anticoagulant effect [172]. Other antifungals are 10 mg of Clotrimazole (troches dissolving in the mouth 4 to 5 times daily) and Ketoconazole or Itraconazole as systemic medications.

Bacterial infections; *Streptococci mutans* and *Lactobacilli* infection are increased in the radiotherapy patients due to the lost of saliva protective and buffer actions. In myelosuppressed cancer patients, systemic infections of gram-positive organisms including *Streptococci viridans* and *Enterococci* spp. are usually from oral origin. Radiotherapy is also associated with a noticeable increase in oral gram-negative pathogens including *Pseudomonas aeruginosa*, *Neisseria* spp. and *Escherichia coli* of which endotoxins can cause adverse systemic effects [133, 137, 152]. Signs of gingivitis may be seen due to the underlying myelosuppression [141, 172, 173]. Myeloablated cancer patients with chronic periodontal disease may develop acute periodontal infections with associated with systemic sequelae. Extensive ulceration of sulcus epithelium may be not directly noticeable, yet it would be a source of disseminated infections. Prophylactic antimicrobials can be used to prevent dental caries and oral infections, aqueous mouth rinses of 0.12% or 0.2% Chlorhexidine have been demonstrated to be beneficial. Alcohol based Chlorhexidine solutions should be avoided since they exacerbate xerostomia and mucositis. Some clinical studies suggested that topical use of Polymyxin E and Tobramycin 4 times daily have been effective [168, 175].

Viral infection, Herpes simplex virus (HSV) and *Herpes varicella zoster* virus (VZV) are the main symptomatic viral infections affecting in the mouth of cancer patients. However cases of Cytomegalovirus-induced ulceration have been occasionally reported. In chemotherapy children, acute herpetic gingivostomatitis with systemic involvement is considered as medical emergency [152, 176, 177]. Acyclovir is the most useful antiviral agent for HSV and VZV infection. Valacyclovir can reduce the incidence of oral HSV infections. Prophylactic use of Acyclovir and Valacyclovir are effective reducing recurrent viral infections in children and adults who receiving bone marrow transplantation or immunosuppressed cancer patients [178-180].

Dental Procedures during Cancer Therapy

Dental treatment during radiation is not suggested, occasionally when there is an emergency, palliative treatment such as temporary dressing is allowed. Definite dental treatments and removal of teeth during radiation should be delayed until radiotherapy finishes and the mouth has healed from mucositis and dermatitis reaction [154].

Routine dental treatment may be performed as usual in patients under chemotherapy if the granulocyte count is higher than 2,000/mm^3 and the platelet count is higher than 40,000/mm^3 [136]. Supragingival prophylaxis can be performed; however, invasive intervention such as periodontal probing and other procedures to diagnose periodontitis should be avoided [172]. Tooth extraction during chemotherapy is contraindication. If emergency is needed for the patients with very low white blood count and platelet count, all dental procedures can be carefully performed without trauma to the soft tissues, antibiotics prophylaxis should be administered under supervision of the oncologist. Symptomatic treatment should be performed such as pulpectomies and temporary fillings therefore the teeth may be reopened for relief pain whenever needed until extraction is allowed. Platelet infusion may be needed in the patients who undergo invasive dental procedures. Splints made for individual may be required to control hemorrhage [136].

Hyposalivation and Xerostomia

The major salivary glands (parotid, submandibular and sublingual) usually produce up to 90% of salivary secretions [181]. The radiotherapy of head and neck tumors generally damages the salivary glands of which parotids glands are at the highest risk to radiation damage. The magnitude of damage depends on the radiation dose, the volume of irradiated glands and the nature of the irradiated salivary glands. The acute effects are alteration of salivary gland function and reduction of resting and stimulated salivary flows. It was observed that even after low doses of 10-15 Gy, a serious loss of function of parotid gland can be observed. During the first week of radiation, saliva may decreases by 50% to 60%, and basal salivary reach a measurable minimum within 2 to 3 weeks after 23 Gy of fractionated RT [182]. With high doses of 60-70 Gy, there is a rapid decrease of salivary flow up to 90% during the first week; after 5 weeks of treatment the salivary flow has nearly ceased and rarely recovered [133].

The duration of salivary function depression varies among patients, gradually recover of adequate saliva may be above several months, however, with high dose of radiation permanent glandular damage can lead to irreversible loss of salivary gland function.

Impaired salivary gland function can be a remarkable effect on the patients' oral health and the quality of life since many consequences may follow such as difficulty oral function with mastication, deglutition and articulation and impaired speech. Burning sensation and cracked lips can be reported. The susceptibility to dental infections and risk of dental caries are also increased as well as soft tissue breakdown, and bone loss can occur [133, 182-186].

Even though xerostomia is not life threatening, symptoms and signs are irreversible. The patients may complain of increased thirst and dryness, burning sensation of the tongue. Atrophy of dorsal tongue surface, fissures at lip commissures can be observed. They may have difficulty wearing dentures, their quality of life is certainly decreased [182].

Maintainance of good oral hygiene is the first key role of xerostomia management in order to minimize the risk of oral infections. In addition providing moisture to oral soft tissues is also essential. Plaque and food debris can easily accumulate due to the reduction of saliva flow and saliva flushing action. Frequent care of oral hygiene is necessary. Only rinsing the oral cavity may not be sufficient for thorough cleansing of the oral tissues. It is compulsory to use mechanical plaque removal by tooth brushing, flossing and other oral hygiene aids for more adequate cleaning. Water irrigation (Water-Pik®) may be used to help cleaning the teeth.

Rinsing with a solution of salt and baking soda 4 to 6 times a day (mix 0.5 teaspoon of salt and 0.5 teaspoon of baking soda in a cup of warm water) helps cleaning and lubricating the oral tissues as well as buffering the oral environment.

Remineralization the teeth by using fluoridated toothpaste, rinsing with 0.05% fluoride mouthwash and applying high concentration prescription fluorides at bed time are recommended, in children, both of topical and systemic fluoride are necessary [133, 139, 168].

Diet counseling for xerostomia usually recommends soft and moist diet. Cariogenic foods and liquids with high sugar content should be avoided. Dry food such as bread, dry meat, pastries, toast and crackers, snack crispy salty foods are not suggested. If the patients have difficulty chewing and swallowing food, try soaking bread or rolls in milk, drinks or sauces before eating; this will help ease with chewing and swallowing. In the more severe cases liquefying and pureed food are recommended for ingestion [138].

Temporary relief of dryness and the treatment of dry mouth usually focus on palliative measures; drink plenty of fluid up to 8 to12 glasses per day, frequent sip of water during the day is suggested. Ice cubes or ice water may be used to keep the mouth cool and moist [138, 168]. Eating yogurt and non acidic fresh fruits is helpful; however, acidic fruits such as orange and grapefruit, even though they may help stimulate salivary flow should be avoided since they irritate the oral tissue and contribute to the demineralization of the teeth. Diet rich in raw dark green leafy vegetables may help moisturize the mouth. Products containing yeast, molds and fungi, alcohol, soda or carbonated fizzy drink should be avoided. Caffeine products like tea, coffee and colas are diuretics may contribute to dry mouth. Besides, colas are acidic and can lead to teeth sensitivity and demineralization. The patients with comorbid disease, some prescribed medications can worsen dry mouth [141].

Saliva substitutes are used for the lubrication, hydratation of the oral tissues and maintaining oral health and functions. Saliva substitutes usually do not provide the same protective roles as natural saliva, their duration effect is often shortened by swallowing and additionally there are some complain of poor tolerated, oily consistency and sticky feeling. Alternatively, some antibacterial enzymes such as lactoperoxidase, glucose oxidase, lysozyme and lactoferrin as found in natural human saliva have been effectively used in saliva substitutes [187]. There are other oral moisturizers such as rinses containing hydroxyethyl-, hydroxypropyl-, or carboxymethylcellulose [168]. Often apply lip moisturizing to help prevention of dryness and cracked lips.

Stimulation of remaining salivary gland tissue by systemic sialagogues help stimulate saliva production from remaining functional salivary glands. The use of 2.5-10 mg Pilocarpine HCl per oral three times daily for 4-12 weeks has been showed to improve the saliva flow rate although, in some cases the improvement can be observed as late as up to 90 days. In addition, studies using Pilocarpine showed a statistically significant patient-perceived improvement in either the sensation of oral dryness or in the sensation of overall xerostomia. However, there are contraindications and adverse effects with Pilocarpine which should be carefully considered before it being prescribed to the patients, of which the most common are sweating, chills, and nausea. An increase in sweating is observed with a high dose of treatment; 10 mg [139, 168, 188-191]. Sugar-free chewing gum and sugar-free candies or lozenges may help to increase salivary output but they may be inconvenient and effect patients 'compliance particularly in those who wearing full denture [139].

Prophylactic pharmacologic treatment for prevention of radiation-induced xerostomia such as the use of 500 mg Amifostine intravenous 15 to 30 minutes before each fraction of radiotherapy is observed decreasing the severity of radiation-induced xerostomia [168, 192, 193]. It is demonstrated the quality of life in the patients receiving Amifostine had been improved including improving of speech, eating, sleep and overall well-being [194]. Reduction of severe hematologic and high grade mucositis was reported to be reduced with high doses of Aminofostine, 500 mg intravenously during chemotherapy [195]. The administration of Pilocarpine before or during radiation and the beneficial effect to lessen the frequency and severity of xerostomia from radiation-induced remain controversial [168, 187, 196].

Several investigation interventions have been demonstrated as for preserving the normal tissues and reduced toxicity in the treatment of cancer. Some reported show potential effectiveness such as: the use of intensity modulated radiotherapy (IMRT) for preserved salivary gland function especially parotid glands [197], salivary gland transfer technique, the transfer of the submandibular gland to submental space in patients undergoing radiotherapy for preserving salivary function since regularly the submental region is shielded during radiotherapy [181]. The gene therapy and the development of future viral vaccines for cancer therapy and furthermore clinical controlled trial studies should be continued [143, 198, 199].

Patients with xerostomia will have dental prosthesis fitting or functional problems because the loss of saliva adhesive effect, the use of denture adhesive may help retaining the dentures. The use of prostheses soft liner for prevention of tissues trauma from wearing dentures is recommended [136].

Dysgeusia or Taste dysfunctions caused by radiation damage the taste receptors by the first week of radiotherapy and gradually worsen from second week throughout the entire cycle of radiation, in relation to the accumulated dose of radiation. The loss of taste usually involves all 4 tastes: sweet, sour, bitter and salty [200]. Partial improvement for the taste receptors to recover and function can be observed between 3 to 10 weeks after radiotherapy and full recovery within 4 months; however, an increase in taste thresholds up to 1 year or more was observed. Zinc sulfate may be used for preventing, and/or reducing the radiation induced taste alterations. The use of 220 mg zinc sulfate supplements 2 or 3 times a day may help with recovery of the sense of taste [137, 200].

Dysphagia is a common, debilitating and potentially life threatening sequel of chemotherapy and radiotherapy. The patients develop difficulty in swallowing solid foods or liquid because of inhibition of deglutition reflex. The surgical intervention and location of cancer can affect speech and swallowing of the patients by the effects of post surgery complications, and lead to development of severe dysphagia which require prolonged tube feedings for more than 3 months or repeated dilatations. During mucositis and pain, dysphagia may be more severe which may lead to malnutrition, dehydratation and other consequences. Once chronic dysphagia has occurred, swallowing rarely returns to normal. Dysphagia has a profound impact on the quality of life of cancer survivors, as it causes anxiety and depression. In severe cases such as the effect of depressed and the absence of cough reflex, it may be the cause of aspiration in patients which lead to aspiration pneumonia and cause of death [137, 161, 201-203].

Management of patients with dysphagia is to provide adequate oral nutrition and maintain safety when eating and drinking. Dietary modifications are to ease swallowing for the patients vary according to the level and severity of dysphagia. The dysphagia's puree diet are for the patients with minimum chewing ability, semisolid foods for the patients who have some chewing ability and soft solid food for those with greater chewing ability. Posture changes like sitting upright can help the patient focus on eating. Management of environment is to create a calm, quiet atmosphere during meals to help patient relax. [138, 161].

Enteral feeding such as the use of gastrotomy tubes helps preventing malnutrition and prolongs life. However, there are some disadvantages observed in long term tube feeding (over 3 months), the patients become dependent and develop severe dysphagia and chronic aspiration due to excessive fibrogenesis after chemoradiation. Modified barium swallowing may be useful to determine the need for long term tube feedings and for swallowing therapy. Oesophageal dilatation may be required in those who are at risk of oesophageal strictures and need the swallowing therapy [122]. The use of Amifostine during chemoradiation has been observed to significantly reduce the incidence of dysphagia and fibrosis in patients with head and neck cancer; however, further studies should be done [204].

Temporomandibular joint disorder (TMD) or Trismus is a common complication which usually occurs when the mastication muscles and temporomandibular joint capsule are in the radiation field. Within 3 to 6 months after radiation the patients may develop progressive joint stiffness and limitation of mouth opening which due to radiation induced hypovascularity and soft tissue fibrosis or scaring from the surgery. Furthermore some authors suggested TMD may develop due to anxiety, depression or the stress associated with cancer or because of sleep disorder [205]. Treatment of trismus is a very difficult task as the limited mouth opening hampers oral hygiene maintenance; dental procedures are especially complex when if trismus is combined with xerostomia. Impaired nutrition and speech can be experienced.

Prevention of trismus: encourage the patients to practice mouth stretching exercises for jaw range of motion daily before the beginning of radiation and consistently practices throughout treatment and after. A strict regimen of mouth exercises is recommended to minimize the problems. Once the limitation of mouth opening occurs, this may be irreversible. The use of simple wedge made by stacking of tongue blades tapping together for exercise and as the guide to improve the mouth opening by adding up one at a time, practice at least 3 to 4 times a day, or the use of rubber stops to increase the mandible opening. Physical therapy such as massage, moist heat application and gentle stretching are recommended. Medications with muscle relaxants, anti anxiety agents and the use of 400 mg pentoxifylline 2 to 3 times daily have been used to ease mouth opening [148, 152, 205].

Neurotoxicity and Teeth Hypersensitivity: there are reports that chemoradiotherapy can cause direct neurotoxicity and is related with leukemic infiltration of dental pulp tissue and direct jaw infiltration. The patients may have deep seated, throbbing mandible pain and dental hypersensitivity may occasionally occur within weeks or months after chemotherapy [137, 206]. Soft-tissue pain also can be found [207]. Management of neurotoxicity is a supportive treatment for pain. Topical fluoride application and desensitizing toothpaste may reduce the discomfort [137, 208].

Osteoradionecrosis

Osteoradionecrosis (ORN) of the jaw is a severe complication of radiation therapy and expressed as a chronic non-healing wound followed by bone necrosis. Non healing bone may become secondarily infected [208]. High radiation dose produces a significant hypovascularization and hypocellularization, causes tissue hypoxia and compromises the healing of bony tissues. The pathogenesis of ORN currently is considered to occur from a fibroatrophic process rather than from vascular alterations, vascular dysfunctions help to generate the initial prefibrotic phase [209]. The mandible is the most commonly affected area [210, 211]. Recently, modern radiation therapy technique and appropriate management of oral care and meticulous oral hygiene demonstrated a continuous decline in the incidence of ORN [210, 212-214].

There are multiple factors associated with an increased incidence of ORN, as it is known that the tumor location, size of radiation treatment field, dose per treatment, total radiation doses and combination interstitial implant and external beam regimen are associated with the occurrence of radiation related side effects [212, 217, 218]. The process of ORN may be spontaneous or result from induced traumatic to the bone and soft tissues such as tooth extraction and surgical treatment in irradiated field shortly before or after radiation and as well as the surgical technique itself [151, 219, 220]. Poor fitting dentures and improper restorations and sharp edge teeth also can cause trauma to the oral mucosa, and poor oral hygiene accelerates the infections in irradiated patients [218]. Different tissues have various levels of tolerance of radiation damage [212]. Patients who have greater risk of ORN are those with multimodality cancer therapies, compromised nutritional status, substances abuse such as tobacco and alcohol. The patients with comorbid disease and decreasing host immune response also affect the ability to repair tissue damage from radiation [212, 221].

To minimize the risk of developing osteoradionecrosis, optimal precautions should be implemented before radiation, as described previously. When there is a small lesion of ORN of the bone, the recommended treatments are prescriptions of daily saline irrigations and antibiotics. For the advanced stage of ORN with pathologic fracture, fistula, full-thickness devitalization of bone, surgical resection of the mandibular segment with free vascularized bone grafting seems to be the standard of care. Treatment with antioxidants and antifibrotic drugs may be helpful in the case that ORN is of fibroblastic origin [209].

Hyperbaric oxygen therapy (HBO) has been used to help the repair of radiation induced damage including mandibular ORN [212, 214, 221, 222]. The therapeutic effects of HBO are for improving the oxygenation of tissues to help eradicate anaerobic bacteria and using the high oxygen tension promotes neovascularization in damaged tissue of irradiated patients [223]. HBO alone or in combination with surgery seem to be the gold standard for treatment and prevention of ORN in irradiated patients [217]. However, hyperbarics is not the only appropriate treatment of radiated patients for prevention of ORN where there is no possible access (economical and availability factors) [217]. The majority of the patients undergoing post radiation therapy dental extractions were observed do not develop osteoradionecrosis. As Sulaiman et al reported in his study of 951 dental extraction in 187 patients occurred either before or after radiation (57.2% after radiation). Only 7 patients received HBO therapy as a prophylactic protocol. The incidence of ORN observed was 2% [151]. Thus the suggested guidelines for the dental management in the irradiated patient should be considered the use of HBO before extractions as an adjunctive therapy not as a standard of care [151]. The use of HBO should be considered in the following situations; there are poor trabecular pattern of bone in the surgical area, vascularization and density pattern are poorer when compared to the pre-radiation radiograph. Besides, HBO is recommended in the patients with comorbid diseases such as diabetes, hematologic profile or the extracted teeth are in the field of radiation.

Caries or demineralization risk, radiation caries caused by two mechanisms, changes in the chemical composition of saliva; increasing in saliva acidity, decreased buffering activity due to decreased salivary flow and increased amount of cariogenic oral bacteria due to the loss of salivary antibacterial effect, the level of *Streptococcus mutans, Lactobacilli* species increase. The consequences are the rapid decalcification of dental enamel. Radiation caries usually are aggressive and the extension of caries involve all surfaces of the tooth. In addition, radiation damage to the pulp of the tooth causes dry and brittle type of dentine which leads to easily loss of enamel from the dentinoenamel junction [133, 208]. Meticulous oral hygiene, topical fluoride application, avoids cariogenic and acidic food helps preventing dental caries.

Cancer therapy in children may result in a long term complications, and with a similar treatment orofacial complications in children are more severe than in adults. The commonest complications include delay or failure of tooth development and eruption, enamel hypoplasia, microdontia and altered root formation. The cartilaginous growth centres located in the condyles of the mandible and on the sutural growth centres of the maxilla, if are affected by a high dose of radiation, a mal-development or an abnormal growth and maturation of the craniofacial skeletal structures can be anticipated. The radiation effect to condylar cartilage of temporomandibular joint (TMJ) may cause TMJ ankylosis and the consequences effect the growth and movement of the jaw. Craniofacial and dental abnormalities can cause severe cosmetic such as micrognathia and functional sequels like trismus. Growth hormone supplements can prevent cartilaginous deviations in radiated children at an early age by stimulating the growth of the condylar cartilage. Orthodontic treatment and surgery may be necessary [136, 208].

Oral Management after Cancer Therapy

After cancer therapy the dentist should establish dental recall schedule for periodical check up. The assessment of the oral hygiene and existing dental care status is necessary.

Frequently recall of the patient is a must for the encouragement of oral hygiene care and early detection of oral diseases. Early detection and management of dental caries and traumatic dental injuries can prevent the possible of pulpal involvement or periapical lesions of the tooth and the future risk of osteoradionecrosis [152]. Thus, regular dental check up and cleaning is essential part of life-long preventive protocol. A period of 3 months is recommended, however, the more frequent can be done according to the actual needs of the individual [149, 152].

Management of carious teeth; After radiation the conservative treatment is preferred. Tooth restorations should be simple and render the acceptable esthetics and functions. Full coverage crowns and splints are ineffective in the patients with xerostomia since it is difficult to clean especially at the cervical margin which is vulnerable to recurrent caries [148].

Ideally restoration materials used in the xerostomia patients should have fluoride release and be cariostatic. Light-activated glass-ionomers seem to be the suitable because of extension fluoride release and fluoride uptake in the dry oral environment, esthetics and greater resistance to acid attack and dehydration as well as the tooth adhesion. The use of conventional glass-ionomer cement base and dental amalgam are recommended on occlusal surface for the reason that fillings with composite resin have higher risk of marginal leakage and recurrent caries underneath the restorations. In children routine restoration treatment must be delayed until the patient is in remission [149].

Endodontic treatment remains a practical treatment alterative for post radiation therapy especially for the infected pulp if the tooth is restorable. However, avoid pushing debris beyond the apex when doing the instrumentation, and shorter endodontic filled are recommended. Periapical radiolucencies may persist after successful endodontic treatment due to decrease alveolar vascularity and hypocellularity. Do not try endodontic therapy in the poor prognosis case just because the risk of ORN from extraction. There were reported several severe cases of ORN from an improper case selection of endodontic treatment [151].

Tooth extraction after radiation in the irradiated field should be considered at risk of developing osteoradionecrosis in all patients who require extraction. Some authors suggested avoiding post-radiation extraction of teeth in radiation fields for prevention of osteoradionecrosis [154]. However, if the extraction cannot be avoided, it can be performed within the 4 months following the completion of radiation treatment, provided the patient does not suffer from the acute effect of the radiation such as mucositis. The risk of ORN does not diminish with time. The longer the clinicians wait, the lessened the healing capacity, and the greater the risk of ORN [149]. Teeth extraction should be performed with minimum mucoperiostal flap and alveoloplasty and also in an atraumatic approach. Prescribe antibiotics coverage before and after extraction is recommended. Bone exposure after extraction should be treated conservatively such as using local saline irrigation with an occasional use of oral antibiotics [151, 214]. It is recommended the patients who had teeth extracted immediately before radiotherapy wait at least one year before wearing dentures [149].

After initial recovery from radiation effects, non surgical periodontal therapy is appropriate for teeth retained in the radiation field, despite with prophylactic antibiotics coverage [152].

Aids

Acquired immunodeficiency syndrome or AIDS is a disease caused by blood-borne retrovirus, human immunodeficiency virus (HIV) and characterized by profound immunosuppression that leads to opportunistic infections, secondary neoplasms, and neurologic manifestations resulted of decreasing CD4+ lymphocyte and impaired cell mediated immunity A healthy people usually have 800-1,200 CD4+T cell/mm^3 of blood [224-226].

AIDS has been major public health problems worldwide for over two decades. It is not only the physical effects that hassle the patients with HIV infection the psychosocial impact is also wearisome. According to UNAIDS and WHO the approximate infection with HIV was increasing rapidly than previously predicted, by the end of 2006 the estimation of people living with HIV infection were about 39.5 million (34.1- 47.1 million), 4.3 million (3.6 - 6.6 million) were the newly infected, and 2.9 million (2.5 - 3.5 million) were AIDS death. The vast majority of HIV-infected people, more than 90 percent, live in the developing world and most of them were not aware of being infected [227].

Diagnosis of HIV infection usually the test of antibodies such as enzyme-linked immunosorbent assay (ELISA) test which is highly sensitive and specific except during the window period which occurs in first three months of infection and where there are occasionally false positive or false negative results. The result confirmation with a more specific test such as the Western Blot and Polymerase Chain Reaction (PCR) is recommended [226].

At the beginning the patient with HIV infection may develop asymptomatic or transient nonspecific symptoms or acute retroviral syndrome; the asymptomatic period may last months to years in most patients. A majority of patients will have acute retroviral syndrome during initial infection which usually begin within 4-28 days after infection and symptoms persist for 3-14 days. The most common symptoms are fever, malaise, rash, fatigue, arthralagia, diarrhea, oral candidiasis, herpes zoster, diffuse lymphadenopathy, progressive wasting and aseptic meningitis in some patients. Mild to moderate cytopenia (*e.g.* leukopenia, anemia, thrombocytopenia) are also common findings. The development of the subsequent manifestations in immunodeficiency patients is related proportionally to the level of CD4+ lymphocyte. The symptoms become worse when CD4+ count drop less than 200/μL. The deficiency of immune functions might lead to the development of opportunistic infections and such as *pneumocystic carinii* pneumonia and candidia*sis*, the development of certain malignancies i.e. Kaposi sarcoma, cervical cancer, non-Hodgkin's lymphoma, and squamous cell cancer of the anus and vulva [226]. Neurologic dysfunction such as AIDS dementia, cryptococcal meningitis and cytomegalovirus encephalitis may occur in some HIV infection [224, 226]. Other transmitted diseases may become co-infective with HIV such as hepatitis, syphilis and Kaposi's-sarcoma-associated with HPV-8 [224].

The advent of highly active antiretroviral therapy (HAART) has been used as the standard treatment for HIV infection and led to a large reduction in the mortality and morbidity of HIV-infected patients who have access to the treatment which currently is only in the developed country. The incidence rates of many opportunistic infections of HIV-associated have been observed decreasing include the orofacial lesions [228-231].

There are 5 classes of the antiviral drug used in HAART: 1. Nucleoside Reverse Transcriptase Inhibitors (*e.g.* Abacavir, Didanosine etc.), 2. Nucleotide Reverse Transcriptase Inhibitor (Tenofovir), 3. Non-Nucleoside Reverse Transcriptase Inhibitors (e.g. Delavirdine, Efavirenz, etc.), 4. Protease inhibitors (*e.g.* Amprenavir, Indinavir etc.), and 5. fusion inhibitor (Enfuvirtide). Combinations of three or four drugs from different classes are necessary to fully control or suppress the replication of HIV [224, 226, 232, 233]. There are variety of HAART regimens but usually consist of two nucleoside reverse transcriptase inhibitors (NRTI) with either non-NRTI or a protease inhibitor [234].

It is generally recommended that the treatment should be deferred if the patient is asymptomatic (CD4+T cell more than 350 cell/mm^3 and viral load less than 100,000 copies/ml) [224]. The reasons for deferring the treatment are patient readiness, the long-term effects of drug-related toxicity, side effect and interaction; and probability of drug adherence.

The success of HAART is evaluated by the plasma viral (RNA) level which should become undetectable [2]. The plasma viral (RNA) level should be measured every 4-8 weeks for first few months and every 3-4 month thereafter. If patients take their drug consistently more than 95% of the time, the plasma level may be suppressed totally to undetectable levels. Partial suppression due to patient's compliance leads to develop the resistant of HIV infection and makes the treatment more difficult and likely to fail [226]. The earliest sign of treatment failure is the increase of the levels of viral replication. About 2-4% of new HIV infection in the United states become multidrug-resistant HIV [224, 238].

During the oral examination the dentists may come across with and unaware of HIV status in asymptomatic patients who present with a specific oral mucosal complaints. These oral manifestations may be some of the opportunistic infections and cancers associate with HIV infection. At least one oral manifestation has been observed develop during the course of the disease in 70-90% of HIV infected [235, 236]. The prevalence of oral lesions are significantly related to the viral loads of greater than 3,000 copies/ml and CD4 cell count of less than 200 cells /mm^3 [224, 236].

The most common oral lesions have been observed strongly associated with HIV infection are oral candidiasis (OC), oral hairy leukoplakia (OHL), oral Kaposi's sarcoma (OKS), Non- Hodgkins's lymphoma (NHL), as well as acute periodontal infections which include linear gingival erythema, necrotizing ulcerative gingivitis, and necrotizing ulcerative periodontitis. Other oral lesions may be found associated with in AIDS patients such as recurrent aphtous-like ulcers, oral herpes viruses (simplex and zoster), human papillomavirus (wart-like) lesions. In children, the most commonly reported oral manifestations associated with HIV infections are slightly dissimilar to those found in adult such as parotid enlargement (PE), periodontal and gingival disease, herpes simplex infection, and others such as recurrent oral ulceration respectively. In contrast oral Kaposi's sarcoma, non-Hodgkins's lymphoma and oral hairy leukoplakia which commonly found in adults but are rare in children [239].

The dentist should be aware or suspect in patients who present with persistent, unexplained, generalized adenopathy or any symptoms of opportunistic infection or those who present with unusual severity or recurrent infection of herpes zoster, herpes simplex, and oral candidiasis may suggest AIDS [2, 9, 240].

Since the oral cavity is easily accessible to clinical examination, specific orofacial lesions which have been shown strongly associated with HIV infection may be an essential means identifying HIV-infected persons as well as a clinical marker of HIV-disease progression, esp. in resource-poor countries. Baccaglini *et al* emphasized that it was considerably important for oral health care professionals worldwide to be competent in the diagnosis and treatments of HIV-associated oral lesions as well as the appropriate referral of the patients to further medical diagnosis and management [2, 241-243].

The Significance of Oral Conditions in HIV

Oral candidiasis (OC) is a common manifestation of immunocompromized HIV-infected; the prevalence is approximately up to 95% [110, 244]. Candidiasis commonly is due to *Candida albicans* and occasionally by *Candida glabata, Candida tropicalis*, and *Candida Kruseii* [224]. The disease is more extensive and severe in HIV patients than those in other group of morbidity and most likely to recur [224]. Pseudomembranous candidiasis and erythematous candidiasis are the most common subtypes however, other subtypes, such as angular cheilitis may also found [224, 245, 246].

In children, it can cause significant morbidity and mortality. The topical disinfectant such as Chlorhexidine digluconate has been shown to be promising agent for treatment and prevention of OC in HIV infected children [247]. Although, the management of OC is the same as in other patient groups still there are reports about resistance to several antifungal drugs, severe side effects and drug interactions associated to systemic antifungal therapy in AIDS patients [248-251]. The use of prophylactic antifungal in HIV is not common for prevention of OC; however, prophylactic doses of Fluconazole may be prescribed to prevent invasive fungal infections such as cryptococcosis [252]. The treatment regimen recommended for specific type of candidiasis such as; the use of Ketoconazole 2% cream, apply 3-4 times per day for 2 weeks for the treatment of angular cheilitis, Clotrimazole troches 10 mg for 2 weeks or Nystatin oral suspension 500,000 U, 1-2 teaspoons swish in mouth for 5 min 3-4 times per days for 2 weeks for the treatment of erythematous candidiasis. Pseudomembranous candidiasis can be treated by the use of Fluconazole 100 mg, 2 tabs on the first day and then 1 tab before bed time for 2 weeks [224].

Oral hairly leukoplakia (OHL) is white thick patches lesions of the mucosa that cannot be wiped or scraped and the vertical corrugation with a hairy appearance can be observed. The presence of OHL is a sign of severe immuno-suppression and has been described as a significant predictor of HIV disease progression in adults [253]. The lesions usually begin at the lateral margins of the tongue, occasionally inside the cheeks and lower lip can be noticed. They may be unilateral or bilateral, and asymptomatic [253]. Although its etiology is not clear and cannot be classified clinically or diagnostically as any other disease entity; however, it is reported that OHL is probably caused by an Epstein-Barr virus (EBV) infection [242]. In addition, oral candidiasis and low CD4+ count remain the major causes related to the development of OHL [255].

Treatment of OHL usually is not required but in the severe cases systemic antiviral agents are recommended for temporary relief; Acyclovir 800 mg orally every 4 hours for 2 weeks [242]. The topical treatment of OHL with Zidovidine, Interferon and Podophyllum resin (POD) is suggested. At the dosages used of POD, adverse effects observed were mild and transient however, serious systemic adverse effects and fatalities have been reported following the use of larger POD doses or after its ingestion. Toxic reaction may develop several hours after POD use [241]. Topical treatments may be impractical for very large lesions. Recurrence is common after therapy is discontinued . When OHL is associated with OC, therapeutic management of OC is required [242].

Periodontal disease is common among HIV-infected patients. It is characterized by gingival bleeding, tooth mobility, bad breath and pain. If it is left untreated especially in children the disease may progress to life-threatening infections such as Ludwig's angina and noma (Cancrum oris) which is a grangrenous condition. [242, 256, 257].

There are risk factors of HIV associated periodontal diseases including the poor oral hygiene, smoking, chronic malnutrition and preexisting gingivitis combined with decreased CD4+ cell counts as well as unusual forms of gingivitis such as; linear gingival erythema, necrotizing ulcerative gingivitis, necrotizing ulcerative periodontitis, and necrotizing stomatitis [242, 258, 259].

Linear gingival erythema (LGE) is characterized by deep red band of 2-3 mm along the marginal gingiva, associated with diffuse erythematic attached gingiva and oral mucosa. The degree of erythema is excessively and increases risk of gingival bleeding in HIV-infected. It is common on the facial gingiva of anterior teeth [224, 242].

Treatment including improving oral hygiene, professional gingival debridement, and the use of 0.12% Chlorhexidine gluconate mouth rinse 5 ml twice daily [224].

There are two periodontal conditions; the necrotizing periodontal diseases have been identified associated with severe immunosuppression which are necrotizing ulcerative gingivitis (NUG) and necrotizing ulcerative periodontitis (NUP). The bacterial causal of NUG and NUP observed are different [259]. Necrotizing periodontal conditions occur more frequently and progress more rapidly due to herpes virus infection of periodontal tissues [260].

Necrotizing ulcerative gingivitis (NUG) is more common among adults than children. It is characterized by the rapid extensive destruction of soft tissue and teeth loss with the presence of sloughing and necrosis ulcer on some of the interdental papillae gingival. In addition, severe pain, bleeding, and fetid halitosis can be observed. NUP can be differentiated from NUG by rapid periodontal attachment loss secondary to necrosis of alveolar bone.

Necrotizing stomatitis is considered to be a consequence of severe, untreated NUP. It is characterized by acute and painful ulceronecrotic lesions on the oral mucosa that expose underlying alveolar bone [242]. There is insufficient evidence to develop evidence based treatment recommendations for HIV-associated periodontal disease. Some HIV patients with NUG, NUP did not response to any conventional therapy [261-264]. Management and control of HIV-associated periodontal disease mainly begins with the maintenance of a good daily oral hygiene, the adjunctive therapy with systemic antibiotics, and the topical use of Chlorhexidine. The treatments include the use of Amoxicillin/Clavulanic acid 1 g, 1 tab 2 times per day for 7 days, or Metronidazole 250 mg orally every 8 hours for 7-10 days, or Clindamycin 300 mg orally every 8 hours for 7 days. Rigorous debridement, and the use of

0.12% Chlorhexidine gluconate rinse or irrigation with Providon-iodine 10% are recommended [224, 241, 242].

Salivary gland diseases including xerostomia and enlargement of salivary gland are observed in HIV patients.

Parotid enlargement is more commonly associated with HIV infection in the children which may be caused by lymphocytic infiltration of the salivary glands which may be unilateral or bilateral swelling of the patotid glands. It occurs in the late course of HIV infection and associates with a slower rate of HIV disease progression. It is usually asymptomatic and decreased salivary flow can be noticed. Treatment is required only in severe cases and may consist of systemic analgesics, anti-inflammatories, antibiotics, and/or steroids [242, 265, 266].

Xerostomia in HIV possibly due to the side effects from either the proliferation of CD8+ T lymphocyte in salivary gland tissue and often caused by medications used that interfere with salivary secretion, such as antiretroviral drug, antihistamines, and antidepressant as well as anti-anxiety medications [224, 267, 268]. Xerostomia increase the development of dental caries and acute gingivitis and can lead to even poorer quality of oral hygiene in HIV patients [224]. Management of xerostomia has been previously discussed in head and neck cancer.

Mycobacterium tuberculosis (TB) frequently co-exists with HIV and is a special challenge to oral health care practitioners, in terms of prevention and minimizing cross infection as well as patient management [269]. Since disseminated TB (pulmonary and non pulmonary) is common in HIV infected patients, oral TB may be observed. Oral mucosa hyperpigmentation can be observed as the result of tuberculosis adrenalitis which is the most specific sign of adrenal damage (primary adrenal insufficiency or Addison's disease) as well as fatigue and weight loss [269, 270]. Although Addison's disease is rare, in the environment with the pandemic of pulmonary tuberculosis and AIDS it does occur. Disseminated TB can lead to multiple organ failure, with widespread systemic consequences [270].

Oral Kaposi's sarcoma is the most prevalent AIDS-associated intraoral malignancy which common site is hard palate and maxillary gingiva. It is an angioproliferative disease which may develop from a human herpes virus 8 (HH-8) infection of mesenchymal progenitors cells. Kaposi's sarcoma is characterized by mucosal lesions that begin as red or bluish-purple muscular patches and gradually develop to darker color and exophytic with ulcerations as lesions advance. It may resemble bacillary epithelial angiomatosis [224].

Treatments of oral Kaposi's sarcoma include incisional biopsy with follow up with the patients 'physician and possibly of radiotherapy or chemotherapy. The intraoral small lesions may be treated with the use of Vinblastine sulfate or sclerosing solution sodium tetradecyl sulfate intralesions injections. Local anesthesia infiltration is suggested before drug injection to reduce pain from the intralesion chemotherapy [224].

Recurrent Aphtous ulcers (RAU) is the most common of oral ulcers occur of HIV-infected patients [235, 236, 265, 266]. The frequency of occurrence and severity of aphtous ulcers usually increase in HIV positive patients which severe recurrent lesions occur when the CD4+ lymphocyte count is less than 100 cells/mm^3. This may be suggestive of HIV disease progression [224, 242].

The etiology of RAU is not well determined. They are characterized as painful ulcers on the nonkeratinized oral mucosa including labial and buccal mucosa, soft palate, and ventral aspect of the tongue. It may appear as minor, major, or herpetiform aphtae. Minor aphtous ulcers are less than 5 mm in diameter covered by pseudomembrane and surrounded by an erythematous halo. They usually heal spontaneously without scarring. Major aphtous ulcers are larger in diameter of 1-3 cm, more painful, and may persist longer. Scarring is very common. Their presence can interfere with mastication, swallowing, and speaking. Healing occurs over two to six weeks. Herpetiform aphtous ulcers occur as a crop of numerous form lesions of 1-2 mm disseminated on the soft palate, tonsils tongue and/or buccal mucosa [224, 242].

The management of RAU is pain control and prevention of superinfection. Topical and/or systemic steroid agents such as corticosteroids, Thalidomide are recommended depending on the severity of the lesions [224, 242]. Thalidomide is contraindicated in pregnant women as it is teratogenic.

Herpes Simplex Virus (HSV) Infection may either be primary (herpetic gingivo-stomatitis) or secondary (herpes labialis). The prevalence of oral HSV infection is 10-35% in adults and children with HIV infection [235, 236, 265, 266]. The presences of HSV infection for more than one month may suggest an AIDS-defining condition. HSV infection manifests as a crop of vesicles usually localized on the keratinized mucosa including hard palate, gingival and /or vermillion borders of the lips and skin surrounding the mouth. The vesicles rupture and form irregular painful ulcers. They may interfere with mastication and swallowing which result in decreasing oral intake and dehydration [242].

The treatment is more effective in the early stage of HSV infection. Topical or systemic therapy with antiviral agents is recommended.

Human Papilloma virus (HPV) Infection or Oral Warts is an asymptomatic mucocutaneous infection of the skin or oral mucosa caused by Human Papilloma virus, which is a DNA virus containing an epithelium growth factor responsible for inducing distinct squamous cell proliferations [224]. The significantly increased of incidence of oral warts due to human papillomavirus infection has been observed since the use of HAART. The prevalence of lesions is observed in adults more than in children. [224, 235, 236, 265, 266]. Oral warts may appear cauliflower-like, spiked, or raised with multifocal flat lesions resembling focal epithelial hyperplasia (Heck's disease) [268]. Multiple papilloma is typical HPV infections. The most common location is the labial and buccal mucosa, as well as tongue and gingival [224].

There is no therapy to eradicate the infection. Treatment may be required for patients with multiple lesions. Topical and systemic agents and various surgical approaches are available. Surgical removal of papules can be done but the recurrent is likely needed for re-treatment. Topical Podophylin or 5-Fluorouracil has been used to treat lesions [224, 242]. Concurrence therapeutic approaches should be considered [242].

The Comprehensive Consideration of Dental Services in HIV Patients

Quality of life: There are many concerns of oral conditions that affect the quality of life of AIDS patients *e.g.* pain, discomfort, and alteration of facial appearance, impair speech and dysphagia which may lead to significant weight loss. The discomforts may not only burden the health of patients with HIV but also influence their self confidence. It was observed that 16.7% of the patients avoided leaving home because of dental problems [271]. Improvement of oral health brought significant improvements in both physical and mental health [272, 273].

Stigma and unacceptable (discrimination): Although the high rate of oral diseases in HIV infection individuals, many do not have dental care regularly. Non compliance with dental services depends on the patients' characteristics and the availability of dental services. HIV-infected individuals continue to experience unacceptable by health care professionals even though, access to dental treatment has significantly improved recently in many countries [239]. Non attendance at appointments and disclosure of HIV status signify unacceptability of care. There are some common reasons of the patients of not telling HIV status during history taken including fear of refusal or some other negative attitude, and the concern about confidentiality [274]. It is uncertain how many patients disclose their HIV status in their history chart; one reported figure was up to 70% and 30% were uncertain [275]. A lot of efforts needs to be done to diminish the stigma and discrimination of treatment the patients with HIV infected [239, 275].

Comprehensive oral care in HIV infection: Maintenance of oral hygiene and regular visits to the dentist are required not only just for a healthy oral cavity but also should be approached as a part of medical cares. Personal oral-hygiene practices, such as tooth brushing and interdental cleaning, are the most effective ways of maintaining good oral health including emphasize on oral-hygiene awareness through health education. In order to prevent the complicated dental diseases that need of the expensive dental services, it is necessary to treat the oral manifestations of HIV infection at all levels of care [242].

Assessment of oral health status is an important part of routine health care since those with AIDS who has regular dental visit require less restoratives and surgical treatments and show significantly improved oral health, function, and quality of life [242, 276, 277].

The initial assessment should include a thorough medical history taking. A head-neck examination should be performed including examination for enlarged lymph node along with a comprehensive complete oral examination, particularly, the soft and hard tissue as well as periodontal examination [224]. Dental care providers play an important role to identify signs and symptoms of oral conditions associated with HIV-infection or oral opportunistic infections which may be the first sign of HIV infection or clinical treatment failure or non-compliance with antiviral drug therapy. As such, pseudomembranous candidiasis and oral hairy leukoplakia should be monitored carefully because they are the sensitive clinical markers for immunosuppression stage [224, 252].

Modification of treatment is not suggested since the treatment needs in HIV-patients are not different from those non-infected [239]. The dental care management of HIV patients is usually uncomplicated, no need for special facilities or equipments. Most treatments can be performed by general practitioners however, those who require the care of specialists should be referred since the referral criteria is not differences to those with non- HIV [252]. Besides, the clinicians should implement the current universal infection control recommendations with every patient, irrespective of the presence or absence of blood borne disease [252].

The patients in advanced stages with low CD4+ cell counts <200 cells/mm^3 are predisposed to HIV associated oral infections require specific treatments. The first priorities are to relieve pain and control of infections, the prevention of concomitant disease, the restoration of functions so as to maintain the patients' nutrition as well as esthetics restoration to improve self- esteem and psychological health [224]. Antibiotics prophylaxis is not routinely recommended since super infections and microorganism drug resistance may be induced, unless the patient is neutropenia, in which case antibiotic prophylaxis is required [224].

It is very important to include complete blood count and routine laboratory chemistries analysis for HIV patients as a baseline assessment prior to dental treatment. Usually the advantages of dental treatment must be weighed against the risk of infections; elective dental procedures may be contraindicated depending on the neutrophil count. If a neutropenia and thrombocytopenia ($<$50,000 cells/mm^3) an elective dental procedure should be postponed. In case of an emergency dental procedure is necessary, the patients should be hospitalized for antibiotic prophylaxis and preparation for abnormal bleeding. The regimen of a single dose one hour before the dental procedure as suggested by the AHA for the prevention of endocarditis has been used by many clinicians; however, others believe that appropriate antibiotic therapy should be continued for as long as open wounds are presented in the oral cavity, the judgments and evaluations is up to the clinicians' experiences and depend on a case-by- case basis [224, 226, 252].

Comorbidities commonly found in concurrence with HIV are HBV, and HCV and often impaired hepatic function. The side-effects and drug interactions with antiretroviral therapy can be anticipated and make dental treatments more complicated, and a protection against infections is necessary [237, 252]. Some considerations should be taken such as the avoidance of Acetaminophen because of its hepatotoxicity, Aspirin and non-steroidal anti-inflammatory drugs or NSAIDs which can decrease coagulation should not be used in patients with impaired hemostasis [63]. Additionally, antiretroviral therapy possibly increases the patients's risk of occurrence of adverse cardiovascular sequels and the development of diabetes, thus, the dentists should be aware and carefully monitor for related symptoms of CVD and diabetes during dental procedures [252].

The Total Oral Health Care the Considerations for the Systemic Diseases

Usually after the diagnosis, the systemic patients were consulted with the dentists for oral assessment and total oral care when the treatment modalities were done; *e.g.* radiotherapy, chemotherapy and organ transplantations. During the systemic treatment it is the responsibility of the physicians to work together with the dental health providers to motivate the patients in an attempt to improve the quality of health through the good oral care and set up the feasible referral system for the patients.

The oral service is specific for individual. The application of dental services depends on the stages of the diseases when seeing the dentists as it was revealed that no treatment plan fits all [2]. The total oral health care usually includes maintenance the oral health, counseling and prevention of oral diseases, and periodically oral assessment or recall.

Maintenance of the oral health mainly consists of oral assessment, treatment plan, dental procedures including restoration services and rehabilitation services.

Preventive dental services and counseling the preventive strategies play an important role for controlling dental diseases. Diet counseling mainly is meant to reduce dental caries potential, including avoiding highly cariogenic foods and habits of frequent snacking between meals. Meticulous plaque removal is important for optimal oral health and minimizing plaque accumulation is the starting point of preventive dental diseases. There are some changes in the treatment prototype that the prevention should not only emphasize on the reserve of pathogens, but also on intervention with their environment. Since dental plaque cannot be totally eradicated with the oral hygiene measures such as mechanical plaque removal, the rinse with an antimicrobial mouth rinse and applied chemotherapeutic agents are suggested. [278]. In addition, the oral health self-care should be a lifelong consistency approach and unite with the patients' value.

The key role of mechanical plaque removal in the systemic patients is to maximize plaque removal and minimize tissue damage which commonly includes toothbrushing, interdental and soft tissues cleaning.

Tooth brushing; plays an important role for daily personal oral hygiene, toothbrush is an excellent device for effective plaque removal which may be manual or electric or powered. There are several types of toothbrushes manufactured in different sizes, shapes as well as bristle length and hardness, for the purposes of better adapt to oral anatomy of different individuals and cleaning efficiency. Thorough tooth brushing requires a different amount of time vary from individual to individual, depending on such factors as the individual tendency of plaque and debris accumulation, the psychomotor skills and the saliva flushing mechanical for clearance of foods, bacteria, and debris [279]. In patients with poor plaque control, patients with limited motor function or those with orthodontic appliances conventional electric or powered toothbrushes electric seem to have a slight edge in plaque removal [65]. In well motivated patients using either manual or powered toothbrushes, no differences reduction of plaque and inflammation were shown. However, an increased gingival abrasion and recession have been observed associated with the increased use of oscillating powered toothbrushes [2].

In addition, there are some disadvantages to tooth brushing as tooth cleaning is limited only on the accessible surfaces of the tooth and toothbrush can harbor and the oral microorganisms can be transferred to a tooth brush during use and can grow on toothbrushes after use. Contaminated toothbrushes can be sources of repeated oral infections causing the localized oral inflammatory diseases as well as disseminate systemically. Besides, periodontal pathogens were observed could survive on air exposed toothbrushes for the long period of four hours thus, the possibility of re-infection from toothbrushes is likely [280-282]. A more serious concern is that bacterial endocarditis is observed from bacteremia caused by toothbrush [280].

For those with a high risk to infection particularly patients with systemic diseases transmissible by blood or saliva and/or a compromised immune system or low resistance to infection due to treatments modalities as such chemotherapy, radiotherapy, etc., a higher level of caution to prevent exposure to microbes is emphasized. Appropriate care and maintenance of toothbrush are important considerations for those with vulnerable systemic. The American Dental Association common recommendations for tooth brush care include the followings;

Rinse the mouth with an antimicrobial mouth rinse before brushing. Thoroughly rinse toothbrushes with tap water after brushing to remove any remaining toothpaste and debris.

Allow the toothbrush to air dry, store tooth brush separately and do not routinely cover toothbrushes or store them in close containers. Change the toothbrushes between brushings to prevent self-infection is recommended especially the patient with periodontal diseases [280]. Usually the average using time of a manual toothbrush is approximately 3 months since the bristles become frayed and worn with use which will decrease cleaning effectiveness but in the infection prone patients toothbrushes should be replaced more often than 3 months. In addition, it is suggested that after every oral or medical contagious illness, the tooth brush should be replaced [283]. Do not share toothbrushes especially a person with compromised immune systems or those with existing infectious diseases.

Disposable toothbrushes such as disposable foam brushes are frequently provided for institutionalized patients which are helpful in plaque removal for those with limitation of motor skills [284-286]. If foam brush was saturated with Chlorhexidine solution, the achievement of plaque removal and inflammation reduction responses were similar to those with the conventional manual toothbrush [287].

Toothbrushes disinfection had been recommended by soaking toothbrushes in an antimicrobial mouth rinse such as a mouth rinse containing essential oil, it is observed that 100% of the bacteria present were eradicated [288]. Virkon® and Listerine® were shown to destroy all the test species and practically all the microorganisms on the toothbrush bristles and proxabrushes. Contaminated toothbrushes with various test species including *Candida albicans*, *Mycobacterium smegmatis*, *M. bovis*, and *Streptococcus mitis* were tested for the efficacy of a Listerine® soaking regime to prevent the bacterial contamination of toothbrushes. Soaking the toothbrush head (bristles) in Listerine® for 20 minutes after brushing was sufficient to eliminate bacterial contamination [288].

There are several of commercial toothbrush sanitizers available on the market. The use of UV toothbrush-sanitizing devices also has been shown to be effective. The use of a Cetylpyridinium chloride spray with toothbrushes was found to be bactericidal [280].

In addition, it was observed that oral bacteria could also spread by sharing eating utensils contaminated by saliva and transmitted between spouses and siblings [280].

When tooth brushing cannot be done in the patients with some manner compromised such as during mucositis or neutropenia and thrombocytopenia the other oral hygiene aids are suggested for maintenance of hygiene. The suggested devices are foam on a stick device or sponge on stick or toothette® with differences of size and handle length, swab on a stick or cotton swabs which frequently used for oral hygiene in the institutionalized settings and gauze wipe. There are evidences showed the effectiveness of plaque removal using foam stick is not difference from the use of toothbrush. However, tooth brushing is more effective in delay the plaque accumulation [2]. After the systemic impairment are improved the regular tooth brushing should be presumed.

Soft tissues cleaning: thorough cleaning of soft tissues is required such as a coated tongue can be a reservoir of oral microorganisms since the papillae on the tongue contributing to retention of debris and oral microorganisms that could be foci of intraoral infection and re-infection transmitted through toothbrushes [289]. Cleaning the tongue and palate helps reduce debris, plaque and number of microorganisms. Tongue cleaning devices include tongue scraper, tongue brush, powered tongue cleaning device etc. Food retained in the buccal vestibule and between the teeth of the patient can be found in the patients with decreased neuromuscular coordination or decreased salivary flow. Either gauze wipe or sponge on stick or toothette® can be used to clean buccal mucosa, palate, and alveolar ridge [289, 290].

Interdental cleaning is an essential component of a successful of oral self care program which supported by most of the oral health professionals. Since accessible to interproximal areas is complicated plaque removal by tooth brushing thus the cleaning is inadequate. Dental floss is the standard devices for interproximal cleaning and is best for plaque and debris removal from tooth embrasures where interdental papilla gingival fills the interproximal space and the teeth are in contact. However, there are some disadvantages in those who loss gingival attachment, and in the excessive gingival recession; the use of regular dental floss may be ineffective to clean the long expanded of root exposure and so the use of thicker so called Superfloss® is recommended. For the patients who have difficulty of manipulating dental floss, a floss holding device is recommended to ease with regular flossing. The other interproximal devices such as interproximal brushes, toothpicks and rubber tips are recommended to aid in cleaning the area that is difficult to reach [291]. Usually the combination use of tooth brushes, dental floss and other interproximal devices are recommended for more effective cleaning.

Patients with dentures, implants and orthodontics appliances: Patients with dental implants, fixed bridge and fixed orthodontic appliances are at significant risk for oral hygiene problems as well as those who wear removable partial dentures. Tooth brushing can be done in patients with fixed bridge or fixed orthodontic appliances but interproximal cleaning can be problem when using dental floss. The use of floss threader or Superfloss® can help guiding dental floss through interproximal of the teeth and under bridge for cleaning. Orthodontic brush and single tuft brush are suggested; water irrigation may be useful for those with orthodontics appliances.

Systemic compromised patients who wear full or removable partial dentures may need assistance with maintaining proper hygiene of the appliances, the oral soft tissues and any remaining natural teeth. The patients should brush their oral tissues with soft nylon brushes and all the remaining natural teeth after eating every meal and before reinserted the dentures. The dentures should be brushed at all area after eating every meal then rinsed well. The dentures should be left out of the mouth for 6 to 8 hours per days, and left to soak in antimicrobial solutions such as denture cleansing tablet or denture bath during this period of time [2, 136, 137].

Topical applied chemotherapeutic agents: Sometimes the patients have difficulty or are unable to fulfill the exacting level of plaque removal required and to keep the desired level of oral hygiene. This depends on many factors including age, culture, socioeconomic status, level of education, belief and attitudes regarding personal care, domestic circumstances, and dental personnel available and frequency of dental visits [292]. These are the reasons providing the basis for development of chemotherapeutic agents that would enhance the mechanical plaque removal and full mouth disinfection for prevention of bacterial re-colonization especially in patients with periodontal diseases [293].

The ideal chemotherapeutic agents for plaque control should be safe, non-toxic, non-allergenic, and non-irritating and be as effective as possible in reducing plaque and gingivitis, have specific effects on pathogenic flora, have an acceptable taste, be easy to use and be inexpensive [65]. The most common is Chlorhexidine which is available in both toothpaste and rinse formulations. The use of this agent has consistently resulted in significance reductions in plaque deposits and gingival inflammation scores [65]. Tricosan is a phenolic agent that has received extensive attention and is a highly effective anti-plaque agent when combined with copolymer of methoxyethylene and maleic acid or zinc citrate [292, 294]. Tricosan preparation are available in either toothpaste preparations or as prebrush rinsing agents [294-296]. However, it has been observed that neither regular toothpaste nor Tricosan-containing toothpastes appear to inhibit the presence of periodontal pathogens [280].

The mouthrinse compounds also consist of essential oils such as thymol, menthol, eucalyptol and methylsalicylate which has been demonstrated to significantly reduce both gingival inflammation as well as plaque accumulations [292]. Other agents such as Delmopinol is a surface active agent derived from morpholinoethanol which is claimed as the most promising agent for rapid and slow plaque forming and dissolve the already formed plaque when absence of mechanical plaque control [297, 298]. It was observed that Delmopinol has weak antimicrobial properties binding to salivary proteins and altering the cohesive and adhesive properties of biofilm formed [299]. Possibly, as a result of these interferences with the binding of microorganisms, Delmopinol interferes with dental plaque maturation [300]. This agent seems to have significant potential as a preventive agent for both caries and periodontal diseases [65]. It have been observed that the long term (6 months) use of Delmopinol rinse 60 seconds twice daily in conjunction with brushing significantly reduced in both plaque and gingivitis scores [300-302].

The use of fluoride; fluoride is the most important caries protection agent; it has been shown to reduce demineralization and enhance remineralization of the teeth [303, 304]. Usually fluoride toothpaste is an important component of an oral hygiene program, in some of systemic circumstances if the patients have to exclude the routine use of fluoride toothpaste, it can be compensated by using other forms of fluoride [304]. Other than the regular topical fluoride by the dental staff or the application of fluoride varnish which can be used as fluoride supplement as well as a home self-applied fluoride including fluoride mouth rinses, self-applied fluoride gel is considered significantly equivalent particular in those received radiotherapy.

The use of fluoride mouth rinses may be contraindicated in patients who cannot effectively swish the solution around their mouths or those with an incompetent or hypotonic lip seal and cannot keep solutions in their mouths for 1-2 min which may occur in the patients with neurological diseases such as cerebrovascular accident (CVA), muscular dystrophy, and motor neuron disease effect of CVA or diabetes [2].

Fluoride gels applied with custom-made trays provided for each patient or brush on fluoride gel with 1% neutral sodium fluoride gel or 0.4% stannous fluoride gel have been recommended.

Apply fluoride gel to the teeth surface for maximum protection effect for 4 minutes with custom built fluoride tray provided for each patient has been demonstrated difficult for those with active gag reflex and not successful for many compromised patients. Brush on fluoride gel for 2 to 3 minutes may be easier to use especially in the elderly compromised patients. The use of a foam applicator may be done. [137, 152, 304]. In children systemic fluoride is recommended.

Periodically assessment (recall); In order to achieve the optimal long term maintenance of oral health the patients must perform daily plaque control and must attend recommended recall appointments regularly. The objective of periodically oral assessment is to prevent the occurrence of new diseases by prophylactic treatment and early detection, treatment of new and recurring of previous disease and/or minimize the recurrent previous disease. Meticulous plaque removal is important for optimal oral health however, compliance with recommended supportive appointments is more important especially for those who cannot perform adequate plaque removal. Usually 3 months period is recommended for recall appointments however, the systemic patients with other risk factors may require supportive intervals more frequently than 3 months [65].

Conclusion

Meticulous maintenance of oral hygiene is the most important measure for the prevention and care of oral infections. Through good oral hygiene, the incidences and severity of oral complications are significantly reduced. In contrast with the bacterial plaque accumulation and gingivitis, pathogenic organisms may disseminate systemically and cause more risk of septicemia. Even with the daily cleaning activities such as tooth brushing, flossing, using toothpicks as well as chewing, bacteria can be disseminated to other systemic organs. The patients should therefore be motivated to keep their mouths very clean.

The oral assessments and dental care prior during and after systemic treatments is important so as to eliminate predisposing factors of trauma and infections which lead to more severe oral complications.

Palliative and conservative treatments are still the choice of care for oral conditions. Together with mechanical plaque removal such as tooth brushing, teeth interproximal cleaning, and the conjunctive use of topical chemotherapeutic agents applied such as; topical fluoride, anti-plaque agents application.

Periodically oral assessments and care should be performed after cancer treatment for the early detection and interventions of any treatment complications.

Acknowledgements

The authors would like to express our thanks to the following experts for their valuable comments: Professor Alain Kupferman, Dr Mathirut Mungthin, Dr Kednapa Tekarnchanavanich, Dr Francois Le Berre, and Miss Ariane Kupferman-Sutthavong for her superb assistance with the preparation of the manuscript.

References

[1]   Johnson NW, Glick M, Mbuguye TN. Oral health and general health. *Adv. Dent. Res.* 2006;19:118-21.

[2]   Harris NO, Jeffery LH. Preventive Dentistry in a hospital setting. In Harris NO, Garcia-Godoy F, eds. New Jersey Pearson Education, Inc., *Primary preventive dentistry.* 6th ed, 2004;605-43.

[3]   Carroll GC, Sebor RJ. Dental flossing and its relationship to transient bacteremia. *J. Periodontol.* 1980;51:691-2.

[4]   Debelian GJ, Olsen I, Tronstad L. Bacteria in conjunction with endodontic therapy. *Endod. dent. Traumatol.* 1995;11:142-9.

[5]   Debelian GJ, Olsen I, Tronstad L. Anaerobic bacteremia and fungemia in patients undergoing endodontic therapy: an overview. *Ann. Periodontol.* 1998;3:281-7.

[6]   Drinnan AJ, Gogan C. Bacteremia and dental treatment. *J. Am. Dent. Assoc.* 1990;120:378.

[7]   Heimdahl A, Hall G, Hedgerg M, Sandgerg H, Soder PO, Turner K, et al. Detection and quantitation by lysis-filtration of bacteremia after different oral surgical procedures. *J. clin. Microbiol.* 1990;28:2205-9.

[8]   Demmer RT, Desvarieux M. Periodontal infections and cardiovascular disease: the heart of the matter. *J. Am. Dent. Assoc.* 2006;137 Suppl:14S-20S.

[9]   Desvarieux M, Demmer RT, Rundek T, Boden-Albala B, Jacobs DR Jr, Sacco RL, Papapanou PN. Periodontal microbiota and carotid intima-media thickness: the Oral Infections and Vascular Disease Epidemiology Study (INVEST). *Circulation.* 2005;111:576-82.

[10]   Spahr A, Klein E, Khuseyinova N, Boeckh C, Muche R, Kunze M, Rothenbacher D, Pezeshki G, Hoffmeister A, Koenig W. Periodontal infections and coronary heart disease: role of periodontal bacteria and importance of total pathogen burden in the Coronary Event and Periodontal Disease (CORODONT) study. *Arch. Intern. Med.* 2006;166:554-9.

[11]   Li X, Kolltveit KM, Tronstad L, Olsen I. Systemic diseases caused by oral infection. *Clin. Microbiol. Rev.* 2000;13:547-5.

[12]   Beck J, Garcia R, Heiss G, Vokonas PS, Offenbacher S. Periodontal disease and cardiovascular disease. *J. Periodontol.* 1996;67 Suppl:1123-37.

[13]   Forner L, Larsen T, Kilian M, Holmstrup P, Forner L. Incidence of bacteremia after chewing, tooth brushing and scaling in individuals with periodontal inflammation. *J. Clin. Periodontol.* 2006;33:401-7.

[14]   Wilson W, Taubert KA, Gewitz M, Lockhart PB, Baddour LM, Levison M, et al. Prevention of Infective Endocarditis. Guidelines from the American Heart Association. A guideline from the American Heart Association Rhumatic fever, Endocarditis, and Kawasaki Disease Committee, Council on Cardiovascular disease in the Young, and the Council on Clinical Cardiology, Council on Cardiovascular Surgery and Anesthesia, and the Quality of Care and Outcomes Research Interdisciplinary Working Group. *Circulation* published online Apr 19, 2007.

[15] Okabe K, Nakagawa K, Yamamoto E. Factors affecting the occurrence of bacteremia associated with tooth extraction. *Int. J. Oral Maxillofac. Surg.* 1995;24:239-42.

[16] Lofthus JE, Waki MY, Jolkovsky DL, Otomo-Corgel J, Newman MG, Flemming T, et al. Bacteremia following subgingival irrigation and scaling and root planning. *J. Periodontol.* 1991;62:602-7.

[17] Lockhart PB, Durack DT. Oral microflora as a cause of endocarditis and other distant site infections. *Infect. Dis. Clin. North Am.* 1999;13:833-50.

[18] Lockhart PB. The risk for endocarditis in dental practice. *Periodontol* 2000. 2000;23:127-35.

[19] Mattila KJ, Nieminen MS, Valtonen VV, Rasi VP, Kesäniemi YA, Syrjälä SL, Jungell PS, Isoluoma M, Hietaniemi K, Jokinen MJ. Association between dental health and acute myocardial infarction. *BMJ.* 1989;298:779-81.

[20] Braudwald E. Approach to the patient with cardiovascular disease. In:Kasper Dl, Brauwald E, Fauci AS, Hauser SL, Longo DL, Jameson JL, eds. *Harrison's principles of internal medicine* 16[th]ed. New York McGraw-Hill, Inc 2005;130-40.

[21] Desvarieux M, Schwahn C, Völzke H, Demmer RT, Lüdemann J, Kessler C, Jacobs DR, John U, Kocher T. Gender differences in the relationship between periodontal disease, tooth loss, and atherosclerosis. *Stroke.* 2004;35:2029-35.

[22] Desvarieux M.Periodontal disease, race, and vascular disease. *Compend. Contin. Educ. Dent.* 2001;22 Spec No:34-41.

[23] Rose LF, Mealey B, Minsk L, Cohen DW. Oral care for patients with cardiovascular disease and stroke. *J. Am. Dent. Assoc.* 2002;133 Suppl:37S-44S.

[24] Haraszthy VI, Zambon JJ, Trevisan M, Zeid M, Genco RJ. Identification of periodontal pathogens in atheromatous plaques. *J. Periodontol.* 2000;71:1554-60.

[25] Pallasch TJ, Slots J. Antibiotic prophylaxis and the medically compromised patient. *Periodontol* 2000. 1996;10:107-38.

[26] Schlein RA, Kudlick EM, Reindorf CA, Gregory J, Royal GC. Toothbrushing and transient bacteremia in patients undergoing orthodontic treatment. *Am. J. Orthod. Dentofacial Orthop.* 1991;99:466-72.

[27] Roberts GJ. Dentists are innocent! "Everyday" bacteremia is the real culprit: a review and assessment of the evidence that dental surgical procedures are a principal cause of bacterial endocarditis in children. *Pediatr. Cardiol.* 1999;20:317-25.

[28] Mask AG. Medical management of the patient with cardiovascular disease. *Periodontol* 2000. 2000;23:136-41.

[29] Bassi GS, Cousin GC, Lawrence C, Bali N, Lowry JC. Improved resuscitation training of senior house officers in oral and maxillofacial surgery. *Br. J. Oral Maxillofac. Surg.* 2002;40:293-5.

[30] ADA council on scientific affairs. Office emergencies and emergency kits. *J. Am. Dent. Assoc.* 2002;113:364-5.

[31] Fisher NDL, Williams GH. Hypertensive Vascular disease. In: Kasper DL, Brauwald E, Fauci AS, Hauser SL, Longo DL, Jameson JL, eds. *Harrison's principles of internal medicine* 16[th]ed. New York McGraw-Hill, Inc 2005;2:1463-81.

[32] Matsuura H. The systemic management of cardiovascular risk patients in dentistry. *Anesth. Pain Control. Dent.* 1993;2:49-61.

[33] McCarthy FM. Safe treatment of the post-heart-attack patient. *Compendium.* 1989;10:598-604.

[34] Shuman SK. A physician's guide to coordinating oral health and primary care. *Geriatrics.* 1990;45:47-57.

[35] Knoll-Köhler E, Förtsch G. Pulpal anesthesia dependent on epinephrine dose in 2% lidocaine. A randomized controlled double-blind crossover study. *Oral Surg. Oral Med. Oral Pathol.* 1992;73:537-40.

[36] Pérusse R, Goulet JP, Turcotte JY. Contraindications to vasoconstrictors in dentistry: Part II. Hyperthyroidism, diabetes, sulfite sensitivity, cortico-dependent asthma, and pheochromocytoma. *Oral Surg. Oral Med. Oral Pathol.* 1992;74:687-91.

[37] Meyer FU. Haemodynamic changes under emotional stress following a minor surgical procedure under local anaesthesia. *Int. J. Oral Maxillofac Surg.* 1987;16:688-94.

[38] Leviner E, Tzukert AA, Mosseri M, Fisher D, Yossipovitch O, Pisanty S, Markitziu A. Perioperative hemodynamic changes in ischemic heart disease patients undergoing dental treatment. *Spec. Care Dentist.* 1992;12:84-8.

[39] Findler M, Garfunkel AA, Galili D.Review of very high-risk cardiac patients in the dental setting. *Compendium.* 1994;15:58, 60-6.

[40] Luria MH, Debanne SM, Osman MI. Long-term follow-up after recovery from acute myocardial infarction. Observations on survival, ventricular arrhythmias, and sudden death. *Arch. Intern. Med.* 1985;145:1592-5.

[41] Cintron G, Medina R, Reyes AA, Lyman G. Cardiovascular effects and safety of dental anesthesia and dental interventions in patients with recent uncomplicated myocardial infarction. *Arch. Intern. Med.* 1986;146:2203-4.

[42] Gilbert GH, Minaker KL. Principles of surgical risk assessment of the elderly patient. *J. Oral Maxillofac. Surg.* 1990;48:972-9.

[43] Doern GV, Ferraro MJ, Brueggemann AB, Ruoff KL. Emergence of high rates of antimicrobial resistance among viridans group streptococci in the United States. *Antimicrob. Agents Chemother.* 1996;40:891-4.

[44] Lockhart PB, Gibson J, Pond SH, Leitch J. Dental management considerations for the patient with an acquired coagulopathy. Part 2: Coagulopathies from drugs. *Br. Dent. J.* 2003;195:495-501.

[45] Mask AG. Medical management of the patient with cardiovascular disease. *Periodontol 2000.* 2000;23:136-41.

[46] Jeske AH, Suchko GD. Lack of a scientific basis for routine discontinuation of oral anticoagulation therapy before dental threatment. *J. Am. Dent. Assoc.* 2003;134:1492-7.

[47] Deitcher SR. Antiplatelet, Anticoagulant, and fibrinolytic therapy. In:Kasper DL, Brauwald E, Fauci AS, Hauser SL, Longo DL, Jameson JL, eds. *Harrison's principles of internal medicine* 16[th]ed. New York McGraw-Hill, Inc 2005;1:687-93.

[48] George JN, Shattil SJ. The clinical importance of acquired abnormalities of platelet function. *N. Engl. J. Med.* 1991;324:27-39.

[49] Ware JA, Heistad DD. Seminars in medicine of the Beth Israel Hospital, Boston. Platelet-endothelium interactions. *N. Engl. J. Med.* 1993;328:628-35.

[50] Vane JR, Anggård EE, Botting RM. Regulatory functions of the vascular endothelium. *N. Engl. J. Med.* 1990;323:27-36.

[51] Schafer AI. Effects of nonsteroidal antiinflammatory drugs on platelet function and systemic hemostasis. *J. Clin. Pharmacol.* 1995;35:209-19.

[52] Hirsh J, Dalen J, Anderson DR, Poller L, Bussey H, Ansell J, et al. Oral anticoagulants: mechanism of action, clinical effectiveness, and optimal therapeutic range. *Chest.* 2001;119Suppl:8S-21S.

[53] Owens CD, Belkin M. Thrombosis and coagulation: operative management of the anticoagulated patient. *Surg. Clin. North Am.* 2005;85:1179-89.

[54] White RH, McKittrick T, Hutchinson R, Twitchell J. Temporary discontinuation of warfarin therapy: changes in the international normalized ratio. *Ann. Intern. Med.* 1995;122:40-2.

[55] Wells PS, Holbrook AM, Crowther NR, Hirsh J. Interactions of warfarin with drugs and food. *Ann. Intern. Med.* 1994;121:676-83.

[56] Campbell JH, Alvarado F, Murray RA. Anticoagulation and minor oral surgery: should the anticoagulation regimen be altered? *J. Oral Maxillofac. Surg.* 2000;58:131-5.

[57] Webster K, Wilde J. Management of anticoagulation in patients with prosthetic heart valves undergoing oral and maxillofacial operations. *Br. J. Oral Maxillofac. Surg.* 2000;38:124-6.

[58] Aguilar D, Goldhaber SZ. Clinical uses of low-molecular-weight heparins. *Chest.* 1999;115:1418-23.

[59] Johnson-Leong C, Rada RE. The use of low-molecular-weight heparins in outpatient oral surgery for patients receiving anticoagulation therapy. *J. Am. Dent. Assoc.* 2002;133:1083-7.

[60] Roden DM. Principles of clinical pharmacology. In: Kasper DL, Brauwald E, Fauci AS, Hauser SL, Longo DL, Jameson JL, eds. *Harrison's principles of internal medicine* 16[th]ed. New York McGraw-Hill, Inc 2005;13-25.

[61] Zanon E, Martinelli F, Bacci C, Cordioli G, Girolami A. Safety of dental extraction among consecutive patients on oral anticoagulant treatment managed using a specific dental management protocol. *Blood Coagul. Fibrinolysis.* 2003;14:27-30.

[62] Blinder D, Manor Y, Martinowitz U, Taicher S, Hashomer T. Dental extractions in patients maintained on continued oral anticoagulant: comparison of local hemostatic modalities. *Oral Surg. Oral Med. Oral Pathol Oral Radiol. Endod.* 1999;88:137-40.

[63] Blinder D, Manor Y, Martinowitz U, Taicher S. Dental extractions in patients maintained on oral anticoagulant therapy: comparison of INR value with occurrence of postoperative bleeding. *Int. J. Oral Maxillofac. Surg.* 2001;30:518-21.

[64] Slots J. Selection of antimicrobial agents in periodontal therapy. *J. Periodontal. Res.* 2002;37:389-98.

[65] Hancock EB, Newell DH. Preventive strategies and supportive treatment. *Periodontol 2000.* 2001;25:59-76.

[66] Balkau B, Eschwège. The diagnosis and classification of diabetes and impaired glucose regulation. In: Pickup JC, Williams G eds. *Textbook of Diabetes* 3rd ed. Blackwell Science 2003;1:2.1-2.13.

[67] Report of the Expert Committee on the Diagnosis and Classification of Diabetes Mellitus. *Diabetes Care.* 1997;20:1183-97.

[68] Powers AC. Diabetes Mellitus. In: Kasper DL, Brauwald E, Fauci AS, Hauser SL, Longo DL, Jameson JL, eds. *Harrison's principles of internal medicine* 16[th]ed. New York McGraw-Hill, Inc 2005; 2152-82.

[69] Joshi N, Mahajan M. Infection and diabetes. In: Pickup JC, Williams G eds. *Textbook of Diabetes* 3rd ed. Blackwell Science 2003;1:40.1-40.16.

[70] Long RG, Hlousek L, Doyle JL. Oral manifestations of systemic diseases. *Mt. Sinai J. Med.* 1998;65:309-15.

[71] Ryan ME, Carnu O, Kamer A. The influence of diabetes on the periodontal tissues. *J. Am. Dent. Assoc.* 2003;134:34s-40s.

[72] Moore PA, Orchard T, Guggenheimer J, Weyant RJ. Diabetes and oral health promotion: a survey of disease prevention behaviors. *J. Am. Dent. Assoc.* 2000;131:1333-41.

[73] Oliver RC, Tervonen T. Periodontitis and tooth loss: comparing diabetics with the general population. *J. Am. Dent. Assoc.* 1993;124:71-6.

[74] Löe H. Periodontal disease. The sixth complication of diabetes mellitus. *Diabetes Care.* 1993;16:329-34.

[75] Tan WC, Tay FBK, Lim LP. Diabetes as a risk factor for periodontal disease: Current status and future considerations. *Ann. Acad. Med. Singapore* 2006;35:571-81.

[76] Grossi SG, Skrepcinski FB, DeCaro T, Zambon JJ, Cummins D, Genco RJ. Response to periodontal therapy in diabetics and smokers. *J. Periodontol.* 1996;67Suppl:1094-102.

[77] Twetman S, Johansson I, Birkhed D, Nederfors T. Caries incidence in young type 1 diabetes mellitus patients in relation to metabolic control and caries-associated risk factors. *Caries Res.* 2002;36:31-5.

[78] Bjelland S, Bray P, Gupta N, Hirscht R. Dentists, diabetes and periodontitis. *Aust. Dent. J.* 2002;47:202-7.

[79] Moore PA, Weyant RJ, Etzel KR, Guggenheimer J, Mongelluzzo MB, Myers DE, et al. Type 1 diabetes mellitus and oral health: assessment of coronal and root caries. *Community Dent. Oral Epidemiol.* 2001;29:183-94.

[80] Lin BP, Taylor GW, Allen DJ, Ship JA. Dental caries in older adults with diabetes mellitus. *Spec. Care Dentist.* 1999;19:8-14.

[81] Karjalainen KM, Knuuttila ML, Käär ML. Relationship between caries and level of metabolic balance in children and adolescents with insulin-dependent diabetes mellitus. *Caries Res.* 1997;31:13-8.

[82] Ciglar L, Skaljac G, Sutalo J, Keros J, Janković B, Knezević A. Influence of diet on dental caries in diabetics. *Coll Antropol.* 2002;26:311-7.

[83] Tavares M, Depaola P, Soparkar P, Joshipura K. The prevalence of root caries in a diabetic population. *J. Dent. Res.* 1991;70:979-83.

[84] Belazi M, Velegraki A, Fleva A, Gidarakou I, Papanaum L, Baka D, et al. Candidal overgrowth in diabetic patients: potential predisposing factors. *Mycoses.* 2005;48:192-6.

[85] Quirino MR, Birman EG, Paula CR. Oral manifestations of diabetes mellitus in controlled and uncontrolled patients. *Braz. Dent. J.* 1995;6:131-6.

[86] Guggenheimer J, Moore PA, Rossie K, Myers D, Mongelluzzo MB, Block HM, et al. Insulin-dependent diabetes mellitus and oral soft tissue pathologies: II. Prevalence and characteristics of Candida and Candidal lesions. *Oral Surg. Oral Med. Oral Pathol. Oral Radiol. Endod.* 2000;89:570-6.

[87] Manfredi M, McCullough MJ, Al-Karaawi ZM, Hurel SJ, Porter SR. The isolation, identification and molecular analysis of Candida spp. isolated from the oral cavities of patients with diabetes mellitus. *Oral. Microbiol. Immunol.* 2002;17:181-5.

[88] Sreebny LM, Yu A, Green A, Valdini A. Xerostomia in diabetes mellitus. *Diabetes Care.* 1992;15:900-4.

[89] Vitkov L, Weitgasser R, Lugstein A, Noack MJ, Fuchs K, Krautgartner WD. Glycaemic disorders in denture stomatitis. *J. Oral Pathol. Med.* 1999;28:406-9.

[90] Ostrosky-Zeichner L, Rex JH, Bennett J, Kullberg BJ. Deeply invasive candidiasis. *Infect. Dis. Clin. North Am.* 2002;16:821-35.

[91] Jones AC, Bentsen TY, Freedman PD. Mucormycosis of the oral cavity. *Oral Surg. Oral Med. Oral Pathol.* 1993;75:455-60.

[92] Seyhan M, Ozcan H, Sahin I, Bayram N, Karincaoğlu Y. High prevalence of glucose metabolism disturbance in patients with lichen planus. *Diabetes Res. Clin. Pract.* 2007;77:198-202.

[93] Albrecht M, Bánóczy J, Dinya E, Tamás G Jr. Occurrence of oral leukoplakia and lichen planus in diabetes mellitus. *J. Oral Pathol. Med.* 1992;21:364-6.

[94] Ponte E, Tabaj D, Maglione M, Melato M. Diabetes mellitus and oral disease. *Acta Diabetol.* 2001;38:57-62.

[95] Katta R. Lichen planus. *Am. Fam. Physician.* 2000;61:3319-28.

[96] Gibson J, Lamey PJ, Lewis M, Frier B. Oral manifestations of previously undiagnosed non-insulin dependent diabetes mellitus. *J. Oral Pathol. Med.* 1990;19:284-7.

[97] Lalla RV, D'Ambrosio JA. Dental management considerations for the patient with diabetes mellitus. *J. Am. Dent Assoc.* 2001;132:1425-32.

[98] Field EA, Longman LP, Bucknall R, Kaye SB, Higham SM, Edgar WM. The establishment of a xerostomia clinic: a prospective study. *Br. J. Oral Maxillofac. Surg.* 1997;35:96-103.

[99] Chávez EM, Borrell LN, Taylor GW, Ship JA. A longitudinal analysis of salivary flow in control subjects and older adults with type 2 diabetes. *Oral Surg. Oral Med. Oral Pathol Oral Radiol Endod.* 2001;91:166-73.

[100] Gilbert GH, Heft MW, Duncan RP. Mouth dryness as reported by older Floridians. *Community Dent. Oral Epidemiol.* 1993;21:390-7.

[101] Kao CH, Tsai SC, Sun SS. Scintigraphic evidence of poor salivary function in type 2 diabetes. *Diabetes Care.* 2001;24:952-3.

[102] Greenspan D. Xerostomia: diagnosis and management. *Oncology* (Williston Park) 1996;10Suppl:7-11.

[103] Miralles L, Silvestre FJ, Hernández-Mijares A, Bautista D, Llambes F, Grau D. Dental caries in type 1 diabetics: influence of systemic factors of the disease upon the development of dental caries. *Med. Oral Patol Oral Cir. Bucal.* 2006;11:E256-60.

[104] Ship JA. Diabetes and oral health. *J. Am. Dent. Assoc.* 2003;134:4S-10S.

[105] Grushka M, Epstein JB, Gorsky M. Burning mouth syndrome. *Am. Fam. Physician.* 2002;65:615-20.

[106] Kalina RE. Seeing into the future. Vision and aging. *West J. Med.* 1997;167:253-7.

[107] Ship JA, Duffy V, Jones JA, Langmore S. Geriatric oral health and its impact on eating. *J. Am. Geriatr. Soc.* 1996;44:456-64.

[108] Safkan-Seppälä B, Ainamo J. Periodontal conditions in insulin-dependent diabetes mellitus. *J. Clin. Periodontol.* 1992;19:24-9.

[109] McKenna SJ. Dental management of patients with diabetes. *Dent. Clin. North Am.* 2006;50:591-606.

[110] Akpan A, Morgan R. Oral candidiasis. *Postgrad. Med. J.* 2002;78:455-9.

[111] Skorecki K, Screen J, Brenner BM. Chronic renal failure.In: Kasper DL, Brauwald E, Fauci AS, Hauser SL, Longo DL, Jameson JL, eds. *Harrison's principles of internal medicine* 16th ed. New York McGraw-Hill, Inc 2005;1653-63.

[112] Silverberg DS, Wexler D, Blum B, Iaina A. Anemia in chronic kidney disease and congestive heart failure. *Blood Purif.* 2003;21:124-30.

[113] Hamid MJ, Dummer CD, Pinto LS Systemic conditions, oral findings and dental management of chronic renal failure patients: general considerations and case report. *Braz. Dent. J.* 2006;17:166-70.

[114] Naylor GD, Fredericks MR. Pharmacologic considerations in the dental management of the patient with disorders of the renal system. *Dent. Clin. North Am.* 1996;40:665-83.

[115] Proctor R, Kumar N, Stein A, Moles D, Porter S. Oral and dental aspects of chronic renal failure. *J. Dent. Res.* 2005;84:199-208.

[116] Klassen JT, Krasko BM. The dental health status of dialysis patients. *J. Can. Dent. Assoc.* 2002;68:34-8.

[117] Hayes CW, Conway WF. Hyperparathyroidism. *Radiol. Clin. North Am.* 1991;29:85-96.

[118] Tong DC, Walker RJ. Antibiotic prophylaxis in dialysis patients undergoing invasive dental treatment. *Nephrology* (Carlton). 2004;9:167-70.

[119] Scully C, Cawson RA, *Medical problems in dentistry*; 5th edition; Elsevier; New York; 2005;115-22.

[120] Quirk PC, Osborne PJ, Walsh LJ. Australian Dental Research Fund Trebitsch Scholarship. Efficacy of antifungal prophylaxis in bone marrow transplantation. *Aust. Dent. J.* 1995;40:267-70.

[121] Näsström K, Forsberg B, Petersson A, Westesson PL. Narrowing of the dental pulp chamber in patients with renal diseases. *Oral Surg. Oral Med. Oral Pathol.* 1985;59:242-6.

[122] Nguyen NP, Vos P, Smith HJ, Nguyen PD, Alfieri A, Karlsson U, et al. Concurrent chemoradiation for locally advanced oropharyngeal cancer. *Am. J. Otolaryngol.* 2007;28:3-8.

[123] Lockhart PB, Clark J. Pretherapy dental status of patients with malignant conditions of the head and neck. *Oral Surg. Oral Med. Oral Pathol.* 1994;77:236-41.

[124] Mealy BL, Semba SE, Hallmon WW. Dentistry and the cancer patient. Part 1. Oral manifestations and complications of chemotherapy. *Compendium Cont. Educ. Dent.* 1994; 15:1252-6.

[125] Pauloski BR, Logemann JA, Colangelo LA, Rademaker AW, McConnel FM, Heiser MA, et al. Surgical variables affecting speech in treated patients with oral and oropharyngeal cancer. *Laryngoscope.* 1998;108:908-16.

[126] Pauloski BR, Logemann JA. Impact of tongue base and posterior pharyngeal wall biomechanics on pharyngeal clearance in irradiated postsurgical oral and oropharyngeal cancer patients. *Head Neck.* 2000;22:120-31.

[127] Nguyen NP, Sallah S. Combined chemotherapy and radiation in the treatment of locally advanced head and neck cancers. *In Vivo.* 2000;14:35-9.

[128] Nguyen NP, Sallah S, Karlsson U, Antoine JE. Combined chemotherapy and radiation therapy for head and neck malignancies: quality of life issues. *Cancer.* 2002;94:1131-41.

[129] Pauloski BR, Rademaker AW, Logemann JA, McConnel FM, Heiser MA, Cardinale S, et al. Surgical variables affecting swallowing in patients treated for oral/oropharyngeal cancer. *Head Neck.* 2004;26:625-36.

[130] Denittis AS, Machtay M, Rosenthal DI, Sanfilippo NJ, Lee JH, Goldfeder S, et al. Advanced oropharyngeal carcinoma treated with surgery and radiotherapy: oncologic outcome and functional assessment. *Am. J. Otolaryngol.* 2001;22:329-35.

[131] Epstein 11JB, Parker IR, Epstein MS, Stevenson-Moore P. Cancer-related oral health care services and resources: a survey of oral and dental care in Canadian cancer centres. *J. Can. Dent. Assoc.* 2004;70:302-4.

[132] Dobrossy L. Epidemiology of head and neck cancer: magnitude of the problem. *Cancer Metastasis Rev.* 2005;24:9-17.

[133] Scully C, Epstein JB. Oral Health Care for the Cancer Patient. *Oral Oncol. Eur. Cancer* 1996;32:281-92.

[134] Lalla RV, Peterson DE. *Oral Mucositis Dent. Clin. N. Am.* 2005;49:167-184.

[135] Collins R, Flynn A, Melville A, Richardson R, Eastwood A. Effective health care: Management of head and neck cancers. *Qual. Saf. Health Care* 2005;14:144-8.

[136] Sutthavong S, Jansisyanont P, Boonyopastham N. Oral health care in head and neck cancer. *J. Med. Assoc. Thai.* 2005;88 Suppl 3:S339-53.

[137] National Cancer Institute:U.S. National Institutes of Oral Health, Oral Complications of Chemotherapy and Head/Neck Radiation(PDQ®) Health Professional version. http://cancer.gov/cancertopics/pdq/supportivecare/oralcomplications/healthpr.

[138] Hancock PJ, Epstein JB, Sadler GR. Oral and dental management Related to Radiotherapy for head and neck cancer. *J. Can. Dent. Assoc.* 2003;69:585-590.

[139] National Institute of Health census Development Conference on Oral Complications of Cancer Therapies: Diagnosis, Prevention, and treatment. Bethesda, Maryland, April 17-19, 1989, *NCI Monogr.* 1990;9:1-184.

[140] Adi A. Garfunkel. Oral Mucositis-The search for a solution. *N Engl J Med.* 2004 16;351:2649-51.

[141] Scully C. Drug Effect on Salivary Glands: Dry mouth. *Oral. Disease* 2003;9:165-76.

[142] Chang KKF, Molassiotis A, Chang AM, Wai WC, Cheung SS. Evaluation of an oral care Protocol intervention in the Prevention of Chemotherapy-induced oral mucositis in Paediatric cancer patients. *Eur J cancer.* 2001;37:2056-63.

[143] Porceddu SV, Campbell B, Rischin D, Corry J, Weih L, Guerrieri M, et al Postoperative chemoradiotherapy for high-risk head-and-neck squamous cell carcinoma. *Int. J. Radiat. Oncol. Biol. Phys*. 2004;60:365-73.

[144] Joyston-Bechal S, Hayes K, Davenport ES, Hardie JM. Caries incidence, mutans streptococci and lactobacilli in irradiated patients during a 12-month preventive programme using chlorhexidine and fluoride. *Caries Res.* 1992;26:384-90.

[145] Rutkauskas JS, Davis JW. Effects of chlorhexidine during immunosuppressive chemotherapy. A preliminary report. *Oral Surg. Oral Med. Oral Pathol*. 1993;76:441-8.

[146] Scully C, Epstein J, Sonis S. Oral Mucositis: A Challenging complication of radiotherapy, Chemotherapy, and Radiochemotherapy: Part 2: Diagnosis and Management of Mucositis. *Head and Neck* 2004;26:77-84.

[147] Hanna E, Alexiou M, Morgan J, Badley J, Maddox AM, Penagaricano J, et al. Intensive chemoradiotherapy as a primary treatment for organ preservation in patients with advanced cancer of the head and neck: efficacy, toxic effects, and limitations. *Arch. Otolaryngol. Head Neck Surg*. 2004;130:861-7.

[148] Vissink A, Burlage FR, Spitkervet FKL, Jansma J, Coppes RP. Prevention and treatment of the consequences of head and neck Radiotherapy. *Crit. Rev. Oral Biomed*. 2003;14:213-25.

[149] Andrews N, Griffiths C. Dental complications of head and neck radiotherapy: Part 2. *Aust. Dent. J.* 2001;46:174-82.

[150] Epstein JB, Stevenson-Moore P. Periodontal disease and periodontal management in patients with cancer. *Oral Oncol*. 2001;37:613-9.

[151] Sulaiman F, Huryn JM, Zlotolow IM. Dental extractions in the irradiated head and neck patient: a retrospective analysis of Memorial Sloan-Kettering Cancer Center protocols, criteria, and end results. *J. Oral Maxillofac. Surg*. 2003;61:1123-31.

[152] The Research Science and Therapy Committee of the American Academy of Periodontilogy. Position Paper. *J. Periodontol*. 1997;68:791-801.

[153] Wah JM. Osteoradionecrosis Prevention Myths. *Int. J. Radiation Oncology Biol. Phys*. 2006;64:661-9.

[154] Lieblich SE, Piecuch JF. Infections of the jaws, including infected fractures, osteomyelitis, and osteoradionecrosis. *Atlas Oral Maxillofac. Surg. Clin. North Am*. 2000;8:121-32.

[155] Peter E, Monopoli M, Woo SB, Sonis S. Assessment of post-endodontic asymptomatic periapical radiolucencies in bone marrow transplant recipients. *Oral Surg. Oral Med. Oral Path.*1993;76:45-8.

[156] Maxymiw WG, Wood RE and Liu F. Post-radiation dental extractions without hyperbaric oxygen. *Oral Surg. Oral Med. Oral Pathol*. 1991;72:270.

[157] Rugg T, Saunders MI, Dische S. Smoking and mucosal reactions. *Br. J. Radiol*. 1990;63:544-6.

[158] Trotti A, Bellm LA, Epstein JB, Frame D, Fuchs HJ, Gwede CK, et al. Mucositis incidence, severity and associated outcomes in patients with head and neck cancer receiving radiotherapy with or without chemotherapy: a systemic literature review. *Radiother. Oncol*. 2003; 66:253-62.

[159] Cheng KK, Molassiotis A, Chang AM, Wai WC, Cheung SS. Evaluation of an oral care protocol intervention in the prevention of chemotherapy –induced oral mucositis in paediatric cancer patients. *Eur. J. Cancer* 2001;37:2056-63.

[160] Garfunkel AA. Oral Mucositis-The search for a solution. *N Engl J Med.* 2004;351:2649-51.

[161] Dahlin C. Oral Complications at the End of Life. *AJN* 2004;104:40-7.

[162] Boyd LD, Lampi KJ. Importance of nutrition for optimum health of the periodontium. *J. Contemp Dent. Pract.* 2001;2:36-45.

[163] Soini H, Muurinen S, Routasalo P, Sandelin E, Savikko N, Suominen M, et al. Oral and nutritional status--Is the MNA a useful tool for dental clinics. *J. Nutr. Health Aging.* 2006;10:495-9.

[164] Hickson M. Malnutrition and ageing. *Postgrad Med. J.* 2006;82:2-8.

[165] Epstien JB, Schubert MM. Oropharyngeal mucositis in cancer therapy. Review of pathogenesis, diagnosis and management. *Oncology* (Huntingt) 2003;17:1767-79.

[166] Ramirez-Amadorv V, Silverman S Jr, Mayer P, Tyler M, Quivey J. Candidal Colonization and oral candidiasis in patients undergoing oral and pharyngeal radiation therapy. *Oral Surg. Oral Med. Oral Pathol. Oral Radiol. Endod.* 1997;84:149-53.

[167] Bunetel L, Bonnaure-Mallet M. Oral pathoses caysed by C.albicans during chemo-therapy. *Oral Surg. Oral Med. Oral Pathol. Oral Radiol. Endod.* 1996;82:161-5.

[168] Chambers MS, Garden AS, Kies MS, Martin JW. Radiation-induced xerostomia in patients with head and neck cancer: pathogenesis, impact on quality of life, and management. *Head Neck.* 2004;26:796-807.

[169] Kami M, Machida U, Okuzumi K. Effect of Fluconazole prophylaxis on fungal blood cultures an autopsy-based study involving 720 patients with haematological malignancy. *Br. J. Haematol.* 2002;117:40-6.

[170] Epstein JB, Vickars L, Spinelli J. Reece D. Efficacy of Chlorhexidine and nystatin rinses in prevention of oralcomplications in leukemia and bone marrow transplantation. *Oral Surg. Oral Med. Oral Pathol. Oral Radiol. Endod.* 1992;73:682-9.

[171] Barkroll P, Attramadal A. Effect of nystatin and chlorhexidine digluconate on candida albicans. *Oral Surg. Oral Med. Oral Pathol Oral Radiol. Endod.* 1989;67:279-81.

[172] Remberton MN, Sloan P, Ariyaratnam S, Thakker NS, Thornhill MH, Derangement of warfarin anti-coagulation by miconazole oral gel. *BDJ.* 1998;184:68-9.

[173] Raber-Durlacher JE, Epstien JB, Raber J, Jaap van Dissel JT, van Winkelhoff AJ, et al. Periodontal infection in cancer patients treated with high-dose chemotherapy. *Support Care Cancer* 2002;10:466-473.

[174] Akintoye SO, Brennan MT, Graber CJ. A retrospective investigation of advanced periodontal diseases as a risk factor of septicemia in hematopoietic stem cell and bone marrow transplant recipients. *Oral Surg. Oral Med. Oral Pathol. Oral Radiol. Endod.* 2002;94:581-8.

[175] Mathews RH, Ercal N. Prevention of mucositis in irradiated head and neck cancer patients. *J. Exp. Ther. Oncol.* 1996;1:135-8.

[176] Samonis G, Mantadakis E, Maraki S. Orofacial viral infections in the immunocompromised host. *Oncol. Rep.* 2000;7:1389-94.

[177] Vancikova Z, Dvorak P. Cytomegalovirus infection in immunocompetent and immunocompromized individuals. *Curr. Drug Targets Immune Endocr. Metabol. Didord.* 2001;1:179-87.

[178] Leflore S, Anderson Pl, Fletcher CV. A risk-benefit evaluation of aciclovir for the treatment and prophylaxis of herpes simplex virus infections. *Drug. Saf.* 2000;23:131-42.

[179] Gluckman E, Powles RL, Ljungman P, Milpied NJ, Camara R, Mandelli F, et al. Long-term survival in allogeneic bone marrow transplant recipients following acyclovir prophylaxis for CMV infection. The European Acyclovir for CMV Prophylaxis Study Group. *Bone Marrow Transplant.* 1997;19:129-33.

[180] Naesens L, De Clercq E. Recent developments in Herpesvirus therapy. *Herpes* 2001;8:12-6.

[181] Seikaly H, Jha N, McGaw T, Coulter L, Liu R, Oldring D. Submandibular gland transfer: a new method of preventing radiation-induced xerostomia. *Laryngoscope.* 2001;111:347-52.

[182] Bussels B, Maes A, Flamen P, Lambin P, Erven K, Hermans R, et al. Dose-response relationships within the parotid gland after radiotherapy for head and neck cancer. *Radiother. Oncol.* 2004;73:297-306.

[183] Epstein JB, Robertson M, Emerton S, Phillips N, Stevenson-Moore P. Quality of life and oral function in patients treated with radiation therapy for head and neck cancer. *Head Neck.* 2001;23:389-98.

[184] Vissink A, Jansma J, Spijkervet FK, Burlage FR, Coppes RP. Oral sequelae of head and neck radiotherapy. *Crit. Rev. Oral Biol. Med.* 2003;14:199-212.

[185] Möller P, Perrier M, Ozsahin M, Monnier P. A prospective study of salivary gland function in patients undergoing radiotherapy for squamous cell carcinoma of the oropharynx. *Oral Surg. Oral Med. Oral Pathol Oral Radiol. Endod.* 2004;97:173-89.

[186] Konings AW, Coppes RP, Vissink A. On the mechanism of salivary gland radiosensitivity. *Int. J. Radiat Oncol. Biol. Phys.* 2005;62:1187-94.

[187] Warde P, Kroll B, O'Sullivan B, Aslanidis J, Tew-George E, Waldron J, et al. A phase II study of Biotene in the treatment of postradiation xerostomia in patients with head and neck cancer. *Support Care Cancer.* 2000;8:203-8.

[188] Rieke JW, Hafermann MD, Johnson JT, LeVeque FG, Iwamoto R, Steiger BW, et al. Oral pilocarpine for radiation-induced xerostomia: integrated efficacy and safety results from two prospective randomized clinical trials. *Int. J. Radiat. Oncol. Biol. Phys.* 1995;31:661-9.

[189] Valdez IH, Wolff A, Atkinson JC, Macynski AA, Fox PC. Use of pilocarpine during head and neck radiation therapy to reduce xerostomia and salivary dysfunction. *Cancer.* 1993;71:1848-51.

[190] Rode M, Smid L, Budihna M, Soba E, Gaspersic D. The effect of pilocarpine and biperiden on salivary secretion during and after radiotherapy in head and neck cancer patients. *Int. J. Radiat. Oncol. Biol. Phys.* 1999;45:373-8.

[191] Al-Hashimi I, Taylor SE. A new medication for treatment of dry mouth in Sjogren's syndrome. *Texas Dent. J.* 2001;118:262-6.

[192] Buntzel J, Glatzel M, Kuttner K, Weinaug R, Frohlich D. Amifostine in simultaneous radiochemotherapy of advanced head and neck cancer. *Semin. Radiat. Oncol.* 2002 12:4-13.

[193] Koukourakis MI. Amifostine in clinical oncology: current use and future applications. *Anticancer Drugs*. 2002;13:181-209.

[194] Wasserman T, Mackowiak JI, Brizel DM, Oster W, Zhang J, Peeples PJ, et al. Effect of amifostine on patient assessed clinical benefit in irradiated head and neck cancer. *Int. J. Radiat. Oncol. Biol. Phys*. 2000;48:1035-9.

[195] Nguyen NP, Sallah S, Karlsson U, Antoine JE. Combined chemotherapy and radiation therapy for head and neck malignancies: quality of life issues. *Cancer*. 2002;94:1131-41.

[196] Warde P, O'Sullivan B, Aslanidis J, Kroll B, Lockwood G, Waldron J, et al. A Phase III placebo-controlled trial of oral pilocarpine in patients undergoing radiotherapy for head-and-neck cancer. *Int. J. Radiat. Oncol. Biol. Phys*. 2002;1:9-13.

[197] Saarilahti K, Kouri M, Collan J, Hamalainen T, Atula T, Joensuu H, et al. Intensity modulated radiotherapy for head and neck cancer: evidence for preserved salivary gland function. *Radiother. Oncol.* 2005;74:251-8.

[198] Badaracco G, Venuti A. Human papillomavirus therapeutic vaccines in head and neck tumors. Rev Anticancer Ther. 2007;7:753-66.

[199] Harrington KJ, Nutting CM, Pandha HS. Gene therapy for head and neck cancer. *Cancer Metastasis Rev.* 2005;24:147-64.

[200] Ripamonti C, Zecca E, Brunelli C, Fulfaro F, Villa S, Balzarini A, et al. A randomized, controlled clinical trial to evaluate the effects of zinc sulfate on cancer patients with taste alterations caused by head and neck irradiation. *Cancer* 1998;82:1938-45.

[201] Biron P, Sebban C, Gourmet R, Chvetzoff G, Philip I, Blay JY. Reseach Controversies in management of oral mucositis. *Support Care Cancer* 2000;8:68-71.

[202] Nguyen NP, Moltz CC, Frank C, Karlsson U, Smith HJ, Nguyen PD, et al. Severity and duration of chronic dysphagia following treatment for head and neck cancer. *Anticancer Res*. 2005;25:2929-34.

[203] Nguyen NP, Frank C, Moltz CC, Vos P, Smith HJ, Karlsson U, et al. Impact of dysphagia on quality of life after treatment of head-and-neck cancer. *Int. J. Radiat. Oncol. Biol. Phys*. 2005;61:772-8.

[204] Büntzel J, Glatzel M, Kuttner K, Weinaug R, Fröhlich D. Amifostine in simultaneous radiochemotherapy of advanced head and neck cancer. *Semin. Radiat. Oncol.* 2002;12 Suppl1:4-13.

[205] Scully C, Ward-Booth P. Detection and treatment of early cancers of the oral cavity. *Crit. Rev. Oncol.* 1995;21:63-75.

[206] Schbert MM, Peterson DE, Lloid ME. Oral complications. In Thomas ED, Blume KG, Forman SJ eds: *Hematopoitic Cell Transplantation*. 2nd ed. Malden, Mass:Blackwell Science Inc, 1999:751-63.

[207] Epstein JB, Elad S, Eliav E, Jurevic R, Benoliel R. Orofacial pain in cancer: part II--clinical perspectives and management. *J. Dent. Res.* 2007;86:506-18.

[208] Otmani N. Oral and maxillofacial side effects of radiation therapy on children. *J. Can. Dent. Assoc.* 2007;73:257-61.

[209] Teng MS, Futran ND. Osteoradionecrosis of the mandible. *Curr. Opin. Otolaryngol. Head Neck Surg.* 2005;13:217-21.

[210] Oh HK, Chambers MS, Garden AS, Wong PF, Martin JW. Risk of osteoradionecrosis after extraction of impacted third molars in irradiated head and neck cancer patients. *J. Oral Maxillofac. Surg.* 2004;62:139-44.

[211] Keller EE. Placement of dental implants in the irradiated mandible: a protocol without adjunctive hyperbaric oxygen. *J. Oral Maxillofac. Surg.* 1997;55:972-80.

[212] Bui QC, Lieber M, Withers HR, Corson K, van Rijnsoever M, Elsaleh H. The efficacy of hyperbaric oxygen therapy in the treatment of radiation-induced late side effects. *Int. J. Radiat. Oncol. Biol. Phys.* 2004;60:871-8.

[213] Jereczek-Fossa BA, Orecchia R. Radiotherapy-induced mandibular bone complications. *Cancer Treat. Rev.* 2002;28:65-74.

[214] Curi MM., Dib LL, Kowalski LP. Management of refractory osteoradionecrosis of the jaws with surgery and adjunctive hyperbaric oxygen therapy. *Int. J. Oral Maxillofac. Surg.* 2000;29:430–4.

[215] Sanger JR., Matloub HS., Yousif NJ, Larson DL. Management of osteoradionecrosis of the mandible. *Clin. Plast. Surg.* 1993;20:517-30.

[216] Tong AC, Leung AC, Cheng JC, Sham J. Incidence of complicated healing and osteoradionecrosis following tooth extraction in patients receiving radiotherapy for treatment of nasopharyngeal carcinoma. *Aust. Dent. J.* 1999;44:187-94.

[217] Chavez JA, Adkinson CD. Adjunctive hyperbaric oxygen in irradiated patients requiring dental extractions: outcomes and complications. *J. Oral Maxillofac. Surg.* 2001;59:518-22.

[218] Niewald M, Barbie O, Schnabel, K. Risk factors and dose-effect relationship for osteoradionecrosis after hyperfractionated and conventionally fractionated radiotherapy for oral cancer. *Brit. J. Radiol.* 1996;69:847–51.

[219] Maxymiw WG, Wood RE and Liu F. Post-radiation dental extractions without hyperbaric oxygen. *Oral Surg. Oral Med. Oral Pathol.* 1991;72:270.

[220] Assael LA. New foundations in understanding osteonecrosis of the jaws. *J. Oral Maxillofac Surg.* 2004;62:125-6.

[221] David LA., Sandor GK, Evans AW, Brown DH. Hyperbaric oxygen therapy and mandibular osteoradionecrosis: A retrospective study and analysis of treatment outcomes. *J. Can. Dent. Assoc.* 2001;67:384.

[222] Maier A, Gaggl A, Klemen H. Review of severe osteoradionecrosis treated by surgery alone or surgery with postoperative hyperbaric oxygenation. *Br. J. Oral. Maxillofac. Surg.* 2000;38:173–6.

[223] Marx RE, Ehler WJ, Tayapongsak P, Pierce LW. Relationship of oxygen dose to angiogenesis induction in irradiated tissue. *Am. J. Surg.* 1990;160:519-24.

[224] Mosca NG, Hathorn AR. HIV-Positive Patients: Dental Management Considerations. *Dent. Clin. N. Am.* 2006;50:635-57.

[225] Barlett JG, Gallant JE. *Medical Management of HIV Infection.* Baltimore: John Hopkins University. 2003.

[226] Beers MH, Porter RS, Jones TV, Kaplan JL, Berkwits M. Infectious diseases: Human Immunodeficiency Virus (HIV). *The Merck manual of diagnosis and therapy*. 18th ed. Staton: Merck research laboratories, 2006;1625-42.

[227] UNAIDS/WHO. *AIDS epidemic update*. Geneva, Switzerland. December, 2006.

[228] Schmidt-Westhausen AM, Priepke F, Bergmann FJ, Reichart PA. Decline in the rate of oral opportunistic infections following introduction of highly active antiretroviral therapy. *J. Oral Pathol. Med.* 2000;29:336-41.

[229] Darbyshire J. Therapeutic interventions in HIV infection - a critical view. *Darbyshire J. Trop Med. Int. Health*. 2000;5:A26-31.

[230] Scully C, Diz Dios P. Orofacial effects of antiretroviral therapies. *Oral Dis.* 2001;7:205-10.

[231] Department of Health and Human Services (DHHS), Guidelines for the use of Antiretroviral Agents in HIV-1-infected Adults and Adolescents. Washington DC: DHSS. 2003.

[232] Palella FJ, Delaney KM, Moorman AC, Loveless MO, Fuhrer J, Satten GA et al. Declining morbidity and mortality among patients with advanced human immunodeficiency virus infection. *N. Engl. J. Med.* 1998; 338:853-60.

[233] Mocroft A. Vella S. Benfield TL, Chiesi A, Miller V, Gargalianos P et al. Changing patterns of mortality across Europe in patients infected with HIV-1-EuroSIDA Study Group. *Lancet* 1998; 352:1725-30.

[234] Luzzi GA, Peto TE, Weiss RA, Conlon CP. HIV and AIDS. In DA Warrell, TM Cox, JD Firth, EJ Benz Jr(ed.) *Oxford Textbook of Medicine*, Oxford: Oxford University Press.4th ed, 2003;431.

[235] Weinert M, Grimes RM, Lynch DP. Oral manifestations of HIV infection. *Ann. Intern. Med.* 1996;125:485-96.

[236] Patton LL, Phelan JA, Ramos-Gomez FJ, Nittayananta W, Shiboski CH, Mbuguye TL. Prevalence and classification of HIV-associated oral lesions. *Oral Dis*. 2002;8 Suppl 2:98-109.

[237] DePaola L and Silva A. HIV infection/AIDS. In Davies A. ed. *Oral cares in advance disease*. New York: Oxford University Press, 2005:185-98.

[238] Tappuni AR, Fleming GJ. The effect of antiretroviral therapy on the prevalence of oral manifestations in HIV-infected patients: a UK study. *Oral Surg. Oral Med. Oral Pathol. Oral Radiol. Endod*. 2001; 92:623-8.

[239] Hodgson TA, Naidoo S, Chidzonga M, Ramos-Gomez F, Shiboski C. (A1) Identification of oral health care needs in children and adults, management of oral diseases. *Adv. Dent. Res*. 2006;19:106-17.

[240] Ito HO. Infective endocarditis and dental procedures: evidence, pathogenesis, and prevention. *J. Med. Invest.* 2006;53:189-98.

[241] Baccaglini L, Atkinson JC, Patton LL, Glick M, Ficarra G, Peterson DE. Management of oral lesions in HIV-positive patients. *Oral Surg. Oral Med. Oral Pathol. Oral Radiol. Endod*. 2007 Mar;103 Suppl:S50.e1-23.

[242] Vaseliu N, Kamiru H, Kabue M. Oral manifestations of HIV infection: HIV curriculum for the health professional. BIPAI's 3rd ed.173-85. http://bayloraids.org/curriculum/files/15.pdf.

[243] Feigal DW, Katz MH, Greenspan D, Westenhouse J, Winkelstein W Jr, Lang W, et al. The prevalence of oral lesions in HIV-infected homosexual and bisexual men: three San Francisco epidemiological cohorts. *AIDS*. 1991;5:519-25.

[244] Patton LL, Phelan JA, Rumos Gomez FJ, Nittayananta W, Shiboski CH, Mbuguve TI Prevalence and classification of HIV associated oral lesions. *Oral Dis*. 2002;8:98-109.

[245] Casiglia JW, Woo S. Oral manifestations of HIV infection. *Clin. Dermatol.* 2000;18:541-51.

[246] Laskris G. Oral manifestations of HIV disease. *Clin. Dermatol.* 2000; 18:447-55.

[247] Barasch A, Safford MM, Dapkute-Marcus I, Fine DH. Efficacy of chlorhexidine gluconate rinse for treatment and prevention of oral candidiasis in HIV-infected children: a pilot study. *Oral Surg. Oral Med. Oral Pathol. Oral Radiol. Endod.* 2004; 97:204-7.

[248] Foster H, Fitzgerald J. Dental disease in children with chronic illness. *Arch. Dis. Child.* 2005 ;90:703-8.

[249] Baily GG, Perry FM, Denning DW, Mandal BK. Fluconazole-resistant candidosis in an HIV cohort. *AIDS*. 1994;8:787-92.

[250] Redding SW, Kirkpatrick WR, Dib O, Fothergill AW, Rinaldi MG, Patterson TF. The epidemiology of non-albicans Candida in oropharyngeal candidiasis in HIV patients. Redding SW. *Spec. Care Dentist*. 2000;20:178-81.

[251] Johnson EM, Warnock DW, Luker J, Porter SR, Scully C. Emergence of azole drug resistance in Candida species from HIV-infected patients receiving prolonged fluconazole therapy for oral candidosis. *J. Antimicrob. Chemother*. 1995;35:103-14.

[252] DePaola LG. Managing the care of patients infected with bloodborne diseases. *J. Am. Dent. Assoc*. 2003;134:350-8.

[253] Lifson AR, Hilton JF, Westenhouse JL, Canchola AJ, Samuel MC, Katz MH, et al. Time from HIV seroconversion to oral candidiasis or hairy leukoplakia among homosexual and bisexual men enrolled in three prospective cohorts. *AIDS*. 1994;8:73-9.

[254] Hahn AM, Huye LE, Ning S, Webster-Cyriaque J, Pagano JS. Interferon regulatory factor 7 is negatively regulated by the Epstein-Barr virus immediate-early gene, BZLF-1. *J. Virol*. 2005;79:10040-52.

[255] Lilly EA, Cameron JE, Shetty KV, Leigh JE, Hager S, McNulty KM, et al. Lack of evidence for local immune activity in oral hairy leukoplakia and oral wart lesions. *Oral Microbiol. Immunol.* 2005;20:154-62.

[256] Berthold P. Noma: a forgotten disease. *Dent. Clin. North Am*. 2003;47:559-74.

[257] Enwonwu CO, Falkler WA Jr, Idigbe EO, Savage KO. Noma (cancrum oris): questions and answers. *Oral Dis*. 1999;5:144-9.

[258] Kroidl A, Schaeben A, Oette M, Wettstein M, Herfordt A, Häussinger D. Prevalence of oral lesions and periodontal diseases in HIV-infected patients on antiretroviral therapy. *Eur. J. Med. Res.* 2005;10:448-53.

[259] Paster BJ, Russell MK, Alpagot T, Lee AM, Boches SK, Galvin JL, et al. Bacterial diversity in necrotizing ulcerative periodontitis in HIV-positive subjects. *Ann. Periodontol*. 2002;7:8-16.

[260] Slots J. Herpesviruses, the missing link between gingivitis and periodontitis? *J. Int. Acad. Periodontol.* 2004;6:113-9.

[261] Robinson PG, Sheiham A, Challacombe SJ, Zakrzewska JM. Periodontal health and HIV infection. *Oral Dis.* 1997;3 Suppl 1:S149-52.

[262] Robinson PG, Sheiham A, Challacombe SJ, Wren MW, Zakrzewska JM. Gingival ulceration in HIV infection. A case series and case control study. *J. Clin. Periodontol.* 1998;25:260-7.

[263] Patton LL, McKaig R. Rapid progression of bone loss in HIV-associated necrotizing ulcerative stomatitis. *J. Periodontol.* 1998;69:710-6.

[264] Glick M, Muzyka BC, Salkin LM, Lurie D. Necrotizing ulcerative periodontitis: a marker for immune deterioration and a predictor for the diagnosis of AIDS. *J. Periodontol.* 1994;65:393-7.

[265] Ramos-Gomez FJ, Flaitz C, Catapano P, Murray P, Milnes AR, Dorenbaum A. Classification, diagnostic criteria, and treatment recommendations for orofacial manifestations in HIV-infected pediatric patients. Collaborative Workgroup on Oral Manifestations of Pediatric HIV Infection. *J. Clin. Pediatr. Dent.* 1999;23:85-96.

[266] Schiødt M, Pindborg JJ. AIDS and the oral cavity. Epidemiology and clinical oral manifestations of human immune deficiency virus infection: a review. *Int. J. Oral Maxillofac. Surg.* 1987;16:1-14.

[267] Chapple IL, Hamburger J. The significance of oral health in HIV disease. *Sex Transm Infect.* 2000;76:236-43.

[268] Schiødt M. Less common oral lesions associated with HIV infection: prevalence and classification. 31 *Oral Dis.* 1997;3 Suppl 1:S208-13.

[269] Johnson NW, Glick M, Mbuguye TN. (A2) Oral health and general health. *Adv. Dent. Res.* 2006;19:118-21.

[270] Alebiolusu CO, Odusan O. Addison's disease: A case report. *Annals of African Medicine.* 2003;2:85-87.

[271] Coates E, Slade GD, Goss AN, Gorkic E. Oral conditions and their social impact among HIV dental patients. *Aust. Dent. J.* 1996;41:33-6.

[272] Coulter ID, Marcus M, Freed JR, Der-Martirosian C, Cunningham WE, Andersen RM, et al. Use of dental care by HIV-infected medical patients. *J. Dent. Res.* 2000;79:1356-61.

[273] Coulter ID, Heslin KC, Marcus M, Hays RD, Freed J, Der-Martirosia C, et al. Associations of self-reported oral health with physical and mental health in a nationally representative sample of HIV persons receiving medical care. *Qual. Life Res.* 2002;11:57-70.

[274] Robinson PG. Implications of HIV disease for oral health services. *Adv. Dent. Res.* 2006;19:73-9.

[275] Barnes DB, Gerbert B, McMaster JR, Greenblatt RM. Self-disclosure experience of people with HIV infection in dedicated and mainstreamed dental facilities. *J. Public Health Dent.* 1996;56:223-5.

[276] Brown JB, Rosenstein D, Mullooly J, O'Keeffe Rosetti M, Robinson S, Chiodo G. Impact of intensified dental care on outcomes in human immunodeficiency virus infection. *AIDS Patient Care STDS.* 2002;16:479-86.

[277] Hastreiter RJ, Jiang P. Do regular dental visits affect the oral health care provided to people with HIV? *J. Am. Dent. Assoc.* 2002;133:1343-50.

[278] Thomas JG, Nakaishi LA. Managing the complexity of a dynamic biofilm. *J. Am. Dent. Assoc.* 2006;137 Suppl 3:10S-15S.

[279] Yankell SL, Saxer UP. Toothbrushes and toothbrushing methods in Harris NO, Garcia-Godoy F, eds. New Jersey Pearson Education, Inc., *Primary preventive dentistry.* 6th ed, 2004;93-117.

[280] Warren DP, Goldschmidt MC, Thompson MB, Adler-Storthz K, Keene HJ. The effects of toothpastes on the residual microbial contamination of toothbrushes. *J. Am. Dent. Assoc.* 2001;132:1241-5.

[281] Haffajee AD, Socransky SS. Microbial etiological agents of destructive periodontal diseases. *Periodontol* 2000. 1994;5:78-111.

[282] Jenkinson HF, Dymock D. *The microbiology of periodontal disease.* Dent Update. 1999;26:191-7.

[283] ADA Division of Communications for the dental patient. Tooth brush care, cleaning and replacement. *J. An. Dent. Assoc.* 2006;137: 415.

[284] Addems A, Epstein JB, Damji S, Spinelli J. The lack of efficacy of a foam brush in maintaining gingival health: a controlled study. *Spec. Care Dentist.* 1992;12:103-6.

[285] Lefkoff MH, Beck FM, Horton JE. The effectiveness of a disposable tooth cleansing device on plaque. *J. Periodontol.* 1995;66:218-21.

[286] Pearson LS. A comparison of the ability of foam swabs and toothbrushes to remove dental plaque: implications for nursing practice. *J. Adv. Nurs.* 1996;23:62-9.

[287] Eley BM, Cox SW. The relationship between gingival crevicular fluid cathepsin B activity and periodontal attachment loss in chronic periodontitis patients: a 2-year longitudinal study. *J. Periodontal. Res.* 1996;31:381-92.

[288] Caudry SD, Klitorinos A, Chan EC. Contaminated toothbrushes and their disinfection. *Pediatr. Dent.* 2000;22:381-4.

[289] Danser MM, Gomez SM, Van der Weijden. Tongue coating and tongue brushing: a literature review. *Int. J. Dent. Hygiene* 2003;1:151-8.

[290] Gil-Montoya JA, de Mello AL, Cardenas CB, Lopez IG. Oral health protocol for the dependent institutionalized elderly. *Geriatr. Nurs.* 2006; 27:95-101.

[291] Warren PR, Chater BV. An overview of established interdental cleaning methods. *J. Clin. Dent.* 1996;7Spec No:65-9.

[292] Hancock EB. Periodontal diseases: prevention. *Ann. Periodontol.* 1996;1:223-49.

[293] Quirynen M, De Soete M, Dierickx K, van Steenberghe D. The intra-oral translocation of periodontopathogens jeopardises the outcome of periodontal therapy. A review of the literature. *J. Clin. Periodontol.* 2001;28:499-507.

[294] Ayad F, Berta R, Petrone M, De Vizio W, Volpe A. Effect on plaque removal and gingivitis of a triclosan-copolymer pre-brush rinse: a six-month clinical study in Canada. *J. Can. Dent. Assoc.* 1995;61:53-61.

[295] Triratana T, Kraivaphan P, Amornchat C, Rustogi K, Petrone MP, Volpe AR. Effect of a triclosan/copolymer pre-brush mouthrinse on established plaque formation and gingivitis: a six-month clinical study in Thailand. *J. Clin. Dent.* 1995;6:142-7.

[296] Worthington HV, Davies RM, Blinkhorn AS, Mankodi S, Petrone M, DeVizio W, et al. A six-month clinical study of the effect of a pre-brush rinse on plaque removal and gingivitis. *Br. Dent. J.* 1993;175:322-6.

[297] Hase JC, Ainamo J, Etemadzadeh H, Astrom M. Plaque formation and gingivitis after mouthrinsing with 0.2% delmopinol hydrochloride, 0.2% chlorhexidine digluconate and placebo for 4 weeks, following an initial professional tooth cleaning. *J. Clin. Periodontol.* 1995;22:533-9.

[298] Moran J, Addy M, Wade WG, Maynard JH, Roberts SE, Aström M, et al. A comparison of delmopinol and chlorhexidine on plaque regrowth over a 4-day period and salivary bacterial counts. *J. Clin. Periodontol.* 1992;19:749-53.

[299] Vassilakos N, Arnebrant T, Rundegren J. In vitro interactions of delmopinol hydrochloride with salivary films adsorbed at solid/liquid interfaces. *Caries Res.* 1993;27:176-82.

[300] Collaert B, Edwardsson S, Attström R, Hase JC, Aström M, Movert R. Rinsing with delmopinol 0.2% and chlorhexidine 0.2%: short-term effect on salivary microbiology, plaque, and gingivitis. *J. Periodontol.* 1992;63:618-25.

[301] Claydon N, Hunter L, Moran J, Wade W, Kelty E, Movert R, et al. A 6-month home-usage trial of 0.1% and 0.2% delmopinol mouthwashes (I). Effects on plaque, gingivitis, supragingival calculus and tooth staining. *J. Clin. Periodontol.* 1996;23:220-8.

[302] Lang NP, Hase JC, Grassi M, Hämmerle CH, Weigel C, Kelty E, et al. Plaque formation and gingivitis after supervised mouthrinsing with 0.2% delmopinol hydrochloride, 0.2% chlorhexidine digluconate and placebo for 6 months. *Oral Dis.* 1998 Jun;4:105-13.

[303] Riordan PJ. The place of fluoride supplements in caries prevention today. *Aust. Dent. J.* 1996;41:335-42.

[304] Mulligan R, Sobel S. Preventive oral health care for compromised individuals. In: Harris NO, Garcia-Godoy F, eds. New Jersey Pearson Education, Inc., *Primary preventive dentistry.* 6th ed, 2004;559-88.

In: Hygiene and Its Role in Health
Editors: P. L. Anderson and J. P. Lachan

ISBN 978-1-60456-195-1
© 2008 Nova Science Publishers, Inc.

Chapter 2

Knowledge and Practical Attitudes Towards Gloves Use in Dental Practice

Fethi Maatouk[*1] *and Afef Zribi*[2]

[1]Paediatric Dentistry, Dentistry School of Monastir, TUNISIA
[2]Private practice, Tunis, TUNISIA

Résumé

De nos jours, l'hygiène et l'asepsie tiennent une place prépondérante dans le domaine médical et particulièrement en médecine dentaire où la « main du dentiste » constitue une importante source de contamination. L'une des mesures de base de prévention des infections nosocomiales comprend donc le lavage des mains et le port de gants qui forment une barrière physique de protection.

Notre étude réalisée à la Clinique Dentaire Universitaire de Monastir (Tunisie) a pour objectif d'évaluer les connaissances, les attitudes et les pratiques du personnel soignant quant au port des gants (Enquête CAP). Elle consiste en un sondage par questionnaire auto administré à un échantillon de 106 praticiens de la Clinique comprenant 16 enseignants, 26 résidents, 32 internes et 32 étudiants en médecine dentaire.

Les résultats révèlent que 78.3% des dentistes utilisent régulièrement des gants, 21.7% portent des masques et 2% des lunettes de protection. Les étudiants disposent d'un minimum de connaissances à propos des gants mais ne possèdent pas une pratique correcte alors que les autres praticiens ont de bonnes connaissances et des attitudes pratiques correctes.

De ce fait, il faut améliorer le comportement des étudiants pour un meilleur respect des conditions d'hygiène et de sécurité notamment par des cycles de formation.

---

[*] Address : Pr. Fethi MAATOUK. Paediatric Dentistry Department. Dentistry School Avicenne Avenue 5019 Monastir. TUNISIA. Tel. + 216 73 460 832 / Fax. + 216 73 461 150 / E-Mail fethi.maatouk@fmdm.rnu.tn Web Site: http://maatouk.tripod.com

Abstract

Nowadays hygiene and asepsis took an important place in all the medical fields and particularly in Dentistry, because the "hand of the dentist" can constitute a important source of infection. So, one basic measure of infection control, supposes a careful hand washing and the use of gloves which form a physical barrier and protect the Health Care Workers from occupational exposure to blood and saliva.

Our study carried out with the University Dental Clinic of Monastir (Tunisia) aims to evaluate knowledge in dental practice and to investigate their attitudes and practices toward the use of the gloves. It consists of a survey by auto-administrated questionnaire managed to a sample of 106 dental practitioners including 16 teachers, 26 trainees and 64 dental students.

Findings revealed that about 78.3% of dentists wore gloves, 21.7% wore masks and 2% wore protective eyeglasses. The students have a minimum necessary knowledge about gloves use but do not have a correct practice while the other practitioners have the good knowledge and the good practical attitudes.

Our study shows an important need to improve the students' behaviour with respect of occupational hygiene and safety conditions in order to reduce occupational blood exposure hazards.

Keywords: *MeSH, Asepsis, Dental staff, Dental practice, Nosocomial infection control, Gloves, Protective/utilization.*

The hygiene and the asepsis took today an important place in all the medical fields and particularly in Dentistry. The patients are aware for this problem, which becomes the major concern of our society. This concern is not recent because since the sixteenth century Semmelweiss encouraged the fight against the infection and mortality in maternities by a simple washing of the hands. Later in 1867, "The Lancet" published the article of Lister on the concept of the disinfectant surgery [1, 2]. But at the base of the great principles of asepsis and sterilization, we find the famous work of Louis Pasteur (1822-1895) who wrote: "Instead of effort to eliminate the microbes in the wounds, it would be more reasonable not to introduce some".

Today, the strict hygiene and the nosocomial infections control must be an absolute priority for all the health care workers, especially for the dental care staff because it can constitute a very important link in the transmission of the infections from a patient to another and also towards all the dentist entourage, particularly the family [3]. It is a risk of "cross contamination" complicated and increased by the characteristics of the dentistry practice, in particular, the multiplication and the diversity of care acts, the miniaturization of the instruments... So the respect of the asepsis, which is the guarantee of an optimal quality of care and comfort for the patient and a medico-legal protection for the practitioner, remains a true challenge with the dentistry [4, 5, 6].

It is known that the "hand of the dentist" plays, as a source of infection, a role which should not be underestimated. Indeed the hands are the first vector of the contamination, and it is estimated that 70 to 80% of the infections are carried by hands. So, one basic measure of infection control, supposes firstly a careful hand washing and secondly the use of gloves which are a personal protective equipment (PPE). These two factors constitute an essential elements for the nosocomial infection control since the glove forms a physical barrier which protects the dentist from direct exposure to blood and body fluids like saliva (occupational blood exposure hazards: OBE). In dentistry, the circumstances of gloves use are so varied that only one type of glove cannot satisfy the whole of the dentist needs [7].

In 1889, the American physician "William halsted" used the glove for the first time at the surgical operation [8]. Until the discovery of rubber, the gloves were manufactured from animal bladders, leather or cotton.

Since 1985 with the AIDS epidemic the frequency of the gloves use increased. Indeed the appearance of this affection was a real catalyst which modified the behaviour of the Care health professionals and also at the origin of the concepts of universal precautions against contamination risk from blood and biological products. These standard precautions were stated in 1989 by Occupational Safety and Health Administration (OSHA) and Centers for Disease Control (CDC). Their purpose is to avoid or control the cross infection [9, 10].

The objectives of the present study were to measure knowledge among dental care staff about rational use of gloves in order to prevent nosocomial hazards, to investigate their practice towards the use of the gloves and to look for any relationship between knowledge and practice.

1. Material and Methods

Our investigation carried out with the university dental clinic of Monastir (Tunisia) was conducted between April and May 2006. It consisted of a survey by questionnaire managed to a sample of 106 dental care workers including 16 teachers, 26 trainees, 32 students of last form and 32 students of 5th form.

In fact, the questionnaire was distributed directly to 111 practitioners but despite that anonymity and confidentiality of the answers was guaranteed 5 of them refused to answer it, so the participant rate was about 95.5%.

Study Tool

The self administrated questionnaire with open answers was adapted from the literature that reported on the understanding and attitudes toward the control of nosocomial infection by wearing gloves. The items of the questionnaire were divided in two headings:

–   Knowledge with 7 questions.
–   Practical attitude towards gloves use with 17 questions.

A pilot study with 20 subjects was used to validate the questionnaire which was found to be consistent, reliable and easy to read.

Sample Presentation

The sample presentation given in Table 1 shows that girls constitute 55.6% of studied subjects which age varied from 25 to 50 years with mean of 27.5 ± 4.3 years. Experience duration varied from 0 to 27 years with average of 2.84 ± 5.78 years for all subjects and 15.25 ± 5.71 years for teachers.

Table 1. Sample presentation

Gender	Male		Female		Total	
Variables	N	%	N	%	N	%
Age (years)						
25-29	36	76.6	54	91.5	90	84.9
30-39	4	8.5	3	5	7	6.6
40-50	7	14.9	2	3.4	9	8.5
Level of education						
Student 5th form	15	31.9	17	28.8	32	30.2
Student last form (diploma)	13	27.7	19	32.2	32	30.2
Trainees (University diploma)	8	17	18	30.5	26	24.5
Teacher (Bachelor degree)	11	23.4	5	8.5	16	15.1
Years of experience						
0-5	36	76.6	54	9 1.5	90	84.9
6-10	3	6.4	2	3.4	5	4.7
11-15	3	6.4	1	1.7	4	3.7
>15	5	10.5	2	3.4	7	6.4
Total	47	44.4	59	55.6	106	100

All dental specialties were involved as shown in table 2.

Table 2. Distribution according to specialties

	None	PD	CD	Ortho	Perio	OS	TP	FP	RPP	Total
N	32	12	9	9	9	11	6	9	9	106
%	30.1	11.3	8.5	8.5	8.5	10.4	5.7	8.5	8.5	100

PD: pediatric dentistry CD: conservative dentistry Ortho: orthodontics Perio: periodontology OS: oral surgery CP: complete prosthesis FP: fixed prosthesis RPP: Removable partial prosthesis.

Statistical Analysis

After validation of the forms, the data were collected by computer system and the statistical analysis was performed with the Epi-Info software version 6.04. The Pearson chi-squared test was used at 5% level of significance to compare different percentages [11].

2. Results

2.1. Knowledge

Table 3 summarizes the knowledge of respondents about gloves and gives percentages of correct answers.

- Principal materials of the gloves: 98 subjects (92.4%) knew only latex probably because it is the unique gloves' material used in the university dental clinic. Only two respondents knew also the vinyl and one knew in more the nitril and the neoprene.
- Type of powder used to lubricate the gloves (Starch of corn, talc...): the answers were all for talc and any response for the corn starch.

Table 3. Knowledge about rational gloves use

Items		Students 5th form	Students last form	Trainees	Teachers	Total n = 106
		% correct answers				
1	Do you know principal materials of the gloves?	90.6	97	100*	75	92.5
2	What type of powder is used to lubricate the gloves?	59.4	78	80.7*	75	72.6
3	Which are the types of gloves used in dental practice?	43.7	62.5	53.8	43.7	51.9
4	What do you think about the protection of the gloves? (partial protection)	100	84.4	96.1	81.2	97.2
5	Are there risks related to the use of the gloves for dentist?	81.2	84.4	96.1	81.2	85.8
6	Are there risks related to the use of the gloves for patient?	46.9	34.3	46.1	56.2	44.3
7	Can we wash the gloves?	87.5	90.6	92.3	93.7	90.6
	Evaluation of knowledge (score/6)					
8	Get good knowledge ≥ 3	68.6	78	92.2	81.1	79.2
	Mean score	3.16± 0.9	3.31 ± 1	3.58± 0.8	3.75± 1.3	3.4 ± 1

* Statistical significative difference p ≤ 0.05.

The use of talc is banned since about 15 years for allergic problems and only the modified corn starch is used now.

- Types of gloves used in dental practice (Examination gloves / sterile operating gloves /sterile gloves for surgery): the respondents make the difference between examination gloves and sterile glove of surgery without knowing the sterile glove of care.
- Level of gloves protection
- Complete protection 2- Partial protection 3- Does not protect at all 4- Protection from cuts 5- Protection from the punctures)

The greatest number of practitioners (97.2 %) believed in the true protection of the gloves. That explains the important use for the gloves. Only 3 dentists (2.8 %) have false idea on the protection of the gloves.

In fact the wearing of gloves does not reduce the frequency of sharps injuries, but may confer some protection by virtue of their wiping action on the sharp object on penetration [8].

- Risks related to gloves' use for the dentist and the patient: 86% admitted risk from gloves' wear for dentist and only 44% admitted risk for patients. It was thought that the risk is primarily the allergy to latex and that it is higher for the dentist who is with the direct and close contact with this material.
- Possibility to wash the gloves: those which confirmed the washing of the gloves did it when the gloves are soiled by blood, saliva or impression material. This wrong idea more frequent in students (12.7%) is due to a fact that they must buy gloves.
- Evaluation of knowledge: according to answers' of the 7 preceding questions, knowledge was scored with 1 for a correct answer and 0 for an incorrect one. Scores are ranged from 0 to 7, with a median of 3. A cut-off score was calculated based on the median value. Participants scoring at or above the median value of the total knowledge score were classified as having good knowledge, while those having a total knowledge score less than the median value were considered as having poor knowledge.

The mean knowledge score was about 3.40 ± 1.02.

According to the function, the best marks are recorded among trainees. Indeed 92.2% of them had good knowledge, but the difference is not statistically significative.

2.2. Practical Attitude

Table 4 shows the percentages of correct practical attitude about rational gloves use.

- Frequency and moment of use of personal protective equipment:
  An important and systematic use of the gloves in the University Dental Clinic is noted in 78.3%. About 20% used them irregularly and only 1.9% of the respondents

never used the gloves. They thought that the risk misses out in complete prosthesis because the patients are toothless. Some believed that the gloves' wearing is unpleasant in some acts of prosthesis and in those needing a tactile sensation like acts of endodontics.

The students were the large consumers of the gloves with 87.5% of them that always used gloves.

Among the answers given about the moment of gloves' use, 5 choices were noted:

1.   Face to a patient at risk
2.   When glove is available
3.   In bloody act
4.   In patient with failing oral hygiene
5.   In contact with saliva

The majority of those who wore masks were students of last forms (52.1%) and only 2% wore protective glasses.

• About factors which guide the choice of gloves, the respondents had selected 4 factors:

1. The type of glove
2. The size of glove
3. The act to carry out
4. The medical history of patient.

2.8% of them take in account all these 4 factors in their choice. The majority of the respondents that is 86% chose gloves according to size. In our dental university clinic, except in the oral surgery department, only one type of gloves is available, the examination gloves, therefore the choice according to these parameters remains theoretical.

• Jewels and watches: the majority of the practitioners did not remove their jewels, of which 63.6% were woman. The 7.5% "not specified answers" were to men who did not carry jewels in fact.

• Time of hands washing and gloves wearing:
     61.3% of the respondents washed their hands before and after the gloves' wearing.

     35.8% of them gave a great importance to the handwashing after the use of the gloves since the hands were soiled by the powder and sweating. It is noted that some were rather interested in the visible stain than in the invisible micro-organisms.

     23.6% of the practitioners wore the gloves at one time when it is useless to carry them (with the interrogation) an equivalent number of the practitioners make the clinical examination in mouth naked hands.

- Gloves use factors:

     The majority of the respondents (86.8%) used one pair of gloves for each patient.

     4.7% of them work without gloves for patients whom they judge without risk.

     5.5% of the practitioners wore an overglove (double pair of gloves) when they treated patient at contamination risk but 5.7% of them had the false ideas that it can protected from the punctures.

     40% of the respondents never used an overglove; among them 45.2% were students because they have only one pair of gloves.

     72.6% of the subjects take off the gloves immediately after the care. But 21.7% of the subjects make gestures apart from the mouth with the soiled gloves (wrote the appointments, the prescriptions, the medical certificates, answered to phone call, take X-ray…). More than half of them were students.

- In case of long care procedure (More than 1 hour): Among the 39 practitioners (37%) who wore the gloves for duration longer than one hour, 66.6% were students. That is explained by the fact that the students brought only one pair of gloves for a clinical session of two hours and half.

- In case of an interruption of care: 92 practitioners (86.8%) take off the gloves with the interruption of care but 25 among them (23.6%), whom were mainly students, re-used them when they continued the cares.

- In case of gloves perforation: 11.3% of respondents keep on perforated gloves; more than half of them were students. That is explained in the same way by the fact that they have only one pair of gloves.

- Assistant or co-workers: among the 61 subjects (58%) that assistant did not wear gloves almost half (47.5%) were students who always work in binomial. Of course, in oral surgery the assistants of surgeons always wear sterile gloves.
- Gloves elimination: the major part of the respondents removed and threw the gloves just at the end of the care in dustbin.

- Allergy to latex gloves: The majority of the practitioners (89.6%) didn't ask the patient if it is allergic to latex.

     As the synthetic gloves are not available at the university dental clinic of Monastir, only the 11 dentists (10.4%) which were allergic to latex used synthetic gloves.

     In fact, some complains about reactions of dryness, redness, urticaria or burns are reported but these reactions are rare and it is thought that they are surely due to repeated washings and to the other dental materials used rather than with true allergy to latex [12, 13, 14, 15, 16].

- Evaluation of the practical attitudes: According to answers' of the 18 preceding questions, practical attitudes were scored with 1 for a correct practice and 0 for a wrong one. Then the total score (note/18) was calculated for the evaluation of correct attitudes.

Table 4. Practical attitude about rational gloves use

Items		% correct attitudes				
		Students 5th form	Students last form	Trainees	Teachers	Total
1	Do you always use gloves?	87.5*	81.3	76.9	56	78.3
2	Do you use mask?	9.4	37.5*	19.2	18.8	21.7
3	Do you use protective glasses?	0	0	3.8	6.3*	1.9
4	Which factor does guide your choice of gloves? (size)	65.6	59.4*	57.7	50	85.8
5	Do you remove jewels and watches before wearing the gloves?	43.8	40.6	38.5	37.5	40.6
6	When do you wash your hands? (Before wearing and after removing gloves)	56.3	40.6	80.8	81.3*	61.3
7	At which time do you wear the gloves? Just before examination	53	53	57.7*	18.8	52
8	Do you change gloves in case of long care procedure?	50	65.6	84.6*	62.5	65
9	How long do you keep the gloves? (≤1H)	18.8	84.4	73.1	87.5*	62.3
10	Do you use one pair of gloves for each patient? (Yes)	93.8	90.6	80.8	81.3	86.8
11	When do you remove the gloves? (just after care)	59.4	71.9	77	87.5	72.6
12	Where do you throw the (soiled) removed gloves? (in dustbin)	100	97	96.2	87.5	96.2
13	In case of an interruption of care do you change gloves? (yes)	25	59.4	61.5*	56.3	49
14	Do you change gloves if it is perforated?	75	90.6	96.2*	93.8	87.7
15	Do you sometimes wear an overgloves (double pair)?	40.6	78*	73	37.5	59.4
16	Does your assistant wear gloves?	9.4	28	46.2	56.3*	31
17	Do you ask whether the patient is allergic to latex?	9.4	3	7.7	18.8	8.5
18	What do you make for a patient allergic to latex? (use a synthetic gloves)	87.5	75	53.8	50	69.8
	Evaluation of the practical attitudes (note/18)					
19	Mean note	8.5±2.3	10 ± 2.6	10.6±2.2*	9.7±3.1	9.7± 2.6
	Get at least a note ≥ 8	43.7	72	88.5	75	68
20	Do you have any allergy to the material of the gloves?	6.25	6.25	19.2	12.5	10.4

* Statistical significative difference p ≤ 0.05.

A cut-off score was calculated based on the median value. Participants scoring at or above the median value were classified as having good practical attitudes, while those having a total attitudes score less than the median value were considered as having bad practical attitudes. The average note was about 9.7 ± 2.6; about nearly 68% of the respondents had the average.

According to the function, like as knowledge, the best notes were recorded among trainees. Indeed 88.5% of them had note equal or better than 9. The worst marks are recorded in the students.

3. Analysis and Discussion

The frequency of personal protective equipment (PPE) wearing in our study was about 78.3% for gloves, 21.7% for mask and only 2% for protective glasses. The respondents suppose surely that the glasses of sight are also safety goggles but special protective glasses, or goggles are required to provide sufficient eye protection.

These rates are lower than what was reported by Burke et al 1994 in a 2-year follow-up study of 2000 dentists in England and Wales about glove use in clinical practice, they found that 83% of respondents wore gloves routinely for all patients and all procedures, 15% wore gloves for either selected patients or procedures and 2% never wore gloves [17, 18].

Morris et al.1996 showed that about 90% of dentists in Kuwait wore gloves, 75% wore masks and 52% wore eyeglasses [19].

A study conducted in Canada revealed that in 1994 91.8% of dentists in Ontario always wore gloves, 74.8% always wore masks and 83.6% always wore eye protection [20].
The situation is almost the same in Saudi Arabia where it was found that only 2%–4% of dental professionals never wore gloves when treating patients [21].

Al-Omari MA et al 2005, which reported that among 120 dentists of private practice in Jordan 81.8 % wore and changed gloves during treatment and between patients [22].
Our frequency of gloves wearing is higher than reported by Treasure and Treasure in a New Zealand study, where only 42.0% of dentists wore gloves, 64.8% wore masks and 66.4% wore eye protection [23].

According to gender Motamed N. et al. [24] and McCarthy et al. [25] showed in their study on knowledge and practices, that women had a significant higher level of knowledge and practice toward universal precautions than men. Hellgren 1994 reported that dentists never using loves at all were older, male practitioners [26]. This is in agreement with our results where girls use more gloves than boys respectively 85% and 66% ($p<10^{-2}$). These percentages decrease significantly with age ($p<10^{-9}$) as also reported by McCarthy et al. 1999 [27].

Regarding function, the students are the large users of the gloves (87.5%). This high rate is in relation with the nature of work in the university dental clinic which imposes to the students the use of gloves, but it does not really reflect a true conscience of the importance of gloves use.

It seems that the use of gloves is more related to a fear of the direct occupational blood (OBE) than to a true comprehension of the interests of its use.

Indeed, in comparison with the residents and the teachers a reduced number of students wash their hands before and after gloves wearing.

53% of the students wear the gloves before the clinical examination and 31.2% carry them even before the medical interrogation of the patient. Often, time before clinical examination includes also the call of the patient from the waiting room, the installation of the patient on dental chair, the recovery of the material of work... in fact gestures which do not require gloves wearing.

All the students wear one pair of gloves for each patient, perhaps because the students often treat only one patient by clinical training session. This is in agreement with the results of a study conducted in a province of northern Italy where 99% of the dentists changed gloves after each patient [28].

60% of the students of our study take off their gloves immediately after the end of care. It was supposed that students whose remain keeping on the gloves until patient leaving write the prescriptions, the appointments, the medical certificates... with the soiled gloves.

It is noted that a significant number of students (66.6% $p<10^{-4}$) wear longer than one hour the same gloves. Indeed the gloves are provided to all the practitioners of the university dental clinic except for the students who must bring them themselves and they buy only one pair of glove for a working session of two hours and half.

21.8% of students don't change gloves with the interruption of care.

According to dental specialities the best "practical attitudes scores" are recorded with the departments of periodontology and "oral surgery" which are the departments where the contact with blood and saliva is almost constant with each care. The lowest scores are noted with the prosthesis departments; in the latter the care and the interventions are much less bloody. Also, in these departments the nature of certain acts is incompatible with the gloves wearing like the dental impression, the handling of the wax. The papers of Burke FJ et al 1992 and Epstein JB et al 1995 lead to the same conclusions [29, 30, 31].

In brief, the glove wearing patterns were found to be related to gender, age and function. The reasons given for not wearing gloves routinely included problems of comfort, loss of tactile sensation, cost and the risk of cross-infection, which was perceived to be small. Burke FJ et al. 1994, Gordon BL et al 2001 and Christensen GJ 2001 reported the same reasons in their study [29, 32, 33].

4. Recommendations with Use of the Gloves [34, 35]

- Use a glove for each patient and a glove for each care:
- The gloves must be preserved in their box in a dry place safe from heat, light and x-rays.
- The gloves must be used as supplementary measure of nosocomial infection control, they do not replace hands washing.
- The hand washing both prior to placement and following removal of gloves is necessary.
- The gloves must be used before the clinical examination in the new patient and right before the act to carry out at a second appointment.
- The jewels and the watch must be removed before wearing the gloves.
- An order of care must be respected: from cleanest care to more contaminated one.

- The maximum time of wearing of gloves is between 30 minutes and 2 hours. This time decreases more especially as the act has a high risk of contamination.
- In the event of interruption of care, it is necessary to change the gloves as well as the resumption of the whole procedure of antisepsy of the hands.
- The washing of the gloves is to be proscribed owing to the fact that it affects the integrity of the glove and thus its effectiveness.
- The worn gloves are not reusable.
- The elimination of the gloves must be done immediately at the end of the care, in the nearest adapted dustbin.
- Gloves must be eliminated just at the end of the care and more close possible of the place of care in the adapted die of waste. We must take off a first glove and lock up it in the other hand than take off the second glove. The hands should never return in contact with the external soiled face of the glove to eliminate. The removal of the glove is followed of a simple or disinfectant washing of the hands according to the level of contamination of the care which has been just carried out.

Conclusion

As in all the specialities of medicine, the medical gloves are largely used in dentistry. They form an effective physical barrier and constitute the best protection to our hands and to our patients. A few years ago, the wearing of gloves was badly perceived with the dentist and the patient doesn't perceive his utility. However, nowadays, with the evolution of the medical culture of the patients, it is the opposite phenomenon which occurs and the gloves wearing now is perceived very favourably and even regarded as an element of great professionalism which improves the public image of the dentist. The use of the gloves is of course useful, but it is necessary to know to correctly use them according to the predetermined rules and recommendations. Because misused, the gloves become a vector of the infection. There are various materials of the gloves, but the latex remains more used considering its performance and its qualities.

However the use of the gloves is not completely without risk since certain reactions of allergies especially related to natural latex are reported.

- Our study shows that there is a need to improve the dental health team behaviour with respect of occupational hygiene and safety conditions in order to reduce OBE hazards.
- To lead to the correct practice we must start first of all by offering the gloves to all the practitioners without exception including the students.
- There is also a great need to provide infection control courses and guidelines for the students and cycles of continuous training for other practitioners, in addition to distribution of standard infection control manuals that incorporate current infection control recommendations.

Acknowledgements

The authors would like to express their gratitude to all those who helped them in this study especially the students.

EL= LIOT R.=20, D.D.S., M.S. and WALTER T., M.S.=20. Shulman ER, Brehm WT.

References

[1]   Chin JE. *Control of communicable disease manual*, 17th ed. Washington, American Public Health Association, 2000:1–9.

[2]   Thomas O, Maiza L. Transmission of infectious diseases. Encycl Med Chir (Elsevier Paris) *odontologie*, 23-841-B-10, 1998,10p.

[3]   Hudson-Davies SC, Jones JH, Sarll DW. Cross-infection control in general dental practice: dentists' behaviour compared with their knowledge and opinions. *Br. Dent. J.* 1995 May 20;178(10):365-9.

[4]   Nash KD. How infection control procedures are affecting dental practice today. *J. Am. Dent. Assoc.* 1992 Mar;123(3):67-73.

[5]   CDC. Updated USPHS guidelines for managing occupational exposures to HBV, HCV, and HIV and considerations for dentistry. *Journal of the American Dental Association*, 2002, 133(12):1627–9.

[6]   Stoopler ET. Oral herpetic infections (HSV1-8). *Dent. Clin. N. Am.* 2005; 49:15-29.

[7]   Aubier M, Kleinfinger S. *Protection des mains au cabinet dentaire*. Paris: CdP, 2001 :80p.

[8]   Upton LG, Barber HD. Double-gloving and the incidence of perforations during specific oral and maxillofacial surgical procedures. *J. Oral Maxillofac. Surg.* 1993;51:261–3.

[9]   CDC. Recommended infection-control practices for dentistry. *MMWR* 1993;35:237-42.

[10]   Bolyard EA, Tablan OC, Williams WW et al. Guideline for infection control in health care personnel. *American Journal of Infection Control* (1998;26:289-354).

[11]   Abramson JH, Abramson ZH. *Making Sense of Data: A Self-Instruction Manual on the Interpretation of Epidemiological Data*. Oxford University Press US, 2001.

[12]   Ahmed DD, Sobczak SC, Yunginger JW. Occupational allergies caused by latex. *Immunology Allergy Clin. North Am.* 2003;23:205-19.

[13]   Chardin H. Hypersensibilités en pratique odontostomatologique : cas particuliers de l'allergie au latex et de l'allergie aux métaux. Encycl Med Chir (Elsevier Paris) *odontologie*, 23-841-C-15, 1997,4p.

[14]   Yip E, Cacioli P. The manufacture of gloves from natural rubber latex. J Allergy Clin Immunol 2002;110(2 Suppl):S3-14.

[15]   Barbara J, Santais MC, Levy DA, et al. Immunoadjuvant properties of glove cornstarch powder in latex-induced hypersensitivity. *Clin. Exp. Allergy* 2003;33:106-112.

[16]   Huber MA, Terezhalmy GT. Adverse Reactions to Latex Products: Preventive and Therapeutic Strategies. *J. Contemp. Dent. Pract.* 2006 February;(7)1:097-106.

[17] Burke FJ, Wilson NH, Cheung SW. Glove use by dentists in England and Wales: results of a 2-year follow-up survey. *Br. Dent. J.* 1994 May 7;176(9):337-41.

[18] Burke FJ, Wilson NH, Cheung SW. Trends in glove use by dentists in England and Wales: 1989-1992. *Int. Dent. J.* 1994 Jun;44(3):195-201.

[19] Morris E et al. Infection control knowledge and practices in Kuwait: a survey on oral health care workers. Saudi dental journal, 1996, 8:19–26.

[20] McCarthy GM, MacDonald JK. The infection control practices of general dental practitioners. *Infection control and hospital epidemiology*, 1997;18(10):699–703.

[21] Al-Rabeah A, Mohamed AG. Infection control in the private dental sector in Riyadh. *Annals of Saudi medicine*, 2002, 22(1–2):13–7.

[22] Al-Omari MA, Al-Dwairi ZN. Compliance with infection control programs in private dental clinics in Jordan. *J. Dent. Educ.* 2005 Jun;69(6):693-8.

[23] Treasure P, Treasure ET. Survey of infection control procedures in New Zealand dental practices. *International dental journal,* 1994, 44(4):342–8.

[24] Motamed N, BabaMahmoodi F, Khalilian A, Peykanheirati M and Nozari M Knowledge and practices of health care workers and medical students towards universal precautions in hospitals in Mazandaran Province. *EMHJ*, 2006;12, 5.

[25] McCarthy GM, MacDonald JK. Gender differences in characteristics, infection control practices, knowledge and attitudes related to HIV among Ontario dentists. Community *Dent. Oral Epidemiol.* 1996 Dec;24(6):412-5.

[26] Hellgren K. Use of gloves among dentists in Sweden--a 3-year follow-up study. Swed *Dent. J.* 1994;18(1-2):9-14.

[27] McCarthy GM, Koval JJ, MacDonald JK, John MA. The role of age- and population-based differences in the attitudes, knowledge and infection control practices of Canadian dentists. *Community Dent. Oral Epidemiol.* 1999;27:298–304.

[28] Veronesi L, Bonanini M, Dall'Aglio P, Pizzi S, Manfredi M, Tanzi ML, Health hazard evaluation in private dental practices: a survey in a province of northen Italy. *Acta Bio Medica Ateneo Parmense* 2004; 75; 50-55.

[29] Burke FJ, Wilson NH, Shaw WC, Cheung SW. Glove use by orthodontists: results of a survey in England and Wales. *Eur. J. Orthod.* 1992 Jun;14(3):246-51.

[30] Burke FJ, Wilson NH, Cheung SW, Shaw WC. Glove use by orthodontists in England and Wales: changes since 1989 and comparisons with general dental practitioners. *Eur. J. Orthod.* 1994 Jun;16(3):241-4.

[31] Epstein JB, Mathias RG, Bridger DV. Survey of knowledge of infectious disease and infection control practices of dental specialists. *J. Can Dent. Assoc.* 1995 Jan;61(1):35-7, 40-4.

[32] Gordon Bl, Burke FJT, Bagg J, Marlborough HS, McHugh ES. Systematic review of adherence to infection control. Guidelines in dentistry. J Dent 2001; 29: 509-16.

[33] Christensen G.J : Operating gloves : The good and the bad . *J. Am. Dent. Assoc.,* 2001; 132, 10: 1455-57.

[34] Harte JA, Charlton DG. Characteristics of infection control programs in U.S. Air Force dental clinics. A survey. *J. Am. Dent. Assoc.,* 2005; 136, 7: 885-892.

[35] Kohn WG, Collins AS, Cleveland JL, Harte JA, Eklund KJ, Malvitz DM; Centers for Disease Control and Prevention. Guidelines for infection control in dental health-care settings—2003. *MMWR Recomm. Rep.* 2003;52(RR-17):1–61.

In: Hygiene and Its Role in Health
Editors: P. L. Anderson and J. P. Lachan

ISBN 978-1-60456-195-1
© 2008 Nova Science Publishers, Inc.

Chapter 3

Role of Environmental Contamination in Norovirus Gastroenteritis

Charmaine Gauci[1], Anthony Gatt[1],
Franco Maria Ruggeri[2] and Ilaria di Bartolo[2]
[1]Infectious Disease Prevention and Control Unit, Malta
[2]Istituto Superiore di Sanita, Italy

Abstract

Norovirus disease, a highly infectious gastroenteritis, traditionally known as winter vomiting disease, is spreading rapidly across many countries and continents. Schools, hospitals, hotels, cruise ships and facilities for the elderly are particularly prone to outbreaks of infection. Although few persons die from the infection, the burden of illness is high since many people can be afflicted in outbreaks. Norovirus is known to occur after eating contaminated food however the majority of cases have resulted from person to person transmission and via environmental contamination. This can occur when persons or health care workers have poor personal hygiene or where there is failure to clean common areas properly.

A protracted outbreak of Norovirus occurred in a hotel in Malta between March and October 2006 with four identified outbreaks affecting a total of 337 persons. The recurrent waves of infection in successive cohorts of tourists indicated a source of environmental contamination. Traditional cleaning agents were not sufficient to eliminate the source of infection. The outbreaks were only successfully curtailed with isolation of ill patients; environmental cleaning with appropriate agents; specific prevention strategies including the early identification of patients; contact precautions with patients; enhanced patient and staff hygiene and training and discipline during food preparation and serving.

Environmental contamination has been shown to be implicated in Norovirus outbreaks. Hygiene measures are not a luxury but a necessity to help reduce the burden of this highly contagious infectious disease.

Introduction

Norovirus has played a major role in outbreaks of gastroenteritis (CDC fact sheet: Norovirus activity, 2003; Mounts AW, 1999; Kaplan JE et al, 1982). These outbreaks occur at any place where persons congregate including airplanes, schools, hospitals, nursing homes, residential institutions, cruise ships, hotels and restaurants. It is well known that Norovirus is transmitted via food and water; however environmental contamination can be very extensive especially in crowded places. Such contamination includes environmental contamination of surfaces and fomites and also direct contact from person to person and airborne transmission via ingestion of aerosolized particles from vomitus. Although the individual effects of the infection is often minimal, in the elderly and debilitated it can have serious effects and the burden caused by outbreaks of Norovirus can be large with a high number of persons being affected and other effects on the implicated premises. Hence it is reasonable to understand the virus and its modes of transmission, to learn from previous outbreaks and identify means to prevent and control such illness.

Norovirus

The *Caliciviridae* family includes a wide range of positive-sense, single-stranded RNA viruses, with a non-enveloped icosahedral capsid, and is divided into four genera, *Norovirus, Sapovirus, Lagovirus,* and *Vesivirus* (Pringle, 1998). This classification is based on genome organization and sequence comparisons, and groups all human caliciviruses within the first two genera, whereas most animal caliciviruses are grouped within the other two genera. Noroviruses were discovered in 1972 as the causative agent of a large GE outbreak in a school of Norwalk, in Ohio (Dolin et al., 1972; Kapikian et al., 1972). The Norwalk-agent and other similar viruses found thereafter were initially termed human enteric caliciviruses, small round viruses (SRVs) and small round structured viruses (SRSVs) based on their appearance at the electron microscope. Due to the unavailability of cell culture methods for their isolation, study of these viruses remained only limited until the early '90s when the Norwalk agent was cloned, sequenced and its genome organization discovered (Estes '90). This opened a second era in the study of these viruses, with the development of molecular methods for diagnosis and characterization, the generation of large amounts of Norovirus epidemiological and virological data, the expression of viral antigens helping the implementation of immune diagnostic assays. After 15 years, human caliciviruses are now recognized as the major cause of epidemic non-bacterial gastroenteritis and among them *Sapovirus* infects mostly children whereas *Norovirus* affects both children and adults either in sporadic or epidemic pathways. Members of the genera *Lagovirus* and *Vesivirus* affect only animals causing a variety of host-dependent diseases with consequences which sometimes may be very severe, as is the case of the rabbit hemorrhagic disease of rabbits, caused by the lagovirus RHDV.

Recent studies suggest that some animal caliciviruses may be capable of crossing species barriers and potentially use humans as their hosts. One serotype of the *Vesivirus* San Miguel sea lion virus (SMSV) was reported to apparently infect humans (Chen et al 2004). More interestingly, Norovirus strains named BEC (Bovine Enteric Calicivirus) have been identified in calves affected or not by diarrhea. BEC strains detected in Germany (Liu et al., 1999), in the UK (Oliver et al., 2003), in the Netherlands (van der Poel et al., 2003) and in the US (Smiley et al., 2003) have been found to cluster in the GGIII genogroup of Norovirus, which although distinct is genetically related to human genogroup GGI (Dastjerdi et al., 1999; Liu et al., 1999; van der Poel et al., 2000; Oliver et al., 2003). Sequence comparison has revealed that Norovirus strains can be divided into at least five distinct genogroups (GGI-V), of which GGI, II, and III contain all known human Norovirus strains. Within genogroups, presenting more than 30% nucleotide differences, a continuously increasing number of genotypes are recognized. Although GGV apparently contains a single genotype infecting mice and GGIV a single strain of human origin, variation within the other genogroups is otherwise high with more than 30 known genotypes affecting humans. Genotypes present nucleotide homologies ranging between 15 and 30% from one another, and contain strains with a broad range of genetic diversity. It is not yet clear how genetic diversity may correlate with relevant differences in the antigenic properties of viruses, neither how many serotypes of Norovirus would exist. Recently a Norovirus strain has been identified in pigs and analysis by sequencing revealed that it is strictly correlated to a human genotype. These new data suggest the hypothesis of its possible zoonotic origin and the potential existence of animal reservoirs and interspecies transmission.

Structure of the Virus

Genome Organization

Norovirus is a small, icosahaedral, single-stranded RNA virus whose capsid is formed by multiple copies of a single major structural protein (Estes, M. K., and M. E. Hardy. 1995; Prasad et al., 1999). The viral genome is a plus-sense, single-stranded RNA of ~7.5 kb that is organized into a 5' untranslated region (UTR), three overlapping open reading frames (ORFs), a 3' UTR, and a poly-(A) tail (Harrison, S. C. 1989). ORF1 encodes the nonstructural polyprotein that is cleaved by a viral 3C-like protease into probably 6 proteins, including a helicase, a cysteine proteinase and the RNA-dependent RNA polymerase [RdRp] (Belliot et al., 2003). ORF2 and ORF3 encode the major (VP1) and minor (VP2) capsid proteins, respectively (Green et al., 2001, Jiang et al., 1990 and Jiang et al., 1993). The VP1 protein (50-60 kDa) forms two domains: P (protruding, P1 and P2) and S (shell). The most conserved region is the S domain, whereas the P2 sub-domain is highly variable and the P1 is only moderately conserved (Chen et al., 2004; Chakravarty et al., 2005). The capsid of Noroviruses and other caliciviruses is composed by 180 molecules of the single predominant protein VP1 (Bertolotti et al., 2002). Most part of the cellular interactions and immune recognition features is therefore thought to be located in the VP1, mostly in the P2 sub-domain, which extends above the viral surface and exhibits the most genome sequence divergence (Chakravarty et al., 2005, Nilsson et al., 2003, Prasad et al., 1999). In addition to forming the shell virus structure the capsid protein presumably also contains viral phenotype or serotype determinants and cellular receptor binding sites. Recent studies have shown that

Noroviruses recognize as receptors the human histo-blood group antigens (HBGAs), which are complex carbohydrates present both on red blood cells and mucosal epithelium and as free antigens in biological fluids, such as saliva, milk, and intestinal contents (Le Pendu, 2004; D'Adamo e Kelly, 2001; Thorven et al., 2005). Different host susceptibility to Norovirus infection may thus depend on the histo-blood antigens of each individual (Thorven *et al.*, 2005; Harrington *et al.*, 2002). The recognition of HBGAs by Noroviruses is strain specific, and seems to be mediated in particular by the P2 sub-domain of VP1 (Tan et al., 2003). The function of VP2 is likely associated with up-regulation of VP1 expression and its stabilization in the virus structure (Bertolotti-Ciarlet et al., 2003).

The Norovirus genus presents a high genetic diversity which in addition to genetic drift by accumulation of point mutations, is probably also maintained in part by homologous recombination. In a recent study, it was estimated that approximately 14% of all strains analyzed were newly classified recombinants strains (Reuter et al., 2006). Recombination within the Norovirus genome usually occurs at the Orf1/Orf2 junction (Ambert-Balay et al., 2005 and Rohayem et al., 2005), but recombination has also been reported within the capsid gene either at the interface been the P1 and P2 sub-domains or within the P2 sub-domain (Ambert-Balay et al., 2005). More recently, a Norovirus recombination site has been reported to be localized in the polymerase gene (Waters el al., 2007).

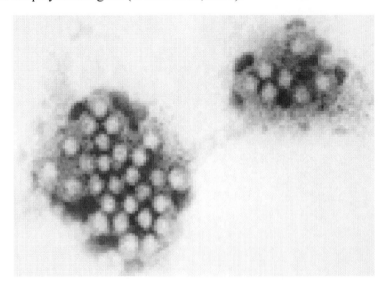

Figure 1. Norovirus.

Taxonomy and Nomenclature

Noroviruses are a group of antigenically and genetically diverse viruses (Ando et al., 2000; Green et al., 1995; Katayama et al., 2002). As Noroviruses are uncultivable viruses, a conventional neutralization test cannot be used for serotyping hence complete information of the existence of multiple serotypes is lacking. However several antigenically distinct viruses have been identified by EM and cross challenge volunteers studies (Katayama et al., 2002).

This antigenic classification scheme is however not exhaustive and not fully reproducible. The recently improved diagnostic molecular method based on reverse transcription-polymerase chain reaction, allowing detection of viral genomic RNA and genomic sequencing, have become the golden standard to characterize the viruses and clarify the relatedness of different strains. Several conserved region have been identified, such as the RdRp gene (RNA-dependent RNA-polymerase, region B) and ORF2 (region C), and have been chosen as suitable to detect the largest number of these diverse viruses. However, such sequences become problematic for studies of phylogenesis because they represent a short stretch of the genome with too limited variation, not sufficient to allow distinguish sequences between each other and assign viruses to the proper cluster (Zheng et al., 2006). To overcome these limitations, phylogenetic analyses are now preferentially performed using the entire ORF2 region whereas analysis of both the RdRp region and ORF2 are considered to be necessary for identification of recombinant strains (produced by recombination of ORF2 and ORF1 of two different strains). Based on these analysis, a genetic classification has been proposed that clusters all human and animal Norovirus strains in 5 genogroups (or genetic cluster G) (Fankhauser et al., 2002; Green et al., 1995; Oliver et al., 2003; Vinje an Koopmans 2000). Strains belonging to GI, GII and GIV are found in humans (with one exception for a GII/11 strain which was identified in pig). G3 and G5 are found in cows and mice, respectively (Zheng et al., 2006). The murine strain MNV-1 is the only Norovirus that can be grown successfully in cell culture and in a small animal model (Karst et al., 2003). Each genogroup is further subdivided into different genotypes based on different criteria, depending on the region analyzed: less than 80% sequence identity in the complete ORF2 or nucleotide sequence similarity of less than 85% (GGI) or 90% (GGII) when considering the polymerase gene in ORF1 (Vinje et al., 2000; Vinje and Koopmans 2000). The name of the "prototype strains" for which sequence information of the entire ORF2 is available in GenBank was initially and is still also used for identification of the genotype or cluster (Ando et al., 2000). The prototype strain of a genetic cluster commonly refers to the first reference strain that was described as being genetically distinct from other reference strains. Examples include the Norwalk (NV), Hawaii (HV), Snow Mountain (SMV), Jena (JV), Southampton (SOV), Toronto (TV), Desert Shield (DSV), and Bristol (BV), and others. More recently, agreement was found to indicate the clusters/genotypes using the abbreviation of the corresponding genogroup, followed by consecutive numbers. Recent phylogenetic studies performed analyzing the entire ORF2 where the hypervariable region is located confirm the existence of a great variability and the proposed classification scheme includes 29 genetic clusters in 5 genogroups, 8 in GI, 17 in GII, 2 in G3, and 1 in G4 and G5 (Zheng et al., 2006). Consistent with the findings of others (Green et al., 1995, Green et al., 2000b, Katayama et al., 2002, Prasad et al., 1999 and Vinjé et al., 2000), in this study the capsid sequences were shown to vary by up to 60% between the five genogroups and 57% among human Norovirus, a level of diversity much higher than that seen for other plus single-stranded RNA viruses). That suggests that the genogroups of Norovirus might be individual species or serotypes (Zheng et al., 2006).

Detection Methods

Noroviruses are considered the most common cause of outbreaks of non-bacterial gastroenteritis worldwide, as well as being an important cause of sporadic gastroenteritis. Noroviruses were discovered by electron microscopy and this method played an important role in the diagnosis of Noroviruses until the introduction of the reverse transcription-polymerase chain reaction procedure in the 1990's. However EM is a time-consuming and relatively insensitive method, and may not recognize the presence of fewer than 10^5 Norovirus particles per ml in biological samples. In addition, stool suspensions may contain a variety of other viruses which may make the recognition of caliciviruses uncertain, and require skilled personnel. ELISAs test is also used to diagnose Norovirus. The method is simple and does not require particular equipment (de Bruin et al., 2006), but may not recognize all Norovirus strains. Among the few commercial kits available in Europe, the first generation tests IDEIA (Dakocytomation Ltd; Ely, UK) and Ridascreen (R-Biopharm AG, Darmstadt, Germany) showed sensitivities as low as 38% and 36% and specificities of 96% and 88% compared to the RT-PCR (de Bruin et al., 2006). Due to large number of genotypes of Norovirus, to the low amount of antigen often present in biological material (faeces, vomitus), the specificity and sensitivity of the commercial tests is not fully satisfactory yet, although they may be helpful to perform a first diagnosis. Newer generations of ELISA platforms are being prepared which may prove quite better than the previous ones, and in the future these may represent the best assay for routine diagnostics in hospital and public health laboratories. A method for hybridization of biotin-labelled viral DNA amplified during diagnostic RT-PCR onto nylon membrane blotted with an array of cold DNA probes (*reverse line blotting hybridization)* has also been conveniently used for diagnosis. This method is rapid, cheap, and allows the simultaneous detection and typing of Norovirus (Vinjé J, Koopmans MP 2000), however it is limited by the steadily increase of newer Norovirus strains with time and the consequent needs for designing and blotting supplemental probes.

Finally, it must be reminded that no attempt of cultivation of Norovirus in cell cultures has so far proven really satisfactory, except for the murine GG.V strains that hinder possible viral isolation techniques, neutralization assays for virus characterization, or serological diagnosis. Currently, the detection method most widely used is reverse transcription polymerase chain reaction (RT-PCR) and most recently real-time PCR which let improve the sensitivity of the test. The limits of PCR is again due to the high numbers of present Norovirus genotypes and their rapid genetic evolution, forcing to either continuously design newer oligonucleotide primers and use as a target for detection the most conserved regions of the genome, such as the RdRp gene. These needs contrast with each other since the amplification of highly conserved regions does not enable easy differentiation between different strains. The targeted regions most widely used for Norovirus molecular detection are named region A (the RdRp gene located in ORF1), region B (the 3'-end of ORF1), region C (a short stretch close to the 5'-end of ORF2), and region D (located at the 3'-end of ORF2) (Ando et al., 2000, Vinjé et al., 2004, Kojima et al., 2002).

The primers in the capsid region allow detection and differentiation of viruses between GI and GII genogroups, and are thus particularly suitable for both accomplishing a first raw genomic characterization of Norovirus and detecting GI - GII mixed infections. Real-time

PCR systems are especially useful, because they are less liable to contamination, and can provide semiquantitative estimates of viral concentration. These methods appear thus both suitable for rapid viral detection in stools and, due to their high sensitivity, for detecting contamination of food, water and environmental samples.

Short conserved sequences have been used successfully for Norovirus detection, especially when applied to multiplex PCR or real-time PCR (Kageyama et al., 2003, Richards et al., 2004 ; Yan et al., 2003), but these sequences present problems for phylogenetic analyses because, in the presence of limited sequence variations, some strains may not be distinguished from each other or even be classified into the proper cluster (Fankhauser et al., 2002, Kageyama et al., 2004). Among recent methods, the technique of nucleic acid sequence-based amplification is also promising (Moore et al., 2004; Patterson et al., 2006) as a method for reliable, sensitive and semi-quantitative detection of Norovirus. Finally, the *Heteroduplex Mobility Assay* (HMA) also constitutes a method allowing direct characterization of the strain genotype without need for sequencing (Mattick *et al.*, 2000).

Clinical Description

The most common symptoms are nausea, abdominal pain, diarrhoea and vomiting. Diarrhoea is one of the commonest symptoms, described in 90.5 % of subjects in one hospital outbreak (Godoy P. et al 2006) and in a number of hospital outbreaks it was described in 80% (Billgren M. et al 2002) of those falling ill. Diarrhoea is described as watery and not bloody.

Vomiting is a predominant symptom (84.2% n=16/19 (Godoy P. et al 2000); 57.9% n=73/126 (Wolf-Dietrich Leers et al 1987) and characteristically can be projectile and explosive (Laila Sekla et al 1989; Dedman D et al 1998; Caul EO 1994) often not permitting those affected from reaching the nearest toilet facilities and thus causing earosol spread to those around them and with consequent contamination of the environment. Nausea may be common (65.9% n=62/94) (Godoy P. et al 2006) and may not be accompanied by vomiting. However an epidemiological study in a gastroenteritis Norovirus outbreak in a Toronto Hospital revealed that only 9.5% (n=126) sufferred from nausea while 57.9% had vomiting (Wolf-Dietrich Leers et al 1987).

Epidemiological investigations of 42 % of acute non-bacterial outbreaks outbreaks in the USA from 1970 to 1980 has shown that vomiting is the predominant symptom among children, while diarrhoea was commoner in adults (Kaplan JE et al 1982).

In a study by Kudaka J et al (2005) in Kyushu, Japan, symptoms caused by several pathogens were compared in 646 cases of gastroenteritis, vomiting was predominant in 71.5% of cases caused by Noroviruses whereas it was present in almost all cases of S. aureus and B. cereus infections and in 22% of C. perfringes and in ETEC and STEC in about 5%.

Many poeple suffering from Noroviral gastroenteritis feel miserable and lethargic and complain of myalgia and some of headaches (CDC Q andA , 2006), but its the vomiting and/or diarrhoea together with the suddeness of the illness that stand out. Abdominal pain can also be a very common symptom but its presence is highly variable: in several outbreaks it was described in 89.5% (n=17/19) (Godoy P. et al 2000), 88.4% (n=84/95) (Godoy P. et al

2006) but only in 27% of those affected in a hospital outbreak (Wolf-Dietrich Leers et al 1987).

The presence of fever is highly variable. It is usually low grade and may be accompanied by chills. In a cohort study conducted in Spain on a small Norovirus outbreak linked to oysters (n=17) fever was present in 17.6% (n=3/17) (Godoy P et al 2000); and in a community outbreak from contaminated potable water in Greece fever was present in 22.3% of the cases (n=709) (Papadopoulos VP et al 2006).

Incubation Period

The incubation period is characteristically short and thought to be 12 – 48 hours. (Wolf-Dietrich Leers et al; CDC; Fact Sheet, 2006⁻). In an international outbreak epidemiologically, statistically and laboratory linked to the consumption of raw oysters in 2002 the mean incubation period was 34 hours (range, 1.5 to 68 hrs) in several clusters in France, while in Italy it was 36 hours (range, 24-48 hrs) (Françoise S. Le Guyader et al 2006).

Infectivity of Noroviruses

It is well known that Noroviuses are hardy, ubiquitous and highly infectious and it is thought that a very low infectivity dose, as few as 10 viral particles may be sufficient to infect an individual (CDC; Fact Sheet 2003).

It is known that not all those exposed to Noroviruses become symptomatic and some are thought to be resistant or immune to these viruses and that this may be strain sepcific, raising the risk of repeated infections to different strains as a reality. Viral shedding in asymptomatic contacts of infected individuals studied in outbreaks has also been recorded suggesting asymptomatic infections (Gallimore CI E et al 2004).

Although presymptomatic viral shedding may occur, shedding usually begins with onset of symptoms and may continue for 2 weeks after recovery. It is unclear to what extent viral shedding over 72 hours after recovery signifies continued infectivity (CDC; Fact Sheet 2003).

Duration of Illness

The illness in helathy persons is usually self limiting and over within 12-72 hours. In a study on the clinical manifestations of Norovirus gastroenteritis in health care settings the median duration of symptoms in hospital, nursing home staff and nursing home residents (n=914) was 2 days with 75% achieving complete recovery within 3 dys. The median duration of symptoms for hospital patients (n=730) was 3 days. 75% of the latter group achieved complete recovery within 5 days, which was significantly longer than that the former groups (P<.001) (Lopman BA et al 2004).

Diagnosis

Generally a physician will make a diagnosis of viral gastroenteritis on the basis of the symptoms and medical examination of the patient. However in order to verify the etiological agent diagnostic tests on stools and vomitus are required. The identification the agent does not change the treatment or outcome much and hence are not routinely used. This limits the data on the burden of the illness especially for sporadic cases. Identification of the pathogen is however important for epidemiological data and will also assist in the control measures in outbreaks.

Stool Sample Collection

Stool specimen collection should occur as soon as possible as the case is detected and the epidemiological investigation is initiated otherwise delay can preclude establishing a diagnosis. If viral gastroenteritis is suspected, samples should be taken immediately and not wait for bacterial and parasitic results of the samples. The highest level of excretion of the virus in the stools is in the acute phase of illness that is within 48 to 72 hours (Goller JL et al, 2004) so ideally a sample is taken in this stage. With improvement in the sensitivity of testing, the pick up rate from stools taken in later stages of the diseases has improved. In outbreaks, ideally 10% of the exposed population is sampled to verify the aetiological agent. Approximately 10-50 ml of stools placed in a stool bottle or urine container are usually required. The softer the stool and the higher the quantity, the higher is the yield. Rectal swabs are of limited or no value due to the limited amount of nucleic acid for amplification. Freezing can destroy the characteristic morphology of the virus which permits diagnosis by electron microscopy hence samples need to be kept refrigerated at 4 °C and tested within 2-3 weeks. If PCR testing will be used, samples can be frozen and tested at a later stage.

Vomitus Sample Collection

Where vomitus is the main symptom, samples of vomitus can be used to supplement the diagnostic yield from the stools. Similar recommendations for the collection, storage and shipment as for stools apply for vomitus.

Environmental Sampling

Norovirus cannot be detected routinely in water, food or environmental samples. However in outbreaks, Norovirus has often been detected from vehicles which have been epidemiologically implicated as the source of infection.

Treatment

As with any other gastroenteritis regardless of the aetiology treatment is symptomatic. Oral rehydration therapy (ORT) is the mainstay of treatment and treatment should be started at home. ORT includes rehydration and maintenance fluids with oral rehydration solutions, combined with continued age-appropriate nutrition (Duggan C et al 1997; Sandhu BK et al 2001). For example infants should be offered more frequent breast or bottle feedings, and older children should be given more fluids. ORT has been instrumental in improving health outcomes among children in developing countries and in preventing millions of deaths worldwide (Kosek M et al 2003; Black RE et al 2003; Parashar U et al 2003).

In healthy older children and adults ORT is sufficient since the illness is usually brief. Young children, the elderly, the sick and those with lowered immune systems are more at risk of developing dehydration and possibly other complications and may require hospitalization. Inpatient treatment may require aggressive treatment with intravenous fluids and correction of electrolyte and metabolic imbalances together with treatment of any other associated conditions those suffering may have.

In general parents of young children and care workers should seek medical review whenever cases of gastroenteritis would not respond to these simple measures and should be trained to recognize early signs of dehydration or when sufferers appear markedly ill or not responding to treatment (Caleb K. King et al 2003).

Immunity

The immune response to a microbe is complex and not well understood. Some people are resistant to the virus however the factors responsible for the resistance or susceptibility to Norovirus have not been identified (Hutson AM et al, 2002). There is evidence for some short term immunity lasting days or weeks however this immunity is partial and reinfection can occur (Parrino TA et al, 1977). Frequent exposure may stimulate a sustained immunity and genetic traits are likely to play an important role (Ewald d et al, 2000). A human challenge model described that a portion of those persons of the susceptible population who encoded a functional FUT2 gene were resistant to infection indicating a memory immune response (Lindesmith L et al, 2003) There is some evidence that blood types B and AB confer partial protection against asymptomatic infection (Miyoshi M et al., 2005; Rockx BH, 2005).

Transmission

Faeco-oral route is probably the main mode of transmission of Norovirus either by the consumption of faecally contaminated food or water or by direct person to person spread (Goodgame,R et al, 2006). Environmental and fomites contamination have also been implicated as a source of infection. Transmission may also occur through aerosolisation of vomitus that presumably results in droplets contaminating surfaces or entering the oral mucosa and swallowed (Marks PJ et al, 2000). There is no evidence of infection occurring through the respiratory system. However several modes of transmission have been documented even for the same outbreak leading to protracted course of infection. For example initial food borne transmission in a restaurant followed by secondary person to person transmission to household contacts. A review of 232 outbreaks reported to the CDC from July 1997 to June 2000, 57% were food borne, 16% were due to person to person spread, and 3% were waterborne, in 23% of the outbreaks, the cause was not determined (Norwalk like viruses CDC report, 2001). Of 1,877 outbreaks in England and Wales in the period 1992-2000, 85% were due to person to person; 5% were food borne; waterborne in one outbreak and unknown in 5% of the outbreaks (Lopman BA et al, 2003).

Food Borne Transmission

Unlike bacteria, viruses cannot "grow" in food. Food is usually contaminated with virus either from a virus infected person who prepares the food (Caceres VM et al, 1998; Bresee JS, 2002; Parshar UD, 1998) or from sewage (Myrmel M, 2006) or contaminated water (Klein G, 2004; Sartorius B, 2004, 2007). No specific food products were associated with Norovirus in a case control study on cases of Norovirus (de Wit MAS et al, 2003). This finding is not remarkable since the virus can survive on almost all food products that are not cooked before consumption and a low dose is required. Most published food borne outbreaks could be traced back to infected foodhandlers at some point in the production chain, suggesting that this is the commonest source of food borne infections. (Frankhauser RL et al, 1998; Daniels NA et al, 2000; Patterson W et al, 1997; Gaulin C et al, 1999). The most common foodstuffs involved in outbreaks are: shellfish such as oysters (Webby RJ, 2007; Le Guyader FS, 2006; Doyle A et al, 2002), mussels and clams; fresh or frozen berries (Hjertqvist M, 2006; Falkenhorst G, 2005; Korsager B, 2005); and vegetables presumably watered with contaminated water; contaminated water (Gallay A, 2006; Pusch D et al, 2005; Brugha R et al, 1999) or ice cubes (Pedalino B, 2003). Shellfish become contaminated when their waters become contaminated from sources such as raw sewage dumped overboard by recreational and/or commercial boats. Shellfish are filter feeders and will concentrate virus particles present in their environment and hence they have been linked to a number of outbreaks.

Food was found to be a source of transmission in a household setting as well apart from direct person to person transmission (Goldman DA, 2000). The impact of food handling hygiene in this setting can be explained by food contamination by a sick household member who prepares meals. However food contamination at an earlier step in the food chain may also be the source. A study estimated that 12-16% of Norovirus gastroenteritis in the households are caused by the introduction of contaminated food or water (de Wit M et al, 2003).

Person to Person Transmission

Frequently, during an outbreak, primary cases result from exposure to a faecally contaminated vehicle (e.g., food or water), whereas secondary and tertiary cases among contacts of primary cases result from person-to-person transmission (Becker et al., 2000; Frankhauser RL, 1998).

During a 1994 study of 50 volunteers exposed to Norovirus, 82% became infected; of these infections, 68% resulted in illness, whereas the remaining 32% were asymptomatic (Graham et al., 1994). Viral shedding in stool began 15 hours after virus administration and peaked 25 to 72 hours after virus administration. Unexpectedly, viral antigen could be detected by ELISA in stool specimens collected 7 days after inoculation in both symptomatic and asymptomatic persons. In a later study of infected volunteers, viral antigen in stool was detected ≤2 weeks after administration of virus (Okhuysen et al., 1995). New, more sensitive molecular assays demonstrated that many infected persons have virus in their stools for several weeks after the resolution of symptoms (Atmar and Estes, 2006; Patterson T et al, 1993; White KE, 1986; Murata T, 2007). During an investigation of a hospital outbreak of Norovirus gastroenteritis, faecal specimens collected tested positive in 26% and 33% from asymptomatic staff and patients respectively. (Gallimore CI et al, 2004).

Environmental Transmission

The potential role of widespread fomite contamination in outbreaks in confined spaces has been described (Jones EL et al, 2007). Norovirus has been demonstarted to survive on environmental surfaces for a long duration increasing the risk of transmission. Both faecal contamination and vomit can contaminate surfaces and delivery of the infectious dose which is very small (up to 100 particles (Atmar and Estes, 2006)) can start off the chain of infection. Large outbreaks occur when viral particles spread in the environment where persons are in close contact. The environment becomes a pathway for infection where Norovirus is introduced; persons, surfaces and objects become contaminated; delivery of an infectious dose to a person leads to infection and consequent symptoms. A number of factors are required for disease transmission and a break in the chain can prevent transmission. These factors are useful to be able to target preventive and control measures (Environ Health Associates, Technical report) . These factors are:

1. *Norovirus infected person present in facility:*The only known reservoir for the virus is the human gastrointestinal tract. It is difficult to ascertain a person who is such a reservoir since the person may not recognise he has such an infection or the person may be asymptomatic.
2. *Virus infected person vomits or defecates at the facility:*Contamination usually occurs when a person defecates or vomits and hence the potential for an asymptomatic person to contaminate the environment is small. During peaks of viral shedding, it is estimated to have up to a billion viral particles per each gram of faeces hence this coupled with the low infectivity dose increase the potential for infection.

Children would be difficult to control and if the symptoms are sudden, it may be difficult to reach appropriate areas in time.

3. *Surfaces exposed to faeces or vomit containing virus:*The environment can become soiled when a person vomits or defecates. If the place has continuous movement, secondary spread can occur to other areas increasing the possibility of spread of infected surfaces and hence the possible exposures. Hands can become infected either by direct contamination or by contamination from the surfaces allowing further dissemination. All types of surfaces can become contaminated including floors, decks, walls, toilet areas and structures. Soft surfaces such as carpeting, rugs, bedding, curtains, furniture, and other objects. Since there is a high release and a minimal amount of contamination is required to cause illness, this route is considered as a major contributing factor to outbreaks.

4. *Virus survives in environment:*The virus has a non enveloped morphology hence it is very difficult to destroy. All objects which are exposed to vomit or faeces are considered as potential sources of infection. Low levels of contamination can persist at levels sufficient to cause disease transmission and infectivity can be maintained for an extended period hence creating a temporary reservoir of contamination in the environment.

5. *Non infected person comes in contact with viable virus:*Movement of persons in areas where contamination is likely to have occurred will result in contact of persons with the virus. Persons who clean up the contaminated areas can also be exposed due to direct contact or aerosolisation or viral matter.

6. *Virus ingested and reaches the alimentary tract:*The portal of entry of the virus is the alimentary tract and the virus must be ingested to produce disease. The infective dose is small so minute quantities of the virus would be enough to cause disease. The person may be exposed through touching the mouth, cigarettes or other objects placed in the mouth. Food and beverage are another source whereby the person comes in contact with the virus.

7. *Norovirus infection occurs in susceptible person :*Susceptibility to the virus is universal. Persons of any gender and age can develop symptoms or become asymptomatic carriers. Since no permanent immunity has been demonstrated, vaccines are not available. The development of such vaccines is hindered by the fact that there are numerous strains of Norovirus with different antigenic properties. Persons at higher risk include children, the elderly and immunocompromised persons.

Once a person is infected, vomiting and defecation occur whereby the cycle of transmission is completed.

Characteristics of Rapid Spread

Characteristics of Norovirus facilitate their spread during epidemics:

- The low infectious dose of less than 100 particles (Kapikian AZ et al, 1996) readily allows spread by droplets, fomites and person to person transmission and environmental transmission.
- Prolonged duration of shedding which can occur in asymptomatic persons increases the risk for secondary spread especially in the food handler setting
- The ability of the virus to survive high levels of chlorine (Keswick BH et al, 1885) and varying temperatures (Kapikian AZ et al, 1996) facilitates spread.
- The diversity of the Norovirus strains, lack of complete cross protection and lack of long term immunity cause repeated infection in life (Parrino TA et al, 1977).

Burden of Illness

Noroviruses are currently recognized as the cause of almost all (96%) outbreaks of non-bacterial gastroenteritis (Mead et al., 1999). All age groups are susceptible to Norvirus disease (Thornton AC et al 2004). and there are no known gender or race differences in susceptibility. Noroviral voluntary laboratory surveillance in Sweden (Martin S et al 2004) over 31 weeks in the winter season 2003-2004 typically revealed two age bands in which such illnesses were more common: those under 5 years and those over 70 years old.

In the younger age group gender distribution was equal whereas in the elderly group more females were affected reflecting the age and gender differences in the Swedish population though some reporting bias may be present in general here. In the other age groups there were almost equal representation between the genders (Figure 2).

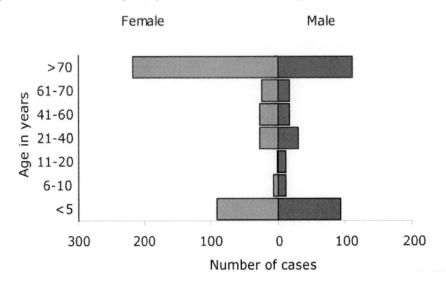

Figure 2. Laboratory confirmed cases of Norovirus by age and sex in Sweden 2003-2004.

However similar laboratory surveillance in England and Wales on the years 1995-October 2002 has shown that the rate of reported Norovirus positive reports showed a tremendous increase in the summer of 2002 over the previous years and that the increase was in those aged 65 years and over. This is thought to be because of a real rise in hospital and health care facilities of Norovirus incidents (Lopman Ben A et al., 2000).

Norovirus deaths are uncommon and relatively rare. Older and frail subjects and those possibly suffering from concomittant diseases raise the susceptibility of these patients to more severe disease and to possible mortality outcome. Noroviruses have been associated with chronic diarrhoea among transplant patients (Kaufman SS et al., 2003).

In the United States of America it is estimated that about 300 people (MMWR CDC 2002) die each year, a small figure when compared to the estimated number of 23 million cases (Mead PS 1999; MMWR CDC 2002) of noroviral infections in the USA per year.

Routine surveillance of Norovirus outbreaks using standardised epidemiological data in England and Wales (Benjamin A. Lopman et al 2003) for the period 1992 to 2000 (1,877 confirmed Norovirus outbreaks affecting a total of 57,060 people) estimated that the rate of hopitalizations in non-hospital outbreaks was 33/10,000 cases (in 52 outbreaks the mean hospitalizations per outbreak was 0.19; range 0-38,). The case fatality rate in 38 hospital and residential-care facilities outbreaks was 7.5/10,000 cases (mean deaths per outbreak 0.07; range 0-2; in which 24 deaths occurred in hospital outbreaks and 19 deaths occurred in residential–care facilities). The conclusion here cannot be missed that deaths are more common in hospital and residential homes outbreaks probably as a consequnce of the fragile nature of patients and residents respectively.

Malta has no specific surveillance system for viral gastroenteritis and laboratory diagnosis is only carried out in a few cases whereby samples are sent abroad. Therefore the knowledge on the impact of Norovirus is limited. A number of identified outbreaks in 2006 attacked closed centres including hotels, hospitals, old peoples' homes and refugee centres (Figure 3).

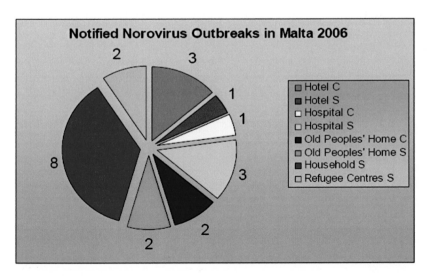

Figure 3. Settings of notified outbreaks in Malta during 2006 (including clinically suspected outbreaks (S) and laboratory confirmed outbreaks (C).

An age stratified random sample of the community in Malta identified Norovirus as being the commonest aetiological agent for the cause of IID in the community (20%, n=6/30) (Gauci C et al, 2007).

Seasonality

Norovirus outbreaks in England and Wales for the period 1992-2000 began to increase in September and peaked in the months of January, February and March. Outbreaks in hospitals and residential facilities occur more commonly in the 6 months from November to April than the rest of the year (994/421 ratio 2.36). Outbreaks in other settings display no winter peak (189/205; ratio 0.92). This difference in the seasonality is significant (p<0.0001). (Lopman BA et al, 2003). However other seasonal peaks have been noted by epidemiological surveillance in Europe. The European Food borne Viruses Network has systematically confirmed the unprecedented spring and summer peaks of noroviral disease in the year 2002 (Lopman BA et al 2004; Leuenberger S et al 2007) followed by winter peaks in the winter of 2002//2003. These peaks were mostly recorded in health care settings. These occurred in several European countries participants of the network. These peaks were caused by a new strain of Norovirus GGII4 which is thought to be more virulent and more stable than previous strains (Leuenberger S et al 2007).

Outbreaks of Norovirus

Outbreaks of Norovirus occur in multiple settings. A review of 348 outbreaks reported to the CDC during January 1996 to November 2000, a total of 39% occurred in restaurants, 29% occurred in nursing homes and hospitals; 12% in schools and day care centers; 10% in vacation settings in including cruise ships and 9% in other settings (Norwalk like viruses CDC report, 2001). Between July 2000 and June 2004, 184 outbreaks of Norovirus were reported to CDC. Of these, nursing homes, retirement centres and hospitals were the most frequent reported settings and person to person contact was the most common mode of transmission followed by food borne spread (Blanton LH, et al., 2006) Of 1,877 outbreaks in England and Wales in the period 1992-2000, 40% occurred in hospitals and 39% in residential care facilities (Lopman BA et al, 2003).

Restaurants and Catered Events

Contaminated food served at restaurants and during events is a common source of outbreaks of Norovirus. A study in the US determined that 41% of 295 outbreaks reported in Minnesota during 1981-1998 met the epidemiological criteria for Norovirus (Deneen VC et al, 2000). Norovirus was detected in 70% of the 23 food borne outbreaks investigated during 1996-1998.

Nursing Homes, Residential Institutions and Hospitals

The importance of Norovirus as a cause of gastroenteritis outbreaks in nursing homes and hospitals has been highlighted (Green et al, 2002; Reuter G et al., 2003; Marx A et al, 1999; Jiang X et al, 1996; Leuenberger L et al, 2007). Norovirus outbreaks occurred in 236 health care facilities for the elderly in Japan during the winter of 2004-2005. These outbreaks were deemed to have been caused by genetically close conventional Norovirus GII-4 strains (Okada M et al, 2006). In some of the outbreaks occurring in institutional settings, the outbreak was caused by a common source exposure initially, e.g. a food or water vehicle. Later spread occurs from person to person which is facilitated by the enclosed living quarters and reduced levels of personal hygiene that result from incontinence, immobility or reduced mental alertness. The impact of a Norovirus outbreak in institutions is high since the affected persons are persons with underlying conditions, elderly or immunocompromised individuals hence the disease is severe or even fatal.

Cruise Ships

Cruise ships were found to be the third most common settings (16%) of Norovirus outbreaks in US, during 1996 to 2004 (Goodgame, 2006). Passengers and crew members on cruise ships and naval vessels are frequently affected by outbreaks of gastroenteritis (Fankhauser RL, et al, 1998; Koo D et al, 1993; McCarthy M et al, 2000, Elmira T et al, 2005; Koopmans M et al, 2006) After a passenger or crew member brings the virus on board, the close living quarters on ships amplify opportunities for person to person transmission. The arrival of new and susceptible passengers every week on the affected ship provides an opportunity for sustained transmission during successive cruises. Outbreaks of gastroenteritis on board of cruise ships is similar to other closed and crowded settings where identifying and interrupting multiple modes of transmission has proved particularly challenging (Green KY et al, 2002; Sharp TW et al, 1995; Kuusi M et al, 2002; Cheesbrough JS et al, 2000).

Hotel Outbreak in Malta

A protracted outbreak of Norovirus occurred in a hotel in Malta between March and October 2006 with four identified outbreaks affecting a total of 337 persons. The recurrent waves of infection in successive cohorts of tourists indicated a source of environmental contamination. Traditional cleaning agents were not sufficient to eliminate the source of infection. The outbreaks were only successfully curtailed with isolation of ill patients; environmental cleaning with appropriate agents; specific prevention strategies including the early identification of patients; contact precautions with patients; enhanced patient and staff hygiene and training and discipline during food preparation and serving.

Methods

The outbreak occurred in a medium sized four star hotel with 116 room availability. This hotel frequently caters for elderly people especially in the off peak season. The outbreak which occurred in this hotel was protracted in the period between March and October with four identified outbreaks. The disease affected mostly people who were on holiday and were staying in the hotel for an average of seven days or more, whereas only few hotel staff members had been affected. Each individual outbreak was propagative in nature with a short incubation period and short symptomatic period for most of the cases.

The Disease Surveillance Unit, which is the national centre for the surveillance and control of communicable diseases, was informed of the outbreak on the 15 th. Of March. An outbreak control team was set up consisting of an epidemiologist, and environmental health inspector and a microbiologist. Inspections were carried out at the implicated hotel and a number of persons residing at the hotel and staff was interviewed in respect of any symptoms and possible exposure factors. A risk assessment of the hotel was carried out by the environmental health inspectors and food samples and environmental samples were taken. Minor deficiencies were noted and they were to be corrected soon after as soon as possible. The clinical picture and course indicated a norovirus aetiology.

A number of stools samples were taken and analysed for bacteriological analysis locally and for Norovirus at the Istituto Superiore Di Sanita (ISS) of Rome.

The hotel management were informed on Norovirus features including the possible causes and the epidemiology of Norovirus. They were also informed on measures to control the outbreak and preventive measures to be taken. Symptomatic foodhandlers were excluded from work with immediate effect up to 48 hrs after cessation of symptoms. They were instructed on hygienic measures to be taken upon their return to work bearing in mind prolonged excretion after symptoms stop.

Results

The first outbreak which occurred in March 2006, affected a total of 66 people; the second outbreak occurred in the beginning of May 2006, lasted 15 days with 105 people being affected, the third outbreak started in mid June and affected 64 persons and the last outbreak occurred in mid October and affected 102 persons. (Table 1)

The affected persons presented with symptoms of nausea, vomiting and diarrhoea and low grade fever. The incubation period was 12 -48 hrs. The duration of illness was variable but the majority of cases have settled down within 12-24hrs. However some of those affected have needed hospital admission because of their frail conditions or associated medical conditions. One fatality was recorded. The ages of the persons affected ranged from 55 to 91 years (median and mean ages not available since age distribution information was not available for all of the cases).

The first outbreak commenced on the 9 th March of 2006 and lasted a total of eight days. The total number of people affected with the illness was 66 with 63 of these being tourists and 3 being hotel staff (a bartender and two food handlers).

Table 1. Number of affected persons in each outbreak by gender and duration of outbreak

Month 2006	No. of People affected	F	M	Duration of Outbreak
March	64	32	32	8 days
April	105	n/a	n/a	15 days
June	87	40	47	23 days
October	102	56	46	13 days

There was no variation in the gender distribution. It was suspected that this outbreak originated from two patrons (a couple) who went ill one to two days before the initiation of the outbreak. It was reported that this couple had left a faecally spoiled bed sheet in the bath at their room on the 7 th. March however they had never requested medical assistance. Their room was cleaned by the housekeepers and it is not known what precautions they had taken during the cleaning procedure. The bed sheets were disposed of. Eight tourists were affected on the first day of the outbreak, with the staff members being affected in the second day. The general distribution of the outbreak was bimodal (Figure 4).

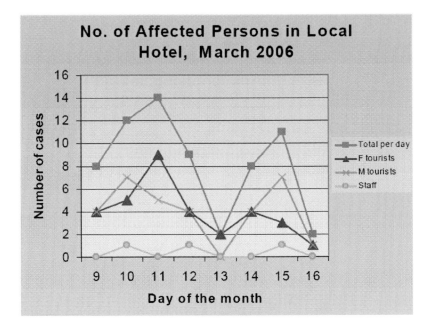

Figure 4. Epidemic curve of the outbreak occurring in March 2006.

The second outbreak started on the 31st of April, 2006. It is highly likely that this outbreak was most probably imported from the UK as the first ill patron became symptomatic 2.5 hrs after arriving at the hotel on the 30th April. He was symptomatic for four days before he called for medical attention. A number of other cases occurred six days within the onset of the first case.

Figure 5 shows the epidemic curve of the May outbreak with a single modal distribution. The nature of the curve gives credence to the above that there was a single source for the outbreak that then transmitted the infection to others. It should be noted that many affected patrons were either spouses or close acquaintances to each other indicating person to person transmission.

Though this outbreak was reported to be larger then the first very few ill patrons necessitated hospital admission, however 7 staff members were affected as follows: one male and one female from the restaurant food handling staff; one male and three females from the housekeeping services; and one male from the front desk. It is important to note that the male housekeeper's job is to count dirty linen and put them into batches for laundering and it is thought that this was the source of his contamination.

This outbreak lasted approximately 3 weeks and ceased by the 20th May. Most of the symptoms were mild to moderate and characteristic of Norovirus. Collection of stool samples from any of the cases for virological studies was unsuccessful.

The third outbreak started on the 13th June i.e. 24 days after the second outbreak, where 6 people fell ill with symptoms of nausea, vomiting, diarrhoea and low grade fever. The average symptomatic period was 24 to 48 hrs. Other characteristics of this outbreak included the propagative nature of the outbreak and the short incubation period which are typical of Norovirus infection. On the second day of the outbreak there were no new cases, however the third and fourth days show a peak of 14 cases on each day. Thereafter there was an average of 4.7 cases a day with a mode of 3 cases daily.

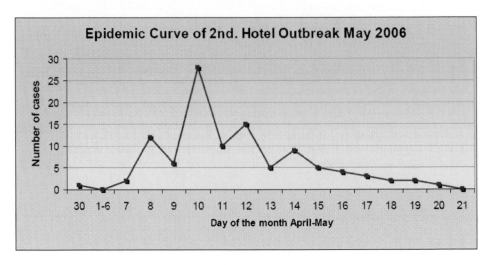

Figure 5. Epidemiological curve of the May outbreak.

The patrons who developed illness on the first day of the June outbreak had been in Malta for a mean of 7.7 days before falling ill indicating that the source of this outbreak was local, possibly within the hotel environment.

The epidemiological curve (Figure 6) of this outbreak shows a trimodal distribution with the peaks getting progressively smaller. A higher proportion of female patrons were affected with 36 females to 28 males; while the first peak consisted mainly of both gender groups, the second peak consisted predominantly of males.

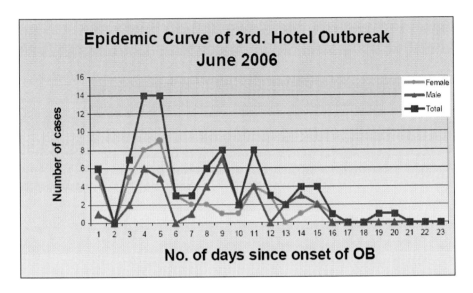

Figure 6. Epidemiological curve of the June outbreak.

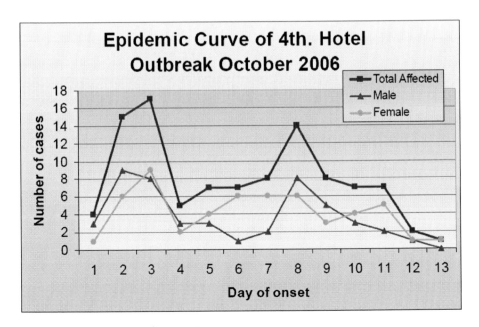

Figure 7. Epidemic curve of the 4th outbreak.

The majority of the afflicted patrons in this outbreaks as in the other outbreaks are either acquaintances or partners who were therefore holidaying together and lodging in the same rooms. Typically and almost invariably the second partner has developed symptoms some 24 -48 hrs after the first patron became ill indicating person to person transmission.

The fourth outbreak started on the 12[th]October of 2006. The clinical features of most of the cases were varying degrees of nausea, vomiting, diarrhea and low grade fever if at all. The symptomatic period lasted between 12 to 48 hrs (Figure 7). Only few become sufficiently ill to need hospitalisation, and this is usually because of the age of those affected and concomitant chronic conditions. Again the short incubation period of 12 to 48 hrs and the clinical features were highly suggestive of Noroviruses. There was no evidence that it was imported. Of the affected cases, one lady passed away as a complication of the disease after suffering from eosophageal rupture during vomiting.

Laboratory Investigations

Samples of food items were analysed bacteriologically in all outbreaks. High E.Coli counts were found in some environmental samples. A food sample (sour cream cucumbers from the hotel kitchen) tested positive for *Salmonella menden* in the last outbreak and action was appropriately taken. In each outbreak a number of stool samples were tested for Salmonella, Campylobacter and E.Coli and resulted negative.

First Outbreak
Seven stool samples were sent for Norovirus testing , 5 of which were positive (Grouping was not performed).

Second Outbreak
No stool samples were collected for virological testing.

Third Outbreak
Samples of swabs from door handle of refrigerator, toilet seat, water tap handle and other swabs were negative for norvirus.

Two stool samples were examined for Norovirus and one tested positive (Grouping was not performed).

Fourth Outbreak
Samples of swabs from hand swab of patient; toilet door hanlde; door handle of room; toilet door handle were negative for norvirus.

The significance of the negative results from the environmental testing is put in doubt because of possible bias including biases in the method of sampling and storage of samples.

General Recommendations and Actions Taken

The outbreaks were confirmed to be Norovirus gastro-enteritis since all of the Kaplan criteria (Turcios RM et al, 2006) were fulfilled as follows:

- Faeces culture negative for bacteria in one or more stool samples
- Vomiting in > 50% of the patients
- Average duration of illness 12-60 hrs
- Incubation period, if known, 15-77 hrs, usually 24-48 hrs

The seriousness of the outbreaks affecting this hotel included the number of persons affected of the outbreaks, the recurrence and propagative factor of the infections and the fact that they have occurred in the same hotel. The tourist industry effect cannot be underestimated. The characteristic of each outbreak had been the propagative manner by which outbreaks have developed in contrast to a point outbreak when there is a point source such as an implicated food item. Prolonged outbreaks of this type have been described in institutions including cruise ships, nursing homes, hospitals and hotels. Ascertainment of the epidemiological data is not complete since it is reliant on self report of the patients however the Disease Surveillance Unit was working in close collaboration with the hotel doctors who notified all the cases seen. Above this in the last outbreak, the hotel management offered medical services free of charge hence most persons would have sought medical help and hence were reported.

Certain factors could have contributed to the large number of guests affected relative to the size of the hotel. These include the rapid turnover of guests, high level of occupancy, the advanced age of the tourists and some degree of disability among the tourists.

The possible routes of transmission included person to person transmission via soiled materials including bed linen, direct contact or aerosolisation between successive cohorts of tourists, spread though hotel staff, spread through contaminated environmental surfaces and reintroduction of new viruses from incoming tourists, possibly even from other countries. These routes could have al played a role at some point in this protracted outbreak. Contaminated food could have played a role as well since some of the foodhandlers were affected however the role would be minimal since there was no indication of a point source outbreaks at any stage and foodhandlers were excluded immediately. Contact with contaminated fomites appears to have played a major role in this outbreak even though this was not confirmed microbiologically. Infection from fomites will directly cause a few cases however these cases will in turn pass on to others by person to person transmission resulting in a larger secondary wave of infection.

Throughout the outbreaks the department has been working in liaison with the hotel management and the hotel physician. Information regarding Norovirus, the illness it can cause and methods to deal with it and prevent it was exchanged with the hotel management.

Advice has been given to the hotel management and the hotel physician included:

- Affected individuals were to be isolated in their rooms until they were free from symptoms;
- Advice given on the importance of proper hand hygiene at all times and use of disposable towels for patrons and staff;
- Advice given on the use and nonuse of bactericidal products and general disinfection;
- Food at the buffet tables was to be served by the staff or else cutlery was to be replaced on very regular basis;
- Any possibility of excretory splashes was to be immediately treated by the hotel cleaning staff and using gloves;
- Persons cleaning areas heavily contaminated with vomitus or faeces were to wear gloves and surgical masks;
- Soiled linen and clothes were to be handled with care and as little as possible and with minimum agitation. They were to be put in plastic bags using gloves. They were to be laundered using hot water at maximum available cycle length and detergent and machine dried (the hotel management agreed to destroy any obviously contaminated linen);
- Affected patrons were not to use the swimming pool;
- Affected food handlers were to be excluded from work and kept on sick leave for 48 hrs following the cessation of symptoms.

The hotel management instituted a package of measures in order to interrupt the chain of infection. After the fourth outbreak the management were advised to close the hotel in order to ensure disinfection to eliminate any pathogens in the environment.

Prevention

Mitigation and control measures to limit the spread and hence the burden imposed upon humans by Norovirus are based on the knowledge of the pathogenesis and epidemiology of the agent. These include:

- Pathogenesis of Norovirus
- Virulence of virus
- Resistance to chlorine and phenol
- Infectious dose
- Stability in environment

The most critical situations for a Norovirus outbreak in a facility are:

- Presence of an infected person
- Poor personal hygiene
- Environmental surfaces and objects contaminated by faeces or vomitus
- Aerosolized Norovirus from vomit

- Ill or asymptomatic employee handling food with bare hands
- Contaminated raw food: shellfish, salads, berries
- Drinking contaminated water, ice
- Contaminated pools, spas
- Cross contamination of foods by infected consumers
- Inadequate cooking of shellfish

Person to person spread and spread via fomites can extend an outbreak however the initiating event is either a person who is symptomatic and is shedding viral particles or more commonly a common food vehicle. Hence in consideration of the mitigation and control efforts, both the initial contamination and the subsequent infection via person to person and via fomites will be required to control the spread of Norovirus.

Prevention and Control of Food Borne Transmission

Any food item can be contaminated with Norovirus, mainly through faecal or vomitus contamination.

Hazard Analysis Critical Control Point (HACCP) is a system to identify hazards and/or critical points and to produce a structured plan to control these situations. The seven HACCP principles can be applied to a food service facility in order to minimize the spread of any food borne illness including Norovirus and include:

(1) Hazard analysis
(2) Critical control point
(3) Critical limits
(4) Monitoring
(5) Corrective action
(6) Verification
(7) Record keeping

A number of outbreaks have been linked to contaminated oysters. Steaming does not kill the virus or prevent its transmission (Kirkland KB et al., 1996) hence one needs to cook them carefully. Other mitigation actions include measures to prevent the contamination of harvest waters with human waste including the surveillance of shoreline for potential sources of faecal contamination and restricting boaters from dumping waste overboard.

Another frequent cause of Norovirus outbreaks is food contamination by infectious food handlers. A small contamination is enough since the infectious dose is low and there is a very high concentration of the virus in the infected person. The most susceptible foods are those foods which are ready to eat requiring handling including salads and sandwiches. Many outbreaks demonstrate a general lack of education regarding Norovirus. This is essential in order to decrease the burden of food borne illness. It is recommended that ill foodhandlers are excluded from work for 48-72 hours however it is known that viral shedding occurs for longer duration after recovery. Despite the fact that the significance in terms of infectivity of this viral antigen shedding is not known, emphasis should be made on hygienic measures including safe food handling practices, strict hygienic measures in the kitchen and proper hand washing. Physicians who suspect a viral gastroenteritis in a food handler should advice on the above recommendations and notify the medical officer of health if food borne illness is suspected.

Water Borne Transmission

Waterborne outbreaks are less common than food borne outbreaks of Norovirus. Monitoring of waters for Norovirus is difficult and the virus usually survives in the chlorine concentration of drinking water. If drinking or recreational water is suspected, high level chlorination up to 10ppm or 10mg/L for more than 30 minutes and yet the efficacy of this method is doubtful.

Person to Person Transmission

Person to person transmission, either directly or via fomites, plays a major role in propagating Norovirus outbreaks especially in closed and semi-closed settings. Although interruption of the chain of infection may be difficult, all the possible measures need to be instituted in order to control the spread.

Hand Washing

Hand washing is the most important means of preventing the transmission of disease. There is strong evidence that the hands are important vehicles for spreading Norovirus since they can easily become contaminated with hundreds of viral particles. The problem is that conventional agents used to control bacterial pathogens such as alcohol based hand disinfectants do not appear to be efficacious in destroying Norovirus. Despite this failure to wash hands increases the biological load in the environment. The use of gloves and other barriers are less important to break the chain of infection. However gloves are required when cleaning up faeces or vomitus. Care must be taken since gloves do get contaminated as well so the risk of transferring the pathogen to other surfaces still exists.

Disinfection

Disinfection of the environment is required in order to stop the circulating pathogen. Initial cleaning of surfaces followed by disinfection must be carefully done to protect the environment. In the event that someone vomits or defecates onto the environmental surfaces, urgent cleaning and disinfection is essential. The areas should be cordoned off to avoid new persons being exposed. The persons carrying out the cleaning and disinfection should be using protective clothing including gloves and masks.

In order to be effective, a disinfectant against Norovirus must:

Provide a broad spectrum of proven activity: The disinfectant must have the necessary spectrum of activity to be effective against Norovirus (non-enveloped).

Demonstrate a reduction in viable organisms: For Viruses, a 4 log (or greater) reduction in titre is the recognized standard required.

Work in a broad temperature range: Generally speaking, the activity of disinfectants increases with temperature. The temperature range the disinfectants are tested in will assist in determining their efficacy for the required cleaning regimes.

Work in a variety of pH conditions: The performance of disinfectants can be affected considerably by pH, e.g. hypochlorite works best under acidic conditions while glutaraldehyde work best under alkaline conditions. Extraneous material present on environmental surfaces may affect the pH conditions in which the disinfectant will be expected to perform.

Work in the presence of organic material: The activity of most disinfectants is reduced in the presence of organic material due to inactivation, absorption or simply due to the presence of a physical barrier. Hypochlorite and formaldehyde are particularly susceptible to inactivation. Testing should indicate if the disinfectant has been tested in the presence of organic materials.

Be easy to mix in the proper concentration: Using the correct concentration is very important.

Work within a reasonable contact time: All disinfectants need time to work. A surface disinfectant will not work if it is rinsed off or dries out before the required contact time is up. If it is not realistic in practice then an alternative disinfectant with shorter contact time should be used.

Be safe to use: Information on health effects of the disinfectant must be available. For example, chlorine dioxide is a strong irritant; phenols are potentially toxic to various organ systems and therefore should only be used under strictly controlled conditions.

Meet all the disinfectant needs of the facility: Ideally, a disinfectant should be able to be used on all surfaces in all environmental areas.

There are no validated studies on the efficacy of disinfectants. It is yet known that a number of products are not effective including: phenolic compounds such as o-benzyl p-cholorophenol and o phenyl phenol; sodium hypochlorite; quaternary ammonia, peroxyacetic acid and iodine in use as per label recommendations. Sodium hypochlorite in concentrations of 500 to 10000 ppm are usually recommended for the decontamination of soiled and potentially contaminated surfaces, however such concentration can cause damage to wood, fabrics and carpets. Accelerated potassium peroxymonosulphate has been proven to be able to reduce Norovirus load by a 1/100,000 fold (Eleraky NZ, 2002). However independent lab tests on feline calcivirus are inconclusive. Table – shows a summary of the commonly used disinfectants against feline calcivirus (Guidance for the Management of Norovirus, Infection in Cruise Ships, HPA, 2007).

Table 2. Summary of commonly used disinfectants against feline calicivirus (as a surrogate for Norovirus)

Product Name	Manufacture	Main active Ingredient	Contact time	Log_{10} Reduction	Effects to health
Accelerated Hydrogen Peroxide™	Virox technologies	0.5% Hydrogen peroxide	5 mins	3.68 @1:16 dilution	Non-toxic
Sodium Hypochlorite	Generic	0.1% Sodium hypochlorite	1 min	>4.0	Irritant
Cryocide 20™	R.P. Adam	0.75% stabilized chlorine Dioxide and QUAT	30 mins	>4.0	Irritant
Mikro-Bac®III	Ecolab	5.32% 0-benzyl-p-chlorophenol 3.55% 0-phenlyphenol	10 mins	>4.0 @1:128 dilution	Corrosive, Harmful
Virkon®	Antec International	21.45% peroxomonosulphate	10 mins	>4.0	Non-toxic
Newgenn High Level Disinfectant	Newgenn Research Ltd	<5% QUAT, <0.5% buffers	1 min	3.3 @ 1:100 dilution	Non-toxic

(Taken from Guidance for the Management of Norovirus, Infection in Cruise Ships,Norovirus Working Group http://www.hpa.org.uk/publications/2007/cruiseliners/cruiseliners.pdf).

(This is not an exhausted list and there may be other brands on the market which are suitable for the purpose).

*Log_{10} reduction is taken fro either published research papers or from efficiency testing undertaken on behalf of the manufacturer.

Screening

Screening of persons in closed environments has been used to identify patients in the initial stage however the effect it may have on the longer term is doubtful.

Closure

In situations where an outbreak is extended by a periodic renewal of susceptible populations, including cruise ships, hotels, camps, the facility will need to be closed down for the premises to be sanitized appropriately. These measures are usually taken as a voluntary measure by the hotel management however in some instances it can be forced by order of the public health authority. An effective environmental mitigation programme should prevent most closures since the environment is the key reservoir of Norovirus.

Specific Settings

Health Care

Prolonged outbreaks of Norovirus occur in institutional setting; hospitals and nursing homes. An additional problem is that persons who are very ill with Norovirus infections often seek medical assistance and many are admitted to hospital.

Control is accomplished primarily by restricting the movements of both ill patients and caregivers in the facility and "universal" precautions. Prompt identification of outbreaks in health care settings is also necessary and infection control personnel should be alerted whenever there are two or more unexplained cases of gastroenteritis. Surveillance should be heightened to rapidly identify any additional cases.

As in any facility, strict measures must be followed when cleaning up vomit or feces. While this seems quite normal in nursing homes and hospitals with incontinent patients, there needs to be a heightened sense of precaution when dealing with outbreaks.

General measures for the control of outbreaks in hospitals and other health care facilities include:

- Isolate or cohort symptomatic individuals
- Emphasize the importance of hand washing and universal precautions
- Wash and dry hands before and after patient contact
- Wear gloves and aprons for contact with infected patients/environment
- Avoid transfer to unaffected floors or departments (unless medically urgent after consultation with infection control staff)
- Minimize movements of staff between affected and unaffected wards
- Exclude affected staff for 48 hours after symptoms cease
- Caution visitors about exposure and insure hand washing
- Exclude children from affected wards
- Advise relatives not to visit if ill
- Use an approved virucide to disinfect any contaminated environmental surface
- Thoroughly clean the ward before reopening to admissions (terminal cleaning is usually 72 hours after last symptom)
- Follow all infection control guidelines

Schools and Child Care Centers

Universal precautions need to be taken in schools especially in outbreaks of Norovirus. If food is delivered, the necessary precautions based on HACCP principles need to be taken. Strict hand washing requirements are necessary and bathrooms used by students must be maintained with the required hand washing essentials and children must be taught to use proper methods in their curriculum.

If the school experiences unexplained acute gastroenteritis in students or staff, surveillance for more cases should be implemented. If more cases develop then a more intensive effort must be made to insure a high degree of sanitation and hygiene, and outbreak protocols as described in this chapter initiated.

Child care centers are more likely to expose both children and workers to fecal contamination as diapered children and those in potty training are just learning about personal hygiene.

It is extremely important that diapering activities be done properly and that hand washing practices be strictly enforced for all workers who diaper children. Diaper waste must be bagged and stored in a covered container away from children and the diaper changing surfaces maintained in a clean and sanitizable condition. Diaper changing stations must be thoroughly cleaned and disinfected between diaper changes using an approved virucidal compound.

Potty chairs must be cleaned and disinfected between children and there must be a dedicated utility sink installed for cleaning potty chairs. Potties should never be cleaned in the sinks used for food and utensils, nor should hand washing be done there.

If an ill child presents at the center with symptoms of gastroenteritis it is best for that child to be sent home and segregated away from other children until the child can be removed.

A child should not return to school for at least 48 hours after the symptoms have subsided, whether or not a diagnosis has been made of Norovirus infection.

Hotels and Cruisers

Usually in a hotel situation or cruise liner a guest or someone else usually introduces the virus and it is passed on from person to person or from person to the environment leading to protracted outbreaks.

In order to control the outbreak the rooms that have accommodated ill guests/residents should be thoroughly cleaned using gloves and hands washed immediately upon entering the next room for service. All windows and doors should be opened. Contaminated bed coverings can be made safe by ordinary laundry processing. Mattresses should be thoroughly aired in bright sunlight. Soft furnishings should be placed in bright sunlight for a few hours. All mattresses and soft furnishings contaminated by vomit should be removed for steam cleaning or discarded. Housekeeping staff can conduct surveillance activities and report evidence of gastroenteritis in a room. Housekeepers must be trained in proper cleaning techniques using the precautions to protect themselves from contamination, and to avoid being vectors for spread or a victim, themselves.

Steam cleaning with temperatures over 60°C may be used for carpets and soft furnishings. Vacuum cleaning carpets and buffing floors during an outbreak have the potential to re-circulate Norovirus and are not recommended.

- The hotel administration should be encouraged create staff health policy
- Ensure that the staff health policy requires staff that is feeling unwell with vomiting, nausea and/or diarrhea do not enter the hotel but report in sick.
- Enquire about similar illness in the families and household contacts of staff.

- Staff sickness reporting logs should be kept recording similar information to the guests/residents sickness
- If staff is affected they should not return to work until 72 hours has elapsed since the last symptom. If ill staff live in the hotel they should remain confined to their quarters until 48hours after the last symptom.
- Controlling Norovirus with HACCP based infection control and environmental health

General Recommendations for the Preventing Infections from Norovirus

- Surveillance and reporting of illness
- Hand washing after using the toilet
- Hand washing before touching any food item
- Hand washing before eating
- Reduce, eliminate or minimize the bare hand contact of food
- Exclude or restrict ill workers from food handling
- Clean and disinfect all surfaces in repeated contact with human hands
- Clean and disinfect all surfaces and objects soiled by vomit or feces
- Educate ill persons concerning transmission
- Exclude or restrict all ill patients through cohorting, quarantine or removal
- Close off areas with excess contamination
- Protective barriers such as gloves and gowns used when cleaning
- Restriction of health care personnel in contact with infected persons
- Sanitary diaper changing and potty training in child care
- Cook all foods, especially shellfish to the temperatures in the food code
- Decontaminate and wash leafy vegetables and berries
- Thoroughly wash all vegetables and fruit before cutting
- Ensure potable water
- Ensure safe sewage disposal
- Protect self-service areas and self-service utensils

Conclusion

Norovirus is difficult to control due to the low infectious dose; the high excretion rate in individuals and the resistances of the virus to the traditionally used disinfectant agents at the normal concentrations. The best mitigation measures is to reduce the circulating load of virus being excreted and being deposited on to the environmental surfaces. To prevent or minimize future outbreaks in confined spaces, the adoption of practices such as surface disinfection and the utilization of methods to identify and exclude those with gastroenteritis may be effective.

The key to success for the prevention of infection and spread of Norovirus gastroenteritis is:

- a clean environment
- early detection of patients who may be symptomatic
- rapid intervention with appropriate precautions
- meticulous attention to hand washing, food discipline, and specialized cleaning
- training for all staff including housekeepers, laundry workers and food handlers
- strict food hygiene practices based on HACCP principles

It is very important that all involved move from being reactive to a proactive preventive approach in planning control and mitigation measures for Norovirus.

References

Ambert-Balay K, Bon F, Le Guyader F, Pothier P, Kohli E.Characterization of new recombinant Noroviruses. *J .Clin. Microbiol.* 2005 Oct;43(10):5179-86.

Ando T., Noel J.S., Fankhauser R.L., Genetic classification of "Norwalk-like viruses", *J. Infec.t Dis.* 2000; 181: 336-48.

Atmar,R.L. and Estes,M.K. The epidemiologic and clinical importance of Norovirus infection *Gastroenterol. Clin. North Am.* 2006, 35: 275-90, viii.

Becker,K.M., Moe,C.L., Southwick,K.L., and MacCormack,J.N. Transmission of Norwalk virus during football game. *N. Engl. J. Med.*, 2000, 343: 1223-1227.

Belliot G., Mitra T., Hammer C., Garfield M., Green K.Y., In vitro proteolytic processing of the MD145 Norovirus ORF1 nonstructural polyprotein yields stable precursors and products similar to those detected in calicivirus-infected cells, *J. Virol.* 2003; 77: 10957-10974.

Benjamin A. Lopman et al Two Eoidemiologic Patterns of Norovius Outbrekas: Surveillanjace in England and Wales, 1992-2000; *Emerg Infect Diseases*; Vol.9,No.1,January 2003. URL: http://www.cdc.gov/ncidod/EID/vol9no1/020175.htm.

Bertolotti-Ciarlet A., White L.J., Chen R., Prasad B.V., Estes M.K., Structural requirements for the assembly of Norwalk virus-like particles, *J. Virol.* 2002; 76: 4044-4055.

Billgren M. et al Epidemiology of Norwalk-like human caliciviruses in hospital outbreaks of acute gastroenteritis in the Stockholm area in 1996. *J. Infect.* 2002 Jan;44(1):26-32.

Black RE, Morris SS, Bryce J. Where and why are 10 million children dying every year? *Lancet* 2003;361:2226--34.

Blanton LH, Adams SM, Beard RS, Wei G, Bulens SN, Widdowson MA, Glass RI, Monroe SS. Molecular and epidemiologic trends of caliciviruses associated with outbreaks of acute gastroenteritis in the United States, 200-2004. *J. Infect. Dis.* 2006; 193(3): 413-21.

Bresee JS, Widdowson MA, Monroe SS, Glass RI. Food borne viral gastroenteritis: challenges and opportunities. *Clin. Infect. Dis.* 2002 Sep 15;35(6):748-53. Epub 2002 Aug 21.

Brugaha R, Vipojnd IB, Evans MR, Sandifer QD, Roberts RJ, Salmon RL, et al A community outbreak of food borne small round structured virus gastroenteritis caused by a contaminated water supply. *Epidemiol. Infect.* 1999; 122:145-54.

Caceres VM, Kim DK, Bresee JS, et al. A viral gastroenteritis outbreak associated with person-to person spread among hospital staff. *Infect. Cont. Hosp. Epidemiol.*, 1998; 19: 162-167.

Caleb K. King et al Managing Acute Gastroenteritis among Children, Oral Rehydration, Maintenance and Nutritional Therapy; CDC *MMWR*, November 21, 2003/ 52(RR16); 1-16. URL: http://www.cdc.gov/mmwr/preview/mmwrhtml/rr5216a1.htm#top

Caul EO. Small round structured viruses: airborne transmission and hospital control. *Lancet* 1994: 343: 1240-2.

CDC "Norovirus activity- United States, *MMWR*, 2002, 52(03):41-45; 2003.

CDC DOCUMENT, 2006 Norovirus question and answer URL: http://www.cdc.gov/ncidod/dvrd/revb/gastro/Norovirus-qa.htm accessed 27/7/2007.

CDC Document Norovirus in Healthcare Facilities Fact Sheet, 2006.

URL: http://www.cdc.gov/ncidod/dhqp/id_NorovirusFS.html accessed 27/7/2007.

CDC: Norovirus: Technical Fact Sheet; August 3rd. 2003; URL: http://www.cdc.gov/ncidod/dvrd/revb/gastro/Norovirus-factsheet.htm accessed 27/7/2007

Chakravarty, S., Hutson A.M., Estes M.K. and Venkataram Prasad B. V. Evolutionary Trace Residues in Noroviruses: Importance in Receptor Binding, Antigenicity, Virion Assembly, and Strain Diversity *J. of Vir.*, 2005, p. 554–568 Vol. 79, No. 1.

Cheesbrough JS, Green J, Gallimore CI, Wright PA, Brown DWG. Widespread environmental contamination with Norwalk-like viruses detected in a prolonged hotel outbreak of gastroenteritis. *Epidemiol. Infect*. 2000, 125: 93-98.

Chen R, Neill JD, Noel JS, Hutson AM, Glass RI, Estes MK, Prasad BV: Inter- and intragenus structural variations in caliciviruses and their functional implications. *J. Virol.* 2004, 78(12):6469-6479.

D'adamo P.J., Kelly G.S., Metabolic and immunologic consequences of ABH secretor and lewis subtype status, *Altern. Med. Rev.* 2001; 4: 390-405.

Daniels NA, Bergmire Sweat DA, Schwab KJ, Hendricks KA, Reddy S, Rowe SM et al . A food borne outbreak of gastroenteritis associated with Norwalk Like viruses: first molecular trace back to deli sandwiches contaminated during preparation. *J. Infect. Dis.* 2000;181:1467-70.

Dastjerdi A.M., Green J., Gallimore C.I., Brown D.W., Bridger J.C., The bovine Newbury agent-2 is genetically more closely related to human SRSVs than to animal caliciviruses, *Virology* 1999; 254: 1–5.

Doyle A, Barrataudi D, Gallay A, Thiolet JM, Le Guyager S, Kohli E, Vaillant V. Norovirus food borne outbreaks associated with the consumption of oysters from the Etang DE Thau, France, December 2002. *Euro Surveill* 2004; 9 (3):24-6.

de Bruin E, Duizer E, Vennema H, Koopmans MP. Diagnosis of Norovirus outbreaks by commercial ELISA or RT-PCR. *J. Virol. Methods*. 2006 Norovirus;137(2):259-64. Epub. 2006 Aug 9.

Dedman D et al Surveillance of small round structured virus (SRSV) infection in England and Wales, 1990–5. *Epidemiol. Infect.* 1998;121:139–49.

Deneen VC, Hunt JM, Paule CR et al. Impact of food borne calcivirus disease: the Minnesota experience. *J. Infect. Dis.* 2000; 181 (suppl 2): S281-3.

de Wit MS, Koopmans M, van Duyhoven Y. Risk factors for Norovirus, sappro-like virus, and Group A Rotavirus gastroenteritis. *Emerg. Infect. Dis.* 2003;9;12 : 1563-1570.

Dolin R., Blacklow N.R., DuPont H., Buscho R.F., Wyatt R.G., Kasel J.A., Hornick R., Chanock R.M., Biological properties of Norwalk agent of acute infectious nonbacterial gastroenteritis, *Proc. Soc. Exp. Biol. Med.* 1972; 140: 578-83.

Eleraky NZ. Virucidal efficacy of four new disinfectants. *Am. Anim. Hosp. Assoc.* 2002; 38:231-234 May/June 2002.

Environ Health Associates, Inc. *Technical Report 1: Norovirus Contamination and Control* http://www.safefoods.tv/9.html accessed on 13/7/07.

Estes, M. K., and M. E. Hardy. 1995. Norwalk virus and other enteric caliciviruses, p. 1009-1034. *In* M. Blaser, P. Smith, J. Ravdin, H. B. Greenberg, and R. Guerrant (ed.), *Infections of the gastrointestinal tract*. Raven Press, New York, N.Y.

Ewald D, Franks C, Thompkins S, Patel MS. Possible community immunity to small round structured virus gastroenteritis in rural aboriginal community. *Comm. Dis. Intell.* 2000; 24:48-50.

Falkenhorst G, Krusell L, Lisby M, Madsen SB, Bottiger B, Molbak K. Imported frozen raspberries cause a series of Norovirus outbreaks in Denmark, *Euro Surveill.* 2005 Sep 22;10(9):E050922.2.

Fankhauser R.L., Monroe S.S., Noel J.S., Ando T.A., Glass R.I., Epidemiologic and molecular trends of Norwalk-like viruses associated with outbreaks of gastroenteritis in the United States, *J. Inf. Dis.* 2002; 186: 1-7.

Frankhauser RL, Noel JS, Monroe S, Ando T, Glass RI. Molecular epidemiology of "Norwalk like viruses" in outbreaks of gastroenteritis in the United States. *J. Infect. Dis.* 1998;178:1571-8.

Françoise S. Le Guyader et al Detection of Multiple Noroviruses Associated with an International Outbreak Linked to Oyster Consumption, *Journal of Clinical Microbiology*, Norovirus. 2006, p. 3878-3882.

Gallay A, De Valk H, Cournot M, Ladeuil B, Hemery C, Castor C, Bon F, Mégraud F, Le Cann P, Desenclos JC; Outbreak Investigation Team A large multi-pathogen waterborne community outbreak linked to faecal contamination of a groundwater system, France, 2000 *Clin. Microbiol. Infect.* 2006 Jun;12(6):561-70.

Gallimore CI, Cubitt D, du Plessis N, Gray JJ. Asymptomatic and symptomatic excretion of Noroviruses during a hospital outbreak of gastroenteritis. *J. Clin. Micro* 2004; 42(5):2271-2274.

Gauci C, Gilles H, O'Brien S, Mamo J. Infectious intestinal disease: do we know it all? Maltese Medical Journal. Dec 2006: 18; 4: 7-12.

Gauci C. Surveillance of IID in Malta. *PhD Thesis*. 2006. University of Malta.

Gaulin C, Frigon M, Poirier D, Fournier C. Transmission of calcivirus by a food handler in the presymptomatic phase of illness. *Epidemiol. Infect.* 1999; 123:475-8.

Godoy P. et al, Norwalk virus-like food poisoning after eating oysters; Facultad de Nedicina, Universidad de Lleida, Spain; *Med. Clin. (Barc).* 2000 May:114(20);765-8.

Godoy P. et al Waterborne outbreak of gastroenteritis caused by Norovirus transmitted through drinking water; Servicios Territoriales del Dipartimento de Salud de Lleida, Lleida, Spain; *Rev. Clin. Esp.* 2006 Oct; 206(9):435-7.

Goldman DA. Introduction : the potential role of hand antisepsis and environmental disinfection in day care and the home. *Paediatr Infect Dis J* 2000; 19:S95-96.

Goller JL, Dimitriadis A, Tan A, Kelly H, Marshall JA. Long-term features of Norovirus gastroenteritis in the elderly. *J. Hosp. Infect.* 2004 Dec;58(4):286-91.

Goodgame,R. (2006) Norovirus gastroenteritis. *Curr. Gastroenterol. Rep.* 8: 401-408.

Graham,D.Y., Jiang,X., Tanaka,T., Opekun,A.R., Madore,H.P., and Estes,M.K. (1994) Norwalk virus infection of volunteers: new insights based on improved assays. *J. Infect. Dis.* 170: 34-43.

Green J., Gallimore C.I., Norcott J.P., Lewis D., Brown D.W., Broadly reactive reverse transcriptase polymerase chain reaction for the diagnosis of SRSV-associated gastroenteritis, *J. Med. Virol.* 1995; 47: 392-8.

Green KJ. Belliot G, Taylor JL, Valdesuso J, lew JF, Kapikian AZ et al. A predominant role for Norwalk like viruses as agents of epidemic gastroenteritis in Maryland nursing homes for the elderly. *J. Infect. Dis.* 2002; 185:133-46.

Green, K. Y., R. M. Chanock, and A. Z. Kapikian. 2001. Human caliciviruses, p. 841-874. *In* D. M. Knipe and P. M. Howley (ed.), *Fields virology*, vol. 1. Lippincott Williams and Wilkins, Philadephia.

Guidance for the Management of Norovirus, Infection in Cruise Ships, Norovirus Working Group http://www.hpa.org.uk/publications/2007/cruiseliners/cruiseliners.pdf.

Harrington P.R., Lindesmith L, Yount B., Moe C.S., Baric R.S., Binding of Norwalk virus-like particles to ABH histo-blood group antigens is blocked by antisera from infected human volunteers or experimentally infected mice, *J. Virol.* 2002; 76: 12335-12343.

Harrison, S. C. 1989. Common features in the design of small RNA viruses, p. 3-19. *In* M. B. A. Oldstone and A. Notkins (ed.), *Concepts in viral pathogenesis*, vol. 3. Springer-Verlag, New York, N.Y.

Hjertqvist M, Johansson A, Svensson N, Abom PE, Magnusson C, Olsson M, Hedlund KO, Andersson Y. Four outbreaks of Norovirus gastroenteritis after consuming raspberries, Sweden, June-August. *Euro Surveill.* 2006 Sep 7;11(9):E060907.1.

Hutson AM et al Norwalk virus infection and disease is associated with ABO histo-blood group type. *J. Infect. Dis.* 2002;185:1335-7.

Jiang X., Wang M., Wang K., Estes M.K., Sequence and genomic organization of Norwalk virus, *Virology* 1993; 195: 51–61.

Jiang, X., D. Y. Graham, K. N. Wang, and M. K. Estes. 1990. Norwalk virus genome cloning and characterization. *Science* 250:1580-1583.

Jiang X, Turf E, Hu J, et al. Outbreaks in elderly nursing homes and retirement facilities associated with human calciviruses. *J. Med. Virol.* 1996; 50:335-41.

Jones EL, Kramer A, Gaither M, Gerba CP. Role of fomite contamination during an outbreak of Norovirus on houseboats. *Int. J. Environ. Health Res.* 2007 Apr;17(2):123-31.

Kapikian A.Z., Wyatt R.G., Dolin R., Thornhill T.S., Kalica A.R., Chanock R.M., Visualization by immune electron microscopy of a 27-nm particle associated with acute infectious nonbacterial gastroenteritis, *J. Virol.* 1972; 10: 1075-81.

Kapikian AZ, Estes MK, Chanock RM. Norwalk group of viruses. In Fields BN, Knipe DM, Howley PM. *Fields Virology* 3rd edition Philadelphia PA. Lippincott- Raven 1996; 783-810.

Kaplan JE, Feldman R, Douglas SC, Lookabaugh C, Gary W. The frequency of a Norwalk-like pattern of illness in outbreaks of acute gastroenteritis. *Am. J. Pub. Health*. 1982; 72 (12): 1329-1332.

Kaplan JE et al Epidemiology of Norwalk gastroenteritis and the role of Norwalk virus in outbreaks of acute non-bacterial gastroenteritis. *Ann. Intern. Med*. 1982 Jun; 96(6 Pt 1):756-61.

Karst S.M., Wobus C.E., Lay M., Davidson J.,Virgin H.W., STAT1-dependent innate immunity to a Norwalk-like virus, *Science* 2003; 299:1575-1578.

Katayama K., Shirato-Horikoshi H., Kojima S., Kageyama T., Oka T., Hoshino F., Fukushi S., Shinohara M., Uchida K., Suzuki Y., Gojobori T., Takeda N., Phylogenetic analysis of the complete genome of 18 Norwalk-like Viruses, *Virology* 2002; 299: 225-239.

Kaufman et al Calicivirus enteritis in an intestinal transplant recipient. *Am. J. Transplant*. 2003;3:764-8.

Keswick BH, Satterwhite TK, Johnson PC et al. Inactivation of Norwalk virus in drinking water by chlorine. *Arch. Int. Medicine* 1997; 157:111-6.

Kirkland KB, Meriwether RA, Leiss JK, MacKenzie WR,. Steaming oysters does not prevent Norwalk-like gastroenteritis. *Pub. Health Rep.*, 1996; 111: 527-30.

Klein G. Spread of viruses through the food chain. *Dtsch Tierarztl Wochenschr*. 2004 Aug;111(8):312-4.

Kojima S, Kageyama T, Fukushi S, Hoshino FB, Shinohara M, Uchida K, Natori K, Takeda N, Katayama K. Genogroup-specific PCR primers for detection of Norwalk-like viruses. *J. Virol. Methods*. 2002 Feb;100(1-2):107-14.

Koopmans M, Harris J, Verhoef L, Depoortere E, Takkinen J, Coulombier D. European investigation into recent Norovirus outbreaks on cruise ships: update. *Euro Surveill* 2006; 11(7): E060706.5.

Korsager B, Hede S, Boggild H, Bottiger BE, Molbak K. Two outbreaks of Norovirus infections associated with the consumption of imported frozen raspberries, Denmark, May-June 2005. *Euro Surveill*. 2005 Jun 23;10(6):E050623.1.

Kosek M, Bern C, Guerrant RL. The global burden of diarrhoeal disease, as estimated from studies published between 1992 and 2000. *Bull. World Health Organ*. 2003;81:197--204.

Koo D, Maloney K, Tauxe R. Epidemiology od diarrhoeal disease outbreaks on cruise ships, 1986 though 1993. *JAMA* 1996; 275:545-7.

Kudaka J et al Symptoms of food borne diseases and gastroenteritis in Kyushu Japan. *Kansenshogaku Zasshi*. 2005 Norovirus;79(11):864-70.

Kuusi M, Nuorti JP, Maunula L, Minh NN, Ratia M, Karlsson J et al. A prolonged outbreak of Norwalk like calcivirus gastroenteritis in rehabilitation centre due to environmental contamination . *Epidemiol. Infect*. 2002; 129:133-8.

Le Guyader FS, Bon F, DeMedici D, Parnaudeau S, Bertone A, Crudeli S, Doyle A, Zidane M, Suffredini E, Kohli E, Maddalo F, Monini M, Gallay A, Pommepuy M, Pothier P, Ruggeri FM. Detection of multiple Noroviruses associated with an international gastroenteritis outbreak linked to oyster consumption. *J. Clin. Microbiol*. 2006 Norovirus;44(11):3878-82.

Duggan C, Nurko S. "Feeding the gut": the scientific basis for continued enteral nutrition during acute diarrhea. *J. Pediatr*. 1997;131: 801--8.

Le Pendu J., Histo-blood group antigen and human milk oligosaccharides, *Adv. Exp. Med. Biol.* 2004; 554: 135-143.

Leuenberger S, Widdowson MA, Feilchenfeldt J, Egger R, Streuli. Norovirus outbreak in a district general hospital –new strain identified. *Swiss Med. Wkly* 2007:137:57-61.

Laila Sekla et al, Foodborne gastroenteritis due to Norwalk virus in a Winnipeg hotel. *CMAJ*, Vol. 140, June 15, 1989.

Leueberger S et al Norovirus outbreak in a district general hospital – new strain identified; *Swiss Medical Weekly*, 2007;137:57-61.

Liu B.L., Viljoen G.J., Clarke I.N., Lambden P.R., Identification of further proteolytic cleavage sites in the Southampton calicivirus polyprotein by expression of the viral protease in *E. coli*, *J. Gen. Virol.* 1999; 80: 291-296.

Lindesmith L. Moe C, Marionnenu S, Ruvoen N, Jiang X, Lindblad L, Stewart P, Le Pendu J, Basic R. Human Susceptibility and resiotance to Norwalk virus infection. *Nat. Med.* 2003 May; 9(5): 548-53.

Lopman BA, Goutam KA, Reacher MH, Brown DWG. Two epidemiologic patterns of Norovirus outbreaks: surveillance in England and Wales, 1992-2000. *Emerg Infect. Dis.* .2003 Jan available at http://www.cdc.gov/ncidod/EID/vol9no1/020175.htm.

Lopman BA et al Clinical manifestation of Norovirus gastroenteritis in health care settings. *Clin. Infect. Dis.* 2004 Aug 1;39(3):318-24.

Lopman BA et al 200 A summertime peak of "winter vomiting disease": Surveillance of Noroviruses in England and Wlaes, 1995 to 2002: *BMC Public Health*:V.3;2003:13.

Lopman BA et al Viral gastroenteritis epidemic of 2002 associated with new Norovirus variant, *Eurosurveillance Weekly* 2004;8 (11); 040311.

Marks PJ et al. Evidence of airborne transmission of Norwalk-like virus in a hotel restaurant. *Epidemiol and Infect.* 2000. 124:481-87.

Martin S et al New Norovirus surveillance system in Sweden. *Eurosurv. Weekly* 2004;8 (39): 040923.

Marx A, Shay DK, Noel JS et al. Outbreak of acute gastroenteritis in a geriatric long term care facility: combined application of epidemiological and molecular diagnostic methods. *Infect. Cont. Hosp. Epidemiol.* 1999;20:306-11.

Mc Carthy M, Esthes MK, Hyams KC. Norwalk like virus infection in military forces: epidemic potential, sporadic disease and the future direction of prevention and control efforts. *J. Infect. Dis.* 2000; 181(suppl):S387-91.

Miyoshi M, Yoshizumi S, Sato C, Okui T, Ogawa H, Honma H. Relationship between ABO histo blood group type and an outbreak of Norovirus gastroenteritis among primary and junior high school students: results of gastroenteritis based questionnaire study. *Kansenshogaku Zasshi.* 2005 sept;79 (9):664-71.

Murata T, Katsushima N, Mizuta K, Muraki Y, Hongo S, Matsuzaki Y. Prolonged norvirus shedding in infants ≤ 6 months of age with gastroenteritis. *Paed Infect. Dis. J.*, 2007;26 (1) 46-49.

Mead PS, Slutsker L, Dietz V, McCaig LF, Bresee JS, Shapiro C et al. Food related illness and death in the United States. *Emerg. Infect. Dis.* 199;5;607-25.

Mounts AW, Holman RC, Clarke MJ, Bresee JS, Glass RI. Trends in hospitalisations associated with gastroenteritis among adults in the United States 1979-1995. *Epidemiol. Infect.* 1999;123:1-8.

Myrmel M, Berg EM, Grinde B, Rimstad E. Enteric viruses in inlet and outlet samples from sewage treatment plants. *J. Water Health.* 2006 Jun;4(2):197-209.

Nilsson M, Hedlund KO, Thorhagen M, Larson G, Johansen K, Ekspong A, Svensson L. Evolution of human calicivirus RNA in vivo: accumulation of mutations in the protruding P2 domain of the capsid leads to structural changes and possibly a new phenotype. *J. Virol.* 2003 Dec;77(24):13117-24.

Okada M, Tanaka T, Oseto M, Takeda N, Shinozaki K. Genetic analysis of Noroviruses associated with fatalities in healthcare facilities. *Arch. Virology* 2006;151(8):1635-1641.

Okhuysen,P.C., Jiang,X., Ye,L., Johnson,P.C., and Estes,M.K. (1995) Viral shedding and fecal IgA response after Norwalk virus infection. *J. Infect. Dis.* 171: 566-569.

Oliver S.L., Dastjerdi A.M., Wong S., El-Attar L., Gallimore C., Brown D.W.G., Green J., Bridger J.C., Molecular characterization of bovine enteric caliciviruses: a distinct third genogroup of Noroviruses (Norwalk-like viruses) unlikely to be of risk to human, *J. Virol.* 2003; 77: 2789-98.

Oliver S.L., Dastjerdi A.M., Wong S., El-Attar L., Gallimore C., Brown D.W.G., Green J., Bridger J.C., Molecular characterization of bovine enteric caliciviruses: a distinct third genogroup of Noroviruses (Norwalk-like viruses) unlikely to be of risk to human, *J. Virol.* 2003; 77: 2789-98.

O'Reilly CE, Bowen AB, Perez NE, Sarisky JP, Shepherd CA, Miller MD, Hubbard BC, Herring M, Buchanan SD, Fitzgerald CC, Hill V, Arrowood MJ, Xiao LX, Hoekstra RM, Mintz ED, Lynch MF; Outbreak Working Group. A waterborne outbreak of gastroenteritis with multiple etiologies among resort island visitors and residents: Ohio, 2004. *Clin. Infect. Dis.* 2007 Feb 15;44(4):506-12. Epub 2007 Jan 8.

Outbreak of Acute Gastroenteritis Associated with Norwalk-Like Viruses among British Military Personnel- Afghanistan, May 2002, *MMWR* Weekly, June 2002/51(22);477-479.

Outbreak of Acute Gastroenteritis Associated with Norwalk-Like Viruses Among British Military Personnel, Afghanistan, May 2002 CDC *MMWR*, June 7, 2002 / 51(22);477-479.URL: http://www.cdc.gov/mmwr/preview/mmwrhtml/mm5122a1.htm.

Papadopoulos VP et al A gastroenteritis outbreak due to Norovirus infection in Xanthi, Northern Greece: management and public health consequences. *J. Gastrointestin. Liver Dis.* 2006 Mar; 15(1):27:30.

Parrino TA, Schreiber DS, Trier JS, Kapikian AZ, Balcklow NR. Clinical immunity in acute gastroenteritis caused by Norwalk agent. *N. Eng. J. Med.* 1997; 297;86-9.

Parshar UD, Dow L, Frabkhauser RL, Humphrey CD, Millert J, Anado T, Williams KS et al. An outbreak of viral gastroenteritis associated with the consumption of sandwiches: implications for the control of transmission by foodhandlers. *Epidemiol. Infect.* 1998; 121: 615-21.

Parashar U, et al Global Illness and deaths caused by rotavirus disease in children. *Emerg. Infect. Dis.* 2003;9:565--72.

Patterson T, Hutchin P, Palmer S. Outbreak of SRSV gastroenteritis at an international conference traced to food handled by a post symptomatic caterer. *Epidemiol. Infect.* 1993, 111; 157-162.

Patterson W, Haswell P, Fryers PT, Green J. Outbreak of small round structured virus gastroenteritis arose after a kitchen assistant vomited. *Comm. Dis. Rep.* 1997;7: R101-3.

Pedalino B, Feely E, McKeown P, Foley B, Smyth B, Moren A. An outbreak of Norwalk-like viral gastroenteritis in holidaymakers traveling to Andorra, January-February 2002. *Euro Surveill.* 2003 Jan;8(1):1-8.

Prasad B.V., Hardy M.E., Dokland T., Bella J., Rossmann M.G., Estes M.K., X-ray crystallographic structure of the Norwalk virus capsid, *Science* 1999; 286: 287–290.

Prasad, B. V. V., M. E. Hardy, T. Dokland, J. Bella, M. G. Rossmann, and M. K. Estes. 1999. X-ray crystallographic structure of the Norwalk virus capsid. *Science* 286:287-290.

Pringle C.R., Virus taxonomy – San Diego 1998, *Arch Virol* 1998; 143: 1449-59.

Pusch D, Oh DY, Wolf S, Dumke R, Schroter-Bobsin U, Hohne M, Roske I, Schreier E. Detection of enteric viruses and bacterial indicators in German environmental waters. *Arch. Virol.* 2005 May;150(5):929-47.

Reuter G, Vennema H, Koopmans M, Szücs G.Epidemic spread of recombinant Noroviruses with four capsid types in Hungary *J. Clin. Virol.* 2006 Jan;35(1):84-8. Epub 2005 Oct 19.

Reuter G, Jiang X, Szucs G. Noroviruses are the most common pathogens causing nosocomial gastroenteritis outbreaks in Hungarian hospitals. *Orv. Hetil.* 2003 Aug 17; 144(33): 1611-6.

Rockx BH, Vennema H, Hoebe OJ, Duizer E, Koopmans MP. Association of histo-blood group santigens and susceptibility to Norovirus infection. *J. Infect. Dis.* 2005 May 1; 191(5): 749-54.

Rohayem J, Munch J, Rethwilm A. Evidence of recombination in the Norovirus capsid gene. *J. Virol.* 2005 Apr;79(8):4977-90.

Sandhu BK; European Society of Paediatric Gastroenterology, Hepatology, and Nutrition Working Group on Acute Diarrhoea. Rationale for early feeding in childhood gastroenteritis. *J. Pediatr. Gastroenterol. Nutr.* 2001;33(Suppl 2):S13--6.

Sartorius B, Andersson Y, Velicko I, De Jong B, Lofdahl M, Hedlund KO, Allestam G, Wangsell C, Bergstedt O, Horal P, Ulleryd P, Soderstrom A. Outbreak of Norovirus in Vastra Gotaland associated with recreational activities at two lakes during August 2004. *Scand. J. Infect Dis.* 2007;39(4):323-31.

Sharp TW, Hyans KC, Watts D, Trofa AF, Martin GJ, Kapikian AZ et al. Epidemiology of Norwalk virus during an outbreak of acute gastroenteritis abroad a US aircraft carrier. *J. Med. Virol.* 1995;45:61-7.

Smiley J.R., Hoet A.E., Traven M., Tsunemitsu H., Saif L.J., Reverse transcription-PCR assays for detection of bovine enteric caliciviruses (BEC) and analysis of the genetic relationships among BEC and human caliciviruses, *J. Clin. Microbiol.* 2003; 41: 3089-99.

Tan M., Huang P., Meller J., Zhong W., Farkas T., Jiang X., Mutations within the P2 Domain of Norovirus Capsid Affect Binding to Human Histo-Blood Group Antigens: Evidence for a Binding Pocket, *J. Virol.* 2003; 77: 12562–12571.

Thornton AC et al Noroviruses: agents in outbreaks of acute gastroenteritis. *Disaster Manag Response*. 2004 Jan-Mar;2(1):4-9.

Thorven M., Grahn A., Hedlund K. O., Johansson H., Wahlfrid C., Larson G., Svensson L., A homozygous nonsense mutation (428G→A) in the human secretor (FUT2) gene provides resistance to symptomatic Norovirus (GGII) infections, *J. Virol.* 2005; 79: 15351-15355.

Turcios RM, Widdowson MA, Sulka AC, Mead PS, Glass RI. Revaluation of epidemiological criteria for identifying outbreaks of acute gastroenteritis due to Norovirus: United States, 1998-2000.

van der Poel WH, van der Heide R, Verschoor F, Gelderblom H, Vinje J, Koopmans MP. Epidemiology of Norwalk-like virus infections in cattle in The Netherlands. *Vet. Microbiol.* 2003 Apr 29;92(4):297-309.

van Der Poel WH, Vinje J, van Der Heide R, Herrera MI, Vivo A, Koopmans MP. Norwalk-like calicivirus genes in farm animals. *Emerg. Infect. Dis.* 2000 Jan-Feb;6(1):36-41.

Vinje J, Koopmans MP. Simultaneous detection and genotyping of "Norwalk-like viruses" by oligonucleotide array in a reverse line blot hybridization format. *J. Clin. Microbiol.* 2000 Jul;38(7):2595-601.

Vinjé J., Green J., Lewis D.C., Gallimore C.I., Brown D.W., Koopmans M.P., Genetic polymorphism across regions of the three open reading frames of "Norwalk-like viruses", *Arch. Virol.* 2000; 145: 223-41.

Vinjé J., Koopmans M.P., Simultaneous detection and genotyping of ''Norwalk-like viruses'' by oligonucleotide array in a reverse line blot hybridization format, *J. Clin. Microbiol.* 2000; 38: 2595–601.

Waters A, Coughlan S, Hall WW. Characterisation of a Norovirus recombination event in the Norovirus polymerase gene. *Virology*. 2007 Jun 20;363(1):11-4.

Webby RJ, Carville KS, Kirk MD, Greening G, Ratcliff RM, Crerar SK, Dempsey K, Sarna M, Stafford R, Patel M, Hall G. Internationally distributed frozen oyster meat causing multiple outbreaks of Norovirus infection in Australia. *Clin. Infect. Dis.* 2007 Apr 15;44(8):1026-31. Epub 2007 Mar 9.

White KE, Osterholm MT, Mariotti JA, Korlath JA, Lawrence DH, Ristinen TL, Greenberg HB. A food borne outbreak of Norwalk virus gastroenteritis. Evidence for post-recovery transmission. *Am. J. Epidemiol.* 1986 Jul;124(1):120-6.

Wolf-Dietrich et al. Leers Norwalk-like Gastroenteritis Epidemic in a Toronto Hospital, *Am. J. Public Health* 1987;77:291-295.

Zheng DP, Ando T, Fankhauser RL, Beard RS, Glass RI, Monroe SS. Norovirus classification and proposed strain nomenclature. *Virology*. 2006 Mar 15;346(2):312-23. Epub 2005 Dec 15.

In: Hygiene and Its Role in Health
Editors: P. L. Anderson and J. P. Lachan

ISBN 978-1-60456-195-1
© 2008 Nova Science Publishers, Inc.

Chapter 4

Risks Associated with Practices, Processes and Environment of Ready-to-Eat and Street-Vended Foods That Lead to Contamination by Common Foodborne Viruses

*Barro Nicolas[*1], M. C. Tahita[2], Traoré Oumar[3], L. Sangaré[4], De Souza Comlan[5] and Traoré Alfred Sababénédjo[6]*

[1, 6]Département de Biochimie-Microbiologie,
UFR-SVT-Université de Ouagadougou
[2]Institut de Recherche en Sciences de la Santé
[3]Institut de l'Environnement et Recherche Agricoles Ouagadougou
[4]Laboratoire de Bactério-Virologie CHU-YO, Ouagadougou
[5]Laboratoire d'analyse médicales et de contrôle de qualité des denrées alimentaires,
BP 1515 Université de Lomé, Togo

Abstract

Street-vended food raises concerns with respect to their potential for serious foodborne bacterial and viral illnesses. Food associated viruses such as gastroenteritis Human calicivirus (HuCV) Norovirus (NLV), Rotavirus (RV), Hepatitis A Virus (HAV), Poliovirus (PV) are responsible for a high number of infectious diseases in human. In addition to foodborne viruses via faecal contamination in the food chain, there are emerging zoonotic viral agents such as Avian Influenza Virus (AIV) H_5N_1 and Severe Acute Respiratory Syndrome Coronavirus: SARS-CoV. Food my be a vetor for this agent associated to raw foodstuffs in primary production level. Epidemiological data on

[*] Author for correspondance: BARRO Nicolas, PhD, Centre de Recherche en Sciences Biologiques, Alimentaires et Nutritionnelles (CRSBAN); Département de Biochimie-Microbiologie; UFR des Sciences de la Vie et de la Terre; Université de Ouagadougou. 03 B.P. 7021 Ouagadougou 03; Burkina Faso. Tel/Fax: (226) 50 33 73 73. e-mail: nicolas_barro@univ-ouaga.bf or barronicolas@yahoo.fr

foodborne viruses analysis shown that one of the most prominent emerging food safety problems stem from viruses because they are not well-known and classical food safety measures are not alsways efficient on them. International concepts such as *Food Safety Objectives* (FSO), *Hazards Analysis and Critical Control Points* (HACCP) and *Behavioral Risk Factors Surveillance System* (BRFS), used for risk assessment were applied to street food process, for indentification of factors playing an important role for contamination by viruses and bacteria during the food processing. These principles were allowed to well-know epidemiology of foodborne pathogens. Epidemiology of foodborne viral diseases is changing, and reemerging viral diseases take place through a complex interaction of social, economic, evolutionary, and ecological factors. They included changes in the pathogens; development, urbanization and new lifestyles; cuts in health systems; unknowledge on viruses, demographic changes, farming system, food handling behaviors, food processing system, environmental conditions, poverty and pollution. As recommends by the Advisory Committee on Microbial Safety of Food to use Kaplan criteria which can give strong circumstantial evidence that an outbreak is attribuable to pathogen agent; these criteria were took into account to give more accurate reflection of the involvement of viruses in incidence of foodborne diseases. Understanding the factors associated with safe street food handling will assist in development of effective safe-street-vended food instruction programs.

Keywords: *Ready-to-eat, street-vended foods, foodborne viruses, factors of viral hazards, risks analysis.*

Introduction

The importance of food safety considering foodborne pathogens bacteria and viruses are increasingly recognized as serious concerns by many public health authorities all over the world. Center of Disease Control (CDC) reports that 79% of outbreaks were due to improper holding temperature, poor hygiene of foodhandlers (Yang et *al.*, 1998). These descriptions were commonly observed with ready-to-eat foods (RTE) and more precisely street-vended foods (SVF) (Barro *et al.*, 2002a; 2002b; Mensah *et al.*, 2002). The World Health Organization (WHO) and Food and Agriculture Organization (FAO) define street foods as foods and beverages prepared and/or sold by vendors in streets and other public places for immediate consumption or at a later time without further processing or preparation (FAO, 1988). With a large proportion of urban dwellers relying heavily on street foods to obtain meals on a daily basis, the street food trade in many cities in developing countries, has grown considerably (Badrie *et al.*, 2005; Ohiokpehai, 2003; Mwangi *et al.*, 2002; Winarno and Allain, 1991). Serveral authors stipulated that ready-to-eat especially street-vended foods raise concerns with respect to their potential for serious foodborne bacterial and viral outbreaks (Bryan, 1978; 1988; Butt *et al.*, 2005; Collins, 1997; Estrada-Garcia *et al.*, 2002; 2004; King *et al.*, 2000; Leclerc *et al.*, 2002; Tjoa *et al.*, 1977; Umoh *et al.*, 1984; Vollaard *et al.*, 2004). This situation is due to the improper food handling practices based on unrespect of good practices as recommended in HACCP principles (Altekruse *et al.*, 1996; Angelillo *et al.*, 2000; Barro *et al.*, 2002b; 2006a; Bidawid *et al.*, 2000b; Canet and N'Diaye, 1996; Yang *et al.*, 2000). In developing countries, fewer cases of foodborne virus outbreaks were reported, because of lack of viruses diagnosis tools, resources for food safety management and food control services (Rutjes *et al.*, 2006; Theron and Cloete, 2002). There are a serious lack of informations and knowledges about viruses as potential dangerous pathogen agents in food industries and in particular street food enterprises (Barro *et al.*, 2007; Rzezutka and Cook, 2004). However, many food safety control efforts are focused on bacterial risks characterization and management. On the other hand, few data were reported on foodborne viruses the viral risks characterization and management. While, viruses are on structural and physiological plan, deeply different from bacteria. Then, methods used to control foodborne bacteria are not always efficient for foodborne viruses. In spite of underreporting increases in foodborne diseases caused by viruses in many parts of the world and the emergence of new or newly recognized foodborne pathogens have been reported (Koopmans and Duizier, 2002). Experts agree that the most common cause of foodborne diseases is microbiological in particular viral (CAC, 2001; Cliver, 1997; Koopmans *et al.*, 2002; 2003; 2004;). However, the situation is more crucial with the RTE and SV foods (Barro *et al.*, 2007; Bryan *et al.*, 1988), thus, increasing many opportunies for contamination (Bryan, 1988; Bryan et *al.*, 1992). The hygienic aspects of RTE and street-vended foods processing and vending operations are a major source of microbial contamination (Barro *et al.*, 2006a; 2007).

In these last years, CDC, Food and Drug Administration (FDA) FAO/WHO, ILSI have developed questions regarding food safety through foodhandling, prepartion, consumption behaviors and others factors acting for contamination (CAC, 2001; 2003; FAO/WHO, 1997; ILSI, 2004; Reij and van schothorst, 2000; Woteki *et al.*, 2001; Yang *et al.*, 1998) and FSO concept (Gorris, 2005). These will help to characterize risk levels for foodborne viral illnsesses and assist in developing food-safety education strategies for those purchase RTE street-vended foods, vendors, foodhandlers that intended to reduce disease.This review considers the use of epidemiological data and farm-to-fork approach, consumers and food handlers behaviors to support FSO, HACCP and risk analysis systems to determine high-risk foods and transmission routes of foodborne viral infections. Paper deal with characterization of the major factors of viral hazards that militating against the production of delivery of Safe Street-vended Foods from food small scale industries.

1. Epidemiological Aspects of Common and Possible Foodborne Viruses

Epidemiological and biological data on viruses show that numerous viruses can be involved in human illness but only a few are commonly recognised as important foodborne pathogens (Koopmans *et al.*, 2002; Koopmans and Duizier, 2002; WHO, 2006; Parashar *et al.*, 1998; Kohli *et al.*, 1999). These viruses transmitted by contaminated food, were classified into three main groups according to the types of illness produce: Viruses that cause gastroenteritis, enterically transmitted hepatitis viruses and viruses that replicate in human intestine but cause illness after they migrate to other organs, suh as the central nervous system or liver (Koopmans and Duizier, 2002). Hepatitis A (HAV) and E (HEV) viruses, Rotaviruses, Norwalk-like (NLV), Adenovirus (AdV, Poliovirus wild type (PV), and Human Astroviruses (HAstV) are among the enteric viruses well-known, responsible of the food and waterborne illness (Appleton, 2000; Berg et al., 2000; Koopmans et al., 2002; Koopmans and Duizier, 2004; Mast and Alter, 1993; Vidal et al., 2005; Nicand et al., 1998; Bishop et al., 1973). However, it seems logical to take into account in the classification of foodborne viruses according their mode of transmission via food chain. In this goal an additional group can be distinguished among the emerging viruses such as Avian Influenza Virus strain H_5N_1 and Severe Acute Respiratory Syndrome Coronavirus (SARS-CoV); Ebola Virus transmissible by raw foodstuffs during the first step of food chain (WHO, 2006). In accordance with these mode of transmission and infection two main groups can be distinguished: (i) the well-know foodborne Viruses which mecanisme of transmission is clearly established; (ii) the group constituted by those the epidemiological aspects of transmission to human through food is not well-know.

The viruses that cause gastroenteritis are spread through close contact with infected persons (by sharing food, water or eating utensils). Individuals may also become infected by eating or drinking contaminated foods or beverages (Nicand et al., 1998; Leclerc et al., 2002; Allwood et al., 2004; Kuzuya et al., 2003; Kapikian and Chanock, 1996). Water is the most common source of outbreaks and may include water from municipal supplies, wells and stored water. Shellfish and salad ingredients are the foods most often implicated in outbreaks (Gilles et al., 2003; Nicand et al., 1998; Leclerc et al., 2002; Allwood et al., 2004; Kuzuya et al., 2003; Butt et al., 2005; Rzezutka and Cook, 2004) Table 1).

1.1. Recognized Coomon Foodborne Viruses

Rotavirus is the most common cause of severe diarrhea among children, resulting in the hospitalization of approximately the death of over 600,000 children annually worldwide (Glass, 2006; Parashar et al., 2003). The disease is characterized by vomiting and watery diarrhea for 3 - 8 days, and fever and abdominal pain occur frequently (Bishop et al., 1973). Rotavirus infection is highly contagious. The primary mode of transmission is fecal-oral, although some have reported low titers of virus in respiratory tract secretions and other body fluids. The virus is stable (remains infective) in the environment, transmission can occur through ingestion of contaminated water or food and contact with contaminated surfaces. Rotavirus can survive for days on hard and dry surfaces, and it can live for hours on human hands (Koopmans and Duizier, 2004). In several countries with a temperate climate, the disease has a winter seasonal pattern, with annual epidemics occurring from November to April. The highest rates of illness occur among infants and young children by 2 years of age. Adults can also be infected, though disease tends to be mild (Parashar et al., 2003; Glass, 2006).

Coxsackieviruses are part of the enterovirus family of viruses (which also includes polioviruses and hepatitis A virus) that live in the human digestive tract. They can spread from person to person, usually on unwashed hands and surfaces contaminated by feces, where they can live for several days. Coxsackievirus can produce a wide variety of symptoms. About half of all kids infected with coxsackievirus have no symptoms. Others suddenly develop high fever, headache, and muscle aches, and some also develop a sore throat, abdominal discomfort, or nausea. A child with a coxsackievirus infection may simply feel hot but have no other symptoms. In most kids, the fever lasts about 3 days, then disappears (Gifford, 1951).

The hepatitis viruses (HVA and HVE) in paricular HVA can be spread by sick person; by eating food contaminated by food sick handlers, not washing their hands properly after using the bathroom. Fresh vegetables and fruits that are generally eaten raw or undercooked shellfish from contaminated water are repeatedly implicated to human viral infections (Berg et al., 2000; Croci et al., 2002). Drinking contaminated water (for example when traveling to underdeveloped areas abroad). Other foods frequently implicated in outbreaks are cold cuts, sandwiches, fruits, fruit juices, milk, milk products, wild boar meat, vegetables, salads, shellfish and iced drinks (Chancellor et al., 2006; Croci et al., 2002; Fiore, 2004; Li et al., 2005; Bidawid, 2000b).

Poliovirus is more common in infants and young children and occurs under conditions of poor hygiene. Poliovirus is spread by the "fecal-oral" route. The virus is excreted from sick person feces. In areas where raw sewage enters a watershed without treatment, poliovirus can be found in rivers, lakes, and streams. When a susceptible person drinks water or eats contaminated cooked foods, raw foods from one of these, the virus enters his digestive tract (Lee and Yap, 1999; Richards, 2001).

Coronaviruses are a cause of diarrhea in animals and have been seen by electron microscopy in human stools, but a causal link to gastroenteritis in humans has not been made. But World Health Organization fear for this virus genus is the recombination between animal strains in some animal species physiological close to human.

Noroviruses are members of a group of viruses called caliciviruses also known previously as "Norwalk-like viruses." Infection with norovirus affects the stomach and intestines, causing an illness called gastroenteritis, or "stomach flu." Noroviruses are found in the stool or vomit of infected people. People can become infected with the virus in several ways, including: eating food or drinking liquids that are contaminated with norovirus; touching surfaces or objects contaminated with norovirus, and then placing their hand in their mouth; having direct contact with another person who is infected and showing symptoms (for example, when caring for someone with illness, or sharing foods or eating utensils with someone who is ill) (Koopman and Duizier, 2004; Wihelmi et al., 2003; Scwartzbrod, 1992).

Food and drinks can very easily become contaminated with norovirus because the virus is so small and because it probably takes fewer than 100 norovirus particles to make a person sick. Food can be contaminated either by direct contact with contaminated hands or work surfaces that are contaminated with stool or vomit, or by tiny droplets from nearby vomit that can travel through air to land on food. Although the virus cannot multiply outside of human bodies, once on food or in water, it can cause illness (WHO, 2002b; Berg et al., 2000).

Some foods can be contaminated with norovirus before being delivered to a restaurant or store. Several outbreaks have been caused by the consumption of oysters harvested from contaminated waters. Other produce such as salads and frozen fruit may also be contaminated at source (Kohli et al., 1999; Klein, 2004; Koopman and Duizier, 2004; Gilles et al., 2003; Vidal et al., 2005).

Astroviruses cause gastroenteritis, predominantly diarrhoea, mainly in children under five years old although it has been reported in adults. Seroprevalence studies show that more than 80% of children between 5 and 10 years old have antibodies to astroviruses. Person to person spread by the faecal-oral route is thought to be the most common route of transmission. Recent work with sensitive assay techniques has shown the prevalence of this virus to be much higher than previously thought: it is endemic all over the world (Parashar *et al.*, 2003).

1.2. Unclearly Recognized as Foodborne Viruses

Avian influenza is on-going outbreak caused by of highly pathogenic strain H_5N_1 in poultry in Asia and, more recently, in Europe and Africa. It has raised concerns about multiple sources of infection and the risk to humans from various exposures. On present evidence, the vast majority of human cases have acquired their infections following direct contact with infected live or dead poultry. WHO is aware of concerns that the virus could also spread to humans through contact with contaminated poultry products such bloods and eggs (WHO, 2006). To date, no epidemiological data suggest that the disease can be transmitted to humans through properly cooked foods. However, in a few instances, cases have been linked to consumption of dishes made of raw contaminated poultry blood. Infection occurs through direct contact between the animals or vectors such as man, utensils, and transport devices such as packaging materials as egg trays. These epidemiological ways made RTE street-vended quicklyroasted chickens à risk product because at each step of processing manual handling operations are predominant, free range chicken slaughter and feather pluck off are done manualy (Barro *et al.*, 2002b; Mensah *et al.*, 1999).

The SARS-CoV global outbreak of 2003 was contained; however, it is possible that the disease could re-emerge. Contamination factors common in retail and food service environments inhibit the effectiveness of alcohol-based hand sanitizers when used in place of hand washing (WHO, 2006). While, considering definition of food chain and taking into account nature of street food enterprise and knowing the SARS-CoV mechanism of transmission, there are risks of contamination during animal slaughter and cut. Indeed, , during animals catch and kill, their body fluids containing virus (SARS-CoV), can contaminated butcher or cross contaminated food via hands or materials (WHO, 2006). It appeared that all the viral contamination take place through the faillure of good hygiene behaviors and good manufacture practices (Koopmans and Duizier, 2002).

1.3. Others Foodborne Viruses

Several other viruses indexed as emerging infectious pathogens were reported (Prashar *et al.*, 1998).

Aichi virus was recognized in 1989 as a cause of oyster associated gastroenteritis in Japan. By age 35, 80% of the surveyed Japanese populations had antibodies. Recently, it has been a cause gastroenteritis outbreak among children in Pakistan. Aichi virus is a species of Kobuvirus, a new genus of Picornaviridae.

Calciviruses other than Noroviruses such as Sapovirus is another genus of the Calicivirus family that can cause gastroenteritis. It is sometimes referred to as classic or morphologically typical calicivirus. The prototype species of this genus is Sapporo virus, and members of the genus have also been referred to as Sapporo-like viruses. These viruses were first described in cases of pediatric diarrhea, but they can also cause disease in adults.

Echovirus 22 (Human Parechovirus 1): Human Parechovirus 1 causes infantile diarrhea and respiratory illness. Echovirus 22 has been placed in a new genus of Picornaviridae called Parechovirus. It has been renamed Human Parechovirus 1.

The Torovirus causes diarrhea in children of all ages. Stools have approximately an 11% chance of being bloody. Enveloped, single stranded positive sense RNA virus from Family Coronaviridae.

Table I. Epidemiological data on recognized foodborne viruses and other possible members

Family/Viruses	Infected organs	Geographic distribution	Hosts / reservoir
1 - Recognized FBV			
Picornavirideae			
Poliovirus	NS	Af, As	Human, mammalia
Hepatitis Virus A	Liver	Af, As, Am, Eu	human
Coxsackie-viruses	NS	Af, As, Am, Eu	human
Human Parechovirus 1	Intestine	Af?, As, Am	Human
Hepeviridae Hepevirus			
Hepatitis Virus E	Liver	Af, As, Am	human
Reovirideae			
Rotavirus	Intestine	Af, As, Am, Eu	Human, mammalia
Calicivirideae			
Norwalk virus	Intestine	Af, As, Am, Eu	Human, mammalia
Sapporo-like virus	Intestine	?	Human, mammalia
Astroviruses	Intestine	Af, As, Am, Eu	Human, mammalia
Adenovirus 40 and 41	Intestine	Af, As, Am, Eu	Human
2 - Unrecognized FBV			
Myxovirus			
Avian influenza virus	respiratory	Af, As, Am, Eu	Human, pigs, birds
Coronavirus			
SARS	respiratory	As	Human, felins
Torovirus	Intestine	?	Human, mammalia
Picornavirus			
Aichi virus	diarrhea	As, ?	Human, mammalia
Filovirus			
Ebolavirus	All organs	Af, Eu	Human, monkeys, bat
Picobirnavirus	diarrhea	?	Human, mammalia

FBV = Foodborne virus, Af= AFrica, As = Asia, Am = America, Eu = Europe.
NS = nervous system, ? = not clearly established.

Picobirnaviruses have been found in the stools of people and animals with and without diarrhea. The significance is unclear. Picobirnaviruses are members of Birnaviridae. They are nonenveloped, have icosahedral capsids and double-stranded RNA genomes that consist of two or three segments.

2. Factors Contributing to Contamination by Foodborne Viruses

The Risk Analysis framework, *Behavioral Risk Factors Surveillance System* (BRFS), *Safe Street vended Food Production* (SSFP) and HACCP principles (CAC, 2004; FAO/WHO, 1997; Reij and Van Schothorst, 2000; Woteki *et al.*, 2001; Barro *et al.*, 2007) were used to identiy the major risk factors of viral contamination. Viral risk analysis in RTE street-vended food industries were done taking into account existing data on the rudimentary aspects of RTE enterprises, lack of regulatory system, the lack of means for efficiently food safety control, unsanitary level of towns in developping countries and social factors (Barro *et al.*, 2002b; 2006c; Mensah *et al.*, 2002; Mosupye and van Holy, 2000).

2.1. Social Change Contributing to Viral Contamination

The urbanization of towns and the associated dietary lifestyles, social and structural changes have caused and increased demand for street foods (Canet and N'Diaye, 1996; Ohiokpehai, 2003; Mwangi *et al.*, 2002; Winarno and Allain, 1991). Dietary preferences and practices and some cultural beliefs and rituals can increase the risk of illness. Food consumption is changing as the result of a variety of factors. Dietary habits may be altered by nutritional recommendations and campaigns; higher living standards have led to greater consumption of animal products; environmental changes increase access to certain foods; habits may be influenced by food policy, production systems and urban lifestyles; and there is an increase in prepacked "convenience" foods, RTE, SV foods and meals consumed in food service establishments. In addition, changing social structures have resulted in a heavier emphasis on the purchase and consumption of food outside the family home. In the context of poverty, street food accounts for a part of the family income, daily diet and so contributes towards meeting nutritionnal requirements (Barro et al., 2002b; Chakravarty et Canet, 1996; van't Riet *et al.*, 2003; Winarno and Allain, 1999). Many traditional "food wisdom's" historically passed down from one generation to the next are being forgotten or becoming obsolete, but some sectors of the general population have been unable to replace that traditional knowledge with modern scientific understanding of food safety and nutrition. As more meals are consumed from street vendors, in restaurants, and other public places it can be difficult for individual consumers to determine if food in public places is safe to eat.

These contemporary ways of food consumption acte as impacting factor on food safety. It is agreed that today, consummers are "time poor" and time spent preparing food is not considered quality time. Consumers place increased emphasis on convenience and speed in preparing meals but, convenience foods need to be correctly stored and prepared in the home

(Cliver, 1997; Collins, 1997; Croci *et al.*, 2002; de Wit *et al.*, 2003). Consumption of raw or lightly cooked food of animal origin is very hazardous. Kurth (2000) reported that the two main issues that arose out were convenience and health. However, consumers could be a great of vendor's behavior change the must exige a right to basic good services which ensure quality of life: adequate food, clothing, shelter, health care, education and sanitation. Considering the number of daily consumers of street foods, the number of sick peoples will be important in case of consumption of contaminated foods. Thus, RTE and SV foods have consequence suh as their association to disease outbreaks (Gilles *et al.*, 2003; Wihelmi *et al.*, 2003; WHO, 2002b; Cheftel *et al.*, 1997).

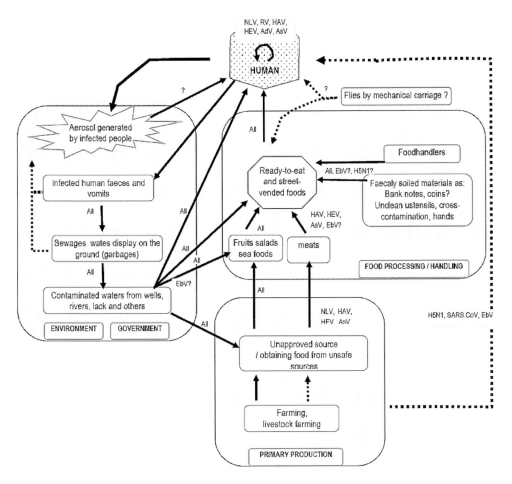

Figure 1. Some common and possible foodborne viruses transmission to human pathways. Continuous lines indicated showing proven modes, dotted lines indicated suggested modes. Norovirus (NLV), Rotavirus (RV), Hepatitis A and E virus (HAV, HEV), Adenovirus causing diarrhoea (AdV), Astrovirus (AsV), Polivirus (PoV), Coxsackie-virus (CxV); Sapporo-like virus (SLV). Influenza virus (H5N1), Severe Acute Respiratory Syndrome Coronavirus (SARS-CoV) Ebola Virus (EbV), All means all the viruses. All: means all the recognized foodborne viruses; ? : Investigations are not proven cleary.

2.2. Farming System and Use of Sick Animal

Most street-vended food products are either produced directly on farms or based on produce derived from agriculture (Barro *et al.*, 2002b). Good agricultural, livestock farming, handling and storage practices are the main determinants of the quality of raw farm-products. Foods may be contaminated by viruses in their growing and harvesting areas. Fruits, vegetables and molluscan shellfish have particularly implicated (Appleton, 2000; Bidawid *et al.*, 2000a; Klein, 2004; Koopman and Duizier, 2002; Theron and Cloete, 2002; Schwartzbrod, 1992; Ward and Irving, 1987). Contamination of fruits and vegetables occurs at every stage of the food chain, from cultivation to processing. Polluted environments during cultivation or poor hygienic conditions in processing increase the risk of contamination by foodborne viruses. Although fruits and vegetables may harbor microorganisms such as HAV, Rotaviruses, good control through ultra-violet irradiation can inactivate viruses and pathogenic microorganisms (Nguyen-the and Carlin, 1994; Steele and Odumeru, 2004).

Animal may carry microorganisms which can cause disease in humans without any evidence of their existence during the animal's life cycle or even after its slaughter. Thus, a special warning must be observed by foodhandlers or butchers during utilization of killed animal, to avoid direct contact with animals fluids or stools. Considering, a influenza virus, previously found only in birds and poultry, crossed the species barrier, infecting some residents of Hong Kong with 'chicken flu' which in some instances resulted in death (WHO, 2006). The key to success in handling of animal disease epidemics is early detection. If a disease can be detected very early in the phase of epidemic development, the possibility exists that it can be arrested and eliminated before it inflicts damage (Van der Poel *et al.*, 2000).

It is not possible to eliminate all pathogens from the current production systems, but producers can do a great deal through good agricultural practices (GAPs) to minimise the risk through systematic and scrupulous adherence to recommended food hygiene practices (FHPs) and the observance of strict good hygienic practices (GHPs) on the farm (FAO/WHO, 1997; Gorris, 2005). Monitoring and surveillance, along with early intervention in the event of a food safety risk becoming apparent is also essential. Without strict control of food preparation, storage and display practices, food-borne illnesses will continue to grow. Farming systems constitute a CCP (Figure 2, steps 1 and 2). Health animal must be used in street food processing to provide safe foods to consumers (Barro *et al.*, 2007).

2.3. Unknowledge of Viruses and Difficulty of Their Detection

RTE and specifically SV foods vendors and handlers are constitued by high rate of illiterates and they are not followed about their health, about viral infection such as HAV and HEV. Thus most people knowledge on viruses as dangerous pathogens date to the recent years with the HIV-AIDS spread and more recently with outbreaks of Avian Influenza Virus H_5N_1 and SARS-CoV. Viruses in most cases seem to be mystic agents and few health services are included virus diagnosis in their routine work on microbial diseases aetiology. Many public and private sector agencies are investigating huge amounts of effort and

Viral hazards and CCP at different steps of street food chain

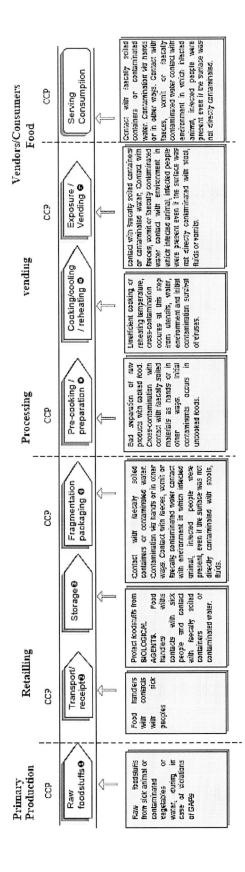

Figure 2. Identification and nature of viral hazards, at different steps of ready-to-eat and street-vended food production chain. CCP = Critical Control Points identified using the decision tree (CAC/RCP, 2003).

resources in the prevention of foodborne illnesses but generally targeting those caused by bacteria. On the other hand, only small parts focused on viruses. However, foodborne viruses are finding in all environments, easly transmitted, dangerous as well as bacteria also responsible for outbreaks (Klein, 2004; Koopmans and Duizier, 2002; Koopmans *et al.*, 2002; Nicand *et al.*, 1998; Wihelmi *et al.*, 2003).

Improving the knowledge on viruses as foodborne pathogens through risk analysis system (CAC, 2004) is absolutely fundamental to avoid viral outbreaks. Foodborne viruses risk management need identification and characterization of viruses and education, information of people about epidemiological aspects of theses viruses

2.4. Ready-to-Eat and Street-Vended Foods Processing Technologies

If viruses are present in foods after processing, they remain infectious in most circumstances and in most foods for several days or weeks, especially if kept cooled at 4 °C (39.2 °F) (Enriquez *et al.*, 1995; Kurdziel *et al.*, 2001) eg: Astroviruses are heat resistant for short periods above 56°C and survive for long periods below -20°C. The fundamental purpose of food processing remains unchanged to make food available and safe when and where it is needed. The use of a greater variety of cooking methods such as micro-waving, barbecuing and slow cooking enhance food variety, but knowledge is required to ensure that these methods are used correctly, and without undermining health and safety of the end-consumer. The ready-to-eat foods that we eat are processed in some form typical methods of food processing. Indeed, street foods are processed manually with rudimentary tools and foods are quality is rarely controlled. In modern insdustries, several technologies such as pasteurisation, refrigeration, sterilisation involve heating to temperatures of at least 120° C (248 °F) or more for a prescribed period of time to kill microbes followed by rapid cooling are used. Radiation processing of food strengthens food conservation, improves food hygiene. Other methods of inactivating viruses within a food are relatively unreliable, but viruses in water and on exposed surfaces can be inactivated with ultraviolet light or with strong oxidizing agents (Cliver, 1997). While, these comodities are unexistant in most RTE food enterprises. RTE Street-vended foods production conditions cannot secure them against viruses and risk of contamination remains (Allwood *et al.*, 2004; Barro *et al.*, 2007; Kurdziel *et al*, 2001; Vollaard *et al.*, 2004). Therefore, it is the key that sufficient attention be given good manufacturing practices (GMPs) to avoid introduction of viruses onto the raw materials and into the food-manufacturing environment during street food preparation, with respect of good hygiene prectices (GHP) at the critical control points (CCP).

People working with food who are sick with Norovirus gastroenteritis are a particular risk to others, because they handle the food and drink many other people will consume. Since the virus is so small, a sick food handler can easily – without meaning to – contaminate the food he or she is handling. Many of those eating the contaminated food may become ill, causing an outbreak.

Outbreaks of norovirus gastroenteritis have taken place in restaurants, cruise ships, nursing homes, hospitals, schools, banquet halls, summer camps, and family dinners – in other words, places where often people have consumed water and/or food prepared or handled by others. It is estimated that as many as half of all food-related outbreaks of illness may be caused by norovirus. In many of these cases, sick food handlers were thought to be implicated.

2.5. Environmental Conditions and Disasters

Viruses pass into the environment from clinically ill or carrier hosts, vomits, stools; although they do not replicate outside living animals or people, they are maintained and transported to susceptible hosts. Population concentrations and movements, both animal and human, have been steadily increasing in this century, enhancing transmission of respiratory and enteric viruses and compounding the difficulty of preventing environmental transmission. In developing countries, the sitaution is worst rapid population increases, particularly in the urban environment further aggravates this problem. Human enteric pathogenic viruses can enter the environment through discharge of waste materials from infected persons, and be transmitted back to susceptible persons to continue the cycle of disease. While epidemic are relied to the general unsanitary level of cities providing harbour to insect vectors and unhygienic behaviour of peoples (Barro *et al.*, 2006a; 2006b; Bryan, 2002). A number of studies have investigated the survival characteristics of several enteric viruses in various environments and foodstuffs, to help explain the transmissibility of these pathogens (Rzezutka and Cook, 2004).

Another factor determining risk contamination of RTE and SV foods is the stability of some of the foodborne viruses in the environment. Studies on environmental survival factors of viruses have been most definitive for polioviruses and others oral-faecal viruses (D'Souza *et al.*, 2006; Kaferstein and Abdussalam, 1999; Pirtle and Beran, 1991; Rzezutka and Cook, 2004; Steele and Odumeru, 2004). During most of RTE street-vended foods processing and vending they are close to these conditions. Rotaviruses in aerosols generated while vomiting were found to survive in the air up to 9 days at 20°C (68 °F) (Sattar *et al.*, 1984). Viruses also may persist for extended periods (1-60 days for 100-fold reduction in infectivity) on severals types of materials commonly found in environment (Abad *et al.*, 1997). Finally, it was shown that viruses may survive for prolonged periods of time, with over 1 year survival of poliovirus and rotavirus in water at 4°C (39.2 °F) (Biziagos *et al.*, 1988).

At last, many disasters contribute to degradation of environmental conditions and increase risk of outbreak. In case of disaster, peoples eat what they have under their hands to survive even contaminated waters froms rivers, lacks and foods prepared under unhygienic conditions and got cheaply in street. For instances these aspects are not well-argued by researchers.

2.6. RTE Foods Handling Conditions

Workers handling food products throughout different steps of food production chain, play a critical role in food quality and safety. Efforts are being made to inform and educate professional food-handlers as well as the consumers about how to avoid foodborne viral illnesses. People known, or suspected, to be suffering from, or to be a carrier of a disease or illness likely to be transmitted through food, should not be allowed to enter any food handling area if there is a likelihood of their contaminating food. Any person so affected should immediately report illness or symptoms of illness to the management.

Attention must pay to foods such as salads, fruits which are intended to be eaten raw. Therefore, raw decorations pose a risk, and the decorative arranging of food can result in food being handled more than is usual to acquire the desired effect. Many infectious virus particles can be transferred from contaminated fingerpads to ham, lettuce, and metal disks. In contrast, few number of virus particles transfer occur, from ham, lettuce, and metal disks to hands (Ansari *et al.*, 1988; Bidawid *et al.*, 2004; Marshall *et al.*, 2001). These data indicate the potential vehicular role for human hands in the spread of viral infections. Under these circumstances, professional food-handlers should take extra precautions to avoid cross-contamination between raw foodstuffs or between raw food and finished products (Cardinale *et al.*, 2005). The consumers must employ special care when purchasing RTE and SV foods.

Most documented foodborne viral outbreaks can be traced to food that has been manually handled by an infected foodhandlers, rather than to industrially processed foods (Mosupye and van Holy, 2000; Mensah *et al.*, 1999). In general microbial contamination of food can occur anywhere in the process, from farm to fork, but most foodborne viral infections can be traced back to infected persons who handle food that is not heated or otherwise treated afterwards (Barro *et al.*, 2007; Cliver, 1997; Koopmans *et al.*, 2003; Bryan, 1988). Therefore, emphasis should be on stringent personal hygiene during preparation. If viruses are present in food preprocessing, residual viral infectivity may be present after some industrial processes. Therefore, it is key that sufficient attention be given to good hygiene practice (GHP) and good manufacturing practice (GMP) to avoid introduction of viruses onto the raw foodstuffs and into the food-manufacturing environment, and to assure adequate management during the manufacturing process. If viruses are present in food after processing, they remain infectious in most circumstances and in most foods for several days or weeks, especially if kept cooled (at 4° C) (Koopman and Duizer, 2004). In addition to common foodborne viruses, there are emerging zoonotic viral agents such as SARS-CoV and H_5N_1 influenza virus for which investigation must be done to clarify all the mechanisms of contamination.

2.7. Governments

Governments must consider the scientifics data of foodborne pathogens and decide how best they should encourage the implementation of these general food safety principles to protect consumers adequately from illness or injury caused by food (CAC, 2003). Policies need to consider the vulnerability of the population, or of different groups within the population; provide health education programmes which effectively communicate the principles of food hygiene to industry and consumers. Consumers should recognize their role by following relevant instructions and applying appropriate food hygiene measures (CAC, 2003; Gorris, 2006; Barro, 2007).

The government and department of health and human services and its public health service must (i) provide leadership in protecting the public health with regard to food issues

(ii) build a policy in a manner that clearly links science to this mission of food safety. Create the lead agency for applied food and environmental laboratory science to support our regulatory and non-regulatory food safety mission. Infectious Diseases control center will had primary responsibility for epidemiology and laboratory science to support infectious and non-infectious disease prevention mission. The National Institutes of Health is the premier agency for basic and clinical biomedical research. Together these agencies promote food safety, prevent foodborne disease, and mitigate the clinical and social impact of infectious and non-infectious illness that occurs as argued by Henney (2002). Accomplishment of these goal are based in sound sience. Advances in food virological techniques are improving the ability to detect and combat the presence of foodborne viruses, such as Hepatitis A virus, in fresh produce as well Risk Assessment is leading the Department's food safety regulation and policy to effective and efficient, science-based solutions to these complex food safety challenges.

Science impact on RTE food safety policy is reflected in new approaches take to solving public health problems (Barro et al., 2007; Mensah et al., 2002; FAO/WHO, 1997). For instance, RTE are an increasingly popular part of the urban population diet, regularly consumed by approximately 80% of the population. (Akinyele, 1998). However, severals departements of food safety are observed an increase in the number of reports of outbreaks of foodborne disease associated with RTE and street-vended foods. The primary problem is that RTE, which are consumed raw can be contaminated with harmful microorganisms, and no steps in the traditional production of street-vended foods provide a means for controlling foodborne pathogens (Estrada-Garcia, et al., 2004, Barro et al., 2007). Indeed a task force of government, university, and industry scientists is to mobilize and develop a coordinated research agenda that would find solutions. Relying on this and other available scientific information, we several authors conducted a risk assessment that will help all the actor on the food safety to develop food safety guidance and polices that reduce the risk of viral diseases.

2.8. Lack of Information, Education and Awareness

Ready-to-eat and street-vended foods should bear appropriate information to ensure that (CAC, 2003):

- adequate and accessible information is available to the next person in the food chain to enable them to handle, store, process, prepare and display the product safely and correctly.
- Insufficient product information, and/or inadequate knowledge of general food hygiene, can lead to products being mishandled at later stages in the food chain. Such mishandling can result in illness, or products becoming unsuitable for consumption, even where adequate hygiene control measures have been taken earlier in the food chain.
- Health education programmes should cover general food hygiene. Such programmes should enable consumers to understand the importance of any product information and to follow any instructions accompanying products, and make informed choices.

In particular consumers should be informed of the relationship between time/temperature control and foodborne illness.

Food hygiene training is fundamentally important. All personnel should be aware of their role and responsibility in protecting food from contamination or deterioration. Food handlers should have the necessary knowledge and skills to enable them to handle food hygienically as recommended by FAO, WHO (FAO/WHO, 1997; CAC, 2001; ILSI, 2004, Gorris, 2005).

3. Viral Hazards and Risk Assessment along RTE and SV Foods Production Chain

By assembling and analyzing the early data collected through the food safety questions, the hazard levels were assessed at every steps of the RTE and SV foods production chain according behavioral risk factors surveillance system (Yang *et al.*, 1998). This method allowed to detect strengths and weaknesses of the RTE and SV foods current safety system used in relation to viral contaminations. According to the risk assessors methodology (Lammerding, 1997; Lammerding and Fazil, 2000; McKone, 1996; Reij and Van Schothorst, 2000; Vose, 1998; Woteki *et al.*, 2001) and in the Food Safety Objectives framework (Gorris, 2005; CAC, 2004), data were processed. Then, it was identified sensitive steps to viral risk, these would give more accurate reflection on implementation of HACCP pre-requisites as GAPs, GHPs GMPs as describe by *Codex Alimentarius* (CAC, 2004), ILSI (ILSI, 2004), ICMSF (2002) and Powell and Attwell (1999). Hazards analysis concisted in processing of existing epidemiological data to determine the level of exposure of street foods to the viral hazards in various situations / circumstances (Koopmans *et al.*, 2003). It is clear that RTE and SV foods requiring either intensive manual handling under poor hygienic conditions, or close-to-fork and end-product manual handling are the products at highest risk (Barro *et al.*, 2007). In spite of various safety assurance measures implemented in throughout the food production chain to prevent RTE and SV foods from being contaminated with bacteria and viruses, CCP and Good Practices (GPs) violations along the RTE and SV foods production chain were always observed (Barro *et al.*, 2006a; FAO, 1997; Mensah *et al.*, 2002, WHO, 2002b). While, violations of these aspects are hazardous and means evidence of risk of viral contamination. As indicated in figure 1, viral contamination can occurs through main steps along the RTE and SV foods production chain. Many small-scale food enterprises like RTE and SV foods industries, operate under a simple organizational structure, consisting of the manager-owner assisted by a few workers, who do not know safety techniques of management (Barro *et al.*, 2006b; Canet and N'Diaye, 1996; Mensah *et al.*, 2002; Mosupye and van Holy, 2000). A poor manufacturing practices and personal hygiene of food handlers, a lacks of good-quality raw foodstuffs materials vegetables for processing are the main characteristics (Barro et *al.*, 2007). These aspects constitute a gap by which viral contamination can occurs. At figure 1, steps 1, 3, 5, 6 and 7 are most important during uncooked foods processing and for cooked foods, steps 5, 6 and 7 are the main critical control points about viral contamination.

The contamination can be of primary or secondary nature. The primary contamination of food occurs when the animal which is going to be killed has already a virus disease. Meat and organs may then carry the virus (Li *et al.*, 2005). Foods may also be contaminated in their growing and harvesting areas by sewage polluted waters, and molluscan shellfishes have been particularly implicated (Appleton, 2000; Bidawid *et al.*, 2000a; Butt *et al.*, 2005; Fiore, 2004; Klein, 2004; Koopmans *et al.*, 2002; 2003; Koopmans and Duizier, 2002; Rzezutka and Cook, 2004; Ward and Irving, 1987). Vegetables and fruits sprinkled by contaminated water carry viruses (Chancellor *et al.*, 2006; Croci et *al.*, 2002; Lee and Yap, 1999; Steele and Odumeru, 2004). The secondary contamination of food occurs during processing, transportation and storage through dirt and smear infections (Koopmans *et al.*, 2003). Foods may be contaminated by infected food-handlers as indicated above, and outbreaks frequently involve cold foods that require much handling during preparation (Koopmans *et al.*, 2003; 2004; Yang *et al.*, 1998; 2000). However, viral contamination of food will never increase during processing, transport or storage and the conatminated products will look, smell and taste normal (D'Souza *et al.*, 2006; Koopmans et *al.*, 2004). Moreever, beacause contamination is often caused by foodhandlers the level of contamination with virus may vary greatly within a product (Koopmans *et al.*, 2004). Water which bears viruses is the most common cause of contamination when used in the production of food or used in cleaning of tools and equipments or rinsing vegetables (Chancellor *et al.*, 2006; Croci *et al.*, 2002; Lee and Yap, 1999; Steele and Odumeru, 2004). In addition, food must be protected from insect as flies which can carry in their legs and proboscis different microorganisms from contaminated environment (Barro *et al.*, 2006b; De jesus *et al.*, 2004; Nichols, 2005). In turn contaminated flies can transfer these microorganisms when landing on food. However, as yet no data was argued specifically transmission of foodborne virus by flies.

Holding cooked and uncooked foods at ambiant temperature for 6 h or longer without any appropiate holding tempertaure (reheating in case of cooked food), do not constitute a major critical control point of street-vending foods about viral risk. Indeed, Viruses do not multiply or produce toxins in foods, and foods merely act as vehicles for their passive transfer. Most foodborne or waterborne viruses unlike vegetative bacteria are intracellular parasites and resistant to clasic heat and pressure treatments (Enriquez *et al.*, 1995; Bidawid *et al.*, 2000a; Hewitt and Greening, 2006; Grove *et al.*, 2006; Kurdziel *et al.*, 2001; Nissen *et al.*, 1996; Wilkinson et *al.*, 2001). But when cooked food is contaminated during viral cross-contamination and contamination from various sources such as utensils, knives raw foodstuffs, flies that sporadically landing on the foods, by vendors bare hands serving and occasional food handling by consumers it become a potential risk for consummers health (Bidawid *et al.*, 2000b; 2003; Klein, 2004; WHO, 1992; Yang *et al.*, 2000). Clearly, the likelihood of virus contamination in primary products will differ for different commodities and is the highest for shellfish and manually handled fruits. For foods contaminated after processing, Kurdziel *et al.* (2001) estimate is that viruses will remain active in most foods.

Although it difficult to anticipate every food safety problem before it happens, policies makers must make sure that prepartors and vendors have a strong science-based food safety system in place that can minimize the harm to public health. By enhancing the science that underpins all of our decision-making in the food safety arena, as well as the rest of the

Agency, we are helping to ensure the level of public health protection that consumers expect and deserve.

Definitions According FAO

Control measure: Any action and activity that can be used to prevent or eliminate a food safety hazard or reduce it to an acceptable level.

Corrective action: Any action to be taken when the results of monitoring at the CCP indicate a loss of control.

Critical Control Point (CCP): A step at which control can be applied and is essential to prevent or eliminate a food safety hazard or reduce it to an acceptable level.

Critical limit: A criterion which separates acceptability from unacceptability.

HACCP: A system which identifies, evaluates, and controls hazards which are significant for food safety.

HACCP plan: A document prepared in accordance with the principles of HACCP to ensure control of hazards which are significant for food safety in the segment of the food chain under consideration.

Hazard: A biological, chemical or physical agent in, or condition of, food with the potential to cause an adverse health effect.

Hazard analysis: The process of collecting and evaluating information on hazards and conditions leading to their presence to decide which are significant for food safety and therefore should be addressed in the HACCP plan.

Step: A point, procedure, operation or stage in the food chain including raw materials, from primary production to final consumption.

Cleaning - the removal of soil, food residue, dirt, grease or other objectionable matter.

Contaminant - any biological or chemical agent, foreign matter, or other substances not intentionally added to food which may compromise food safety or suitability.

Contamination - the introduction or occurrence of a contaminant in food or food environment.

Establishment - any building or area in which food is handled and the surroundings under the control of the same management.

Food hygiene - all conditions and measures necessary to ensure the safety and suitability of food at all stages of the food chain.

Food handler - any person who directly handles packaged or unpackaged food, food equipment and utensils, or food contact surfaces and is therefore expected to comply with food hygiene requirements

Food safety - assurance that food will not cause harm to the consumer when it is prepared and/or eaten according to its intended use.

Food suitability - assurance that food is acceptable for human consumption according to its intended use.

Primary production - those steps in the food chain up to and including, for example, harvesting, slaughter, milking, fishing.

Acknowledgements

The authors would like to thank the International Foundation for Science (IFS) and Sustainable Food Security In Central West Africa (SADAOC) Foundation which have financed the street food project in the CRSBAN, University of Ouagadougou.

References

Abad, F.X.; Pinto, R.M. and Bosch, A. (1997). Disinfection of human enteric viruses on fomits. *FEMS Microbiol. Lett.*, 156: 107-111.

Abdussalam, M. and Kaferstein, F.K. (1993). Safety of street foods. *World Health Forum*, 14: 191-194.

Akinyele, I.O. (1998). Street food and their contribution to the food security and nutritional status of Nigerians. *West Afr. J. Food Nutr*, 3 : 6-20.

Allwood, P.B.; Malik, Y.S.; Maherchandani, S.; Vought, K.; Johnson, L.A.; Braymen, C.; Hedberg, C.W. and Goyal, S.M. (2004). Occurrence of Escherichia coli, noroviruses, and F-specific coliphages in fresh market-ready produce. *J. Food Prot.*; 67: 2387-2390.

Altekruse, S.F.; Street, D.A.; Fein, S.B. and Levy AS. (1996). Consumer knowledge of foodborne microbial hazards and food-handling practices. *J. Food Prot.*, 59: 287-294.

Angelillo, I.F.; Viggiani, N.M.; Rizzo, L. and Bianco, A. (2000). Food handlers and foodborne diseases: knowledge, attitudes, and reported behavior in Italy. *J. Food Prot.*, 63: 381-385.

Ansari, S.A.; Sattar, S.A.; Springthorpe, V.S.; Wells, G.A.; Tostowaryk, W. (1988) Rotavirus survival on human hands and transfer of infectious virus to animate and nonporous inanimate surfaces. *J. Clin. Microbiol.*, 26: 1513-1518.

Appleton, H. (2000). Control of food-borne viruses. *Br. Med. Bull.*, 56: 172-183.

Badrie, N.; Joseph, M. and Darbasie, N. (2005). Nutritive composition of street food "double" chana (Cicer arietinum) burger and its components sold in trinidadn West Indies. *J. Food Comp. Anal.*, 18: 171-179.

Barro, N.; Bello, A.R.; Itsiembou, Y.; Savadogo, A.; Ouattara, C.A.T.; Nikiéma, A.P.; De Souza, C. and Traoré, A.S. (2007). Street-vended Foods Improvement: Contamination Mechanisms and Application of Food Safety Objective Strategy: Critical Review. *Pakistan J. Nutr.*, 6(1): 1-10.

Barro, N.; Bello, A.R.; Savadogo, A.; Ouattara, C.A.T.; Ilboudo, A-J.; and Traoré, A.S. (2006a) Hygienic status assessment of dishwaters, utensils, hands and pieces of money in street foods vending sites in Ouagadougou; Burkina Faso. *Afri J. Biotech.*, 5: 1107-1112.

Barro, N.; Nikiéma, P.; Ouattara, C.A.T. and Traoré, A.S. (2002b). Evaluation de l'hygiène et de la qualité microbiologique de quelques aliments rue et les caractéristiques des consommateurs dans les villes de Ouagadougou et de Bobo-Dioulasso (Burkina Faso). *Rev. Sci. Tech Sci. Santé*, 25: 7-21.

Barro, N.; Ouattara, C.A.T.; Nikiéma, P.; Ouattara, A.S. and Traoré, A.S. (2002a). Evaluation de la qualité microbiologique de quelques aliments de rue dans la ville de Ouagadougou au Burkina Faso. *Cah santé*, 12: 369-374.

Barro, N.; Savadogo, A.; Ouattara, C. A. T. and Traoré, A. S. (2006b). Carriage bacteria by proboscis, legs and faeces of two flies in street food vending sites in Ouagadougou, Burkina Faso. *J. Food Protect.*, 69: 2007-2010.

Berg, D.; Kohn, M. and Farley, T. (2000). McFarland L. Multistate outbreaks of acute gastroenteritis traced to fecal-contaminated oysters harvested in Louisiana. *J. Infect Dis.*, 181: S381–S386.

Bidawid, S.; Farber, J.M. and Sattar, S.A. (2000b). Contamination of foods by foodhandlers: experiments on hepatitis A virus transfer to food and its interruption. *Appl. Environ. Microbiol.*, 66: 2759-2763.

Bidawid, S.; Farber, J.M.; Sattar, S.A. and Hayward, S. (2000a). Heat inactivation of hepatitis A virus in dairy foods. *J. Food Prot.*, 63: 522-528.

Bidawid, S.; Malik, N.; Adegbunrin, O.; Sattar, S.A. and Farber, J.M. (2004). Norovirus cross-contamination during food handling and interruption of virus transfer by hand antisepsis: experiments with feline calicivirus as a surrogate. *J. Food Prot.*, 67: 103-109.

Biziagos, E.; Passagot, J.; Crance, J.M. and Deloince, R. (1988) Long-term survival of hepatitis A virus and poliovirus type 1 in mineral water. *Appl. Environ. Microbiol.*, 54: 2705-2710.

Borchardt, M.A.; Bertz, P.D.; Spencer, S.K. and Battigelli, D.A. (2003). Incidence of enteric viruses in groundwater from household wells in wisconsin. *Appl. Environ. Microbiol.*, 69: 1172-1180.

Bryan, F.L. (1978). Factors that contributs to outbreaks of foodborne disease. *J. Food Prot.*, 41: 816-827.

Bryan, F.L. (1988). Risk associated with practices, procedures and processes that lead to outbreaks of foodborne diseases. *J. Food Prot.*, 51: 663-673.

Bryan, F.L. (2002). Reflections on career in public health: evolving foodborne pathogens, environmental health, and food safety programs. *J. Environ. Health*, 65: 14-24.

Bryan, F.L.; Michanie, S.C.; Alvarez, P. and Paniagua, A. (1988). Critical control points of street-vended foods in dominican republic. *J. Food Prot.*, 51: 373-383.

Bryan, F.L.; Teufel, P.; Riaz, S.; Rooth, S.; Qadar, F. and Malik, Z. (1992). Hazards and critical control points of street-vended chat, a regionally popular food in Pakistan. *J. Food Prot.*, 55: 708-713.

Butt, A.A.; Aldridge, K.E. and Sanders, C.V. (2005). Infections related to the ingestion of seafood Part I: Viral and bacterial infections. *Lancet Infect. Dis.*, 5: 69-70.

CAC (Codex Alimentarius Commission) (2001). Proposed draft revised code of hygenic practices for the preparation and sale of street-vended foods(regional standard-Latin America and Caribbean, CAC/RCP 43-1995. In: *Consideration of the Draft revised code of Hygienic practices for street-vended foods*. Report of the 12th session, Santo Domingo, Dominican Republic 13-16 February, 2001. Joint FAO/WHO stnadard programme, Codex Coordinating committee for Latin American and tthe Caribbean.

CAC (*Codex Alimentarius* Commission) (2004). *Report of the twentieth session of the codex committee on general principles*, paris, France 3-7 may 2004 ALINORM 04/27/331 appendix II pp 37-38. ftp// ftp.fao.org/codex/alinorm04/al0433ae.pdf.

Canet, C. and N'diaye, C. (1996). L'alimentation de rue en Afrique. *Food, Nutrition and Agriculture*, 17/18 : 4-13.

Cardinale, E.; Perrier Gros-Claude, J.D.; Tall, F.; Gueye, E.F. and Salvat G. (2005). Risk factors for contamination of ready-to-eat street-vended poultry dishes in Dakar, Senegal. *Int. J. Food Microbiol*, 25 : 157-165.

Cassin, M.H.; Lammerding, A.M.; Todd, E.D.; Ross, W. and McColl, R.S. (1998). Quantitative risk assessment for Escherichia coli 0157:H7 in ground beef humburgers. *Int J. Food Microbiol.*, 41: 21-44.

Chakravarty, I. and Canet, C. (1996).Street food in Calcutta. *Food, Nutrition and Agriculture,* 17/18: 7.

Chancellor, D.D.; Tyagi, S.; Bazaco, M.C.; Bacvinskas, S.; Chancellor, M.B.; Dato, V.M. and de Miguel, F. (2006). Green onions: potential mechanism for hepatitis A contamination. *J. Food Prot.,* 69: 1468-1472.

Cheftel, E.; Spiegel, A.; Bornet, G.; Morell, E.; Michel, E. and Buisson, Y. (1997). Toxic food infection caused by Shigella flexneri in a military unit. *Cah. Santé,* 7 : 295-299.

Cliver, D.O. (1997). Virus transmission via food. *World Health Stat Q,* 50 : 90-101.

Codex Alimentarius, Committee on Food Hygiene. (1999). Discussion Paper on Viruses in Food. FAO/WHO, document CX/FH 99/11. Rome, Italy.

Collins, J.E. (1997). Impact of changing consumer lifestyles on the emergence/reemergence of foodborne pathogens. *Emerg. Infect. Dis.,* 3: 471-479.

Croci, L.; De Medici ,D.; Scalfaro, C.; Fiore, A.; Toti, L. (2002). The survival of hepatitis A virus in fresh produce. *Int. J. Food Microbiol.,* 73: 29-34.

de Wit, M.A.; Koopmans, M.P.and van Duynhoven YT. (2003). Risk factors for norovirus, Sapporo-like virus, and group A rotavirus gastroenteritis. *Emerg. Infect. Dis.,* 9: 1563-1570.

Doultry, J.C.; Druce, J.D.; Birch, C.J.; Bowden, D.S. and Marshall, J.A. (1999). Inactivation of feline calicivirus, a Norwalk virus surrogate. *J. Hosp. Infect.,* 41:51-57.

D'Souza, D.H.; Sair, A.; Williams, K.; Papafragkou, E.; Jean, J.; Moore, C. and Jaykus, L. (2006). Persistence of caliciviruses on environmental surfaces and their transfer to food. *Int. J. Food Microbiol.,* 108: 84-91.

Enriquez, C.E.; Hurst, C.J. and Gerra, C.P. (1995). Survival of the enteric adenovirus 40 and 41 in tap, sea and waste water. *Water Res.,* 11: 2548-2553.

Estrada-Garcia, T.; Cerna, J.F.; Thompson, M.R. and Lopez-Sancedo, C. (2002). Faecal ciontamination and enterotoxigenic Ecscherichia coli in street-vended chili sauces in Mexico and its public health relevance. *Epidemiol. Infect.,* 129: 223-226.

Estrada-Garcia, T.; Lopez-Sancedo, C.; Zamarripa-Ayala, B.; Thompson, M.R.; Gutierrez-Cogco, L.; Mancera-Martinez, A. and Escobar-Gutierrez, A. (2004). Prevalence of Escherichia coli and Salmonella spp in Street-vended food of open markets (tianguis) and general hygienic and trading practices in Mexico city. *Epidemiol Infect.*; 132: 1181-1184.

FAO. (1988). Street foods. Report of an FAO expert consultation, Yogyakarta, Indonesia. FAO *Food Nutr.,* paper n 46.

FAO/WHO. (1997). Risk Management and Food Safety, Report of the joint FAO/WHO Consultation. FAO *Food Nutr.,* paper n 65.

Fiore, A.E. (2004). Hepatitis A transmitted by food. *Clin. Infect. Dis.,* 38: 705-715.

Gifford, R. (1951). Clinical and epidemiologic observations of Coxsackie virus infection. *N. Engl. J. Med.,* 244:868-873.

Gilles, C.; De Casanove, J-N.; Dubois, E.; Bon, F.; Pothier, P.; Kholi, E. and Vaillant, V. (2003). Epidémie de gastro-entérites à norovirus liée à la contamination d'huître, Somme Janvier 2001. *Bull. Epidemiol. Hebdo,* 8: 47-48.

Glass R.I. (2006). New hope for defeating rotavirus. *Sci. Am.,* 294:46-55.

Gorris, L.G.M. (2005). Food safety Objective: an integral par of food chain management. *Food Contr,* 16: 801-809.

Grove, S.F.; Lee, A.; Lewis, T.; Stewart, C.M.; Chen, H. and Hoover, D.G. (2006). Inactivation of foodborne viruses of significance by high pressure and other processes. *J Food Prot.,* 69: 957-968.

Henney, M.D. (2002). Good science: critical to regulatory decision making *FEMS Microbiol. Rev.,* 26: 187-205.

Hewitt, J. and Greening G.E. (2006). Effect of heat treatment on hepatitis A virus and norovirus in New Zealand greenshell mussels (Perna canaliculus) by quantitative real-time reverse transcription PCR and cell culture. *J. Food Prot.,* 69 : 2217-2223.

ICMSF (International Commission on Microbiological Specification for Food) (2002). Microorganisms in food Book 7 Microbiological testing in food safety management, NY Kluver Academic / Plenum ISBN 0306 472627.

ILSI (International Life Science Institute) (2004). Food safety objective role in microbiological food safety management. ILSI Europe reports series, ISBN 1 578811759.

Kaferstein, F. and Abdussalam, M. (1999). Food safety in 21st century. *Bull. World Health Oragan,* 77: 347-351.

Kapikian, A.Z. and Chanock, R.M. (1996). Rotaviruses. *In* Fields BN, Knipe DM Howley PM Ed. *Virology* 3rd edn. Philadelphia: Lippincott-Raven Press, pp 1657-1708.

King, L.K.; Awumbila, B.; Canacoo, E.A. and Ofosu-Amaah, S. (2000). An assessment of the safety of street foods in the Ga district of Ghana; implication for the spread of zoososes. *Acta tropica,* 76: 39-43.

Klein, G. (2004). Spread of viruses through the food chain. *Dtsch Tierarztl Wochenschr,* 111: 312-314. (Abstract).

Kohli, E.; Bon, F.; Frmantin, C.; Pothier P. (1999). Gastroenterites virales. *Spectra Biol.,* 8: 27-30.

Koopmans, M. and Duizer, E. (2002). Foodborne viruses: an emerging problem http://europe.ilsi.org/NR/rdonlyres/E8E0F6C5-C767-4AA8-B1A7-E62A8BBE1EF9/0/RPFoodbornvirus.pdf visited december 02 /2006.

Koopmans, M. and Duizer, E. (2004). Foodborne viruses: an emerging problem. *Int. J. Food Microbiol,* 90: 23-41.

Koopmans, M.; Vennema, H.; Heersma, H.; van Strien, E.; van Duynhoven, Y.; Brown, D.; Reacher, M. and Lopman, B. (2003). European Consortium on Foodborne Viruses. Early identification of common-source foodborne virus outbreaks in Europe. *Emerg. Infect. Dis.,* 9: 1136-1142.

Koopmans, M.; von Bonsdorff, C.H.; Vinje, J.; de Medici, D. and Monroe, S. (2002). Foodborne viruses. *FEMS Microbiol Rev.,* 26: 187-205.

Kurdziel, A.S.; Wilkinson, N.; Langton, S. and Cook, N. (2001). Survival of poliovirus on soft fruit and salad vegetables. *J Food Prot,* 64:706-709.

Kurth, L. (2000). The futur of meal solution in australia. *Proceeding from the 4th annual meal solutions the next step conference*, 13-14th April, The Grace Hotel, Sydney.

Kuzuya, M.; Fujii, R.; Hamano, M. and Ogura, H. (2003). Outbreak of acute gastroenteritis caused by human group C rotavirus in a youth educational center in Okayama Prefecture. *Kansenshogaku Zasshi, 77*: 53-59.

Lammerding, A.M. and Fazil, A. (2000). Hazard identification and exposure assessment for microbial food safety risk assessment. *Int. J. Food Microbiol., 58*: 147-151.

Lammerding, A.M. (1997). An overview of microbial food safety risk assessment. *J. Food Prot., 11*: 1420-5.

Leclerc, H.; Schwartzbrod, L. and Dei-Cas, E. (2002). Microbial agents associated with waterborne diseases. *Crit. Rev. Microbiol., 28*: 371-409.

Lee, A.S. and Yap, K.L. (1999). Recovery of poliovirus from cut surface of stored fresh papaya fruit. *Southeast Asian J. Trop Med. Public Health, 30*: 280-283.

Li, T.C.; Chijiwa, K.; Sera, N.; Ishibashi, T.; Etoh, Y.; Shinohara, Y.; Kurata, Y.; Ishida, M.; Sakamoto, S.; Takeda, N. and Miyamura, T. (2005). Hepatitis E virus transmission from wild boar meat. *Emerg. Infect Dis., 11*: 1958-60.

Marshall, JA.; Yuen, L.K. and Catton, M.G. (2001). Multiple outbreaks of NLV gastroenteritis associated with a Mediterranean-style restaurant. *J. Med. Microbiol., 50*: 143-151.

Mast, E.E. and Alter, M.J. (1993). Epidemiology of viral hepatitis. *Semin. Virol., 4*: 273-283.

McKone, T.E. (1996). Overview of the risk analysis approach and terminology: the merging of science judgement and values. *Food Contr, 7*: 69-76.

Mensah, P.; Owusu-Darko, K.; Yeboah-Manu, D.; Ablordey, A.; Nkrumah, F.K. and Kamiya, H. (1999). The role of street food vendors in transmission of enteric pathogens. *Ghana Med. J., 33*: 19-29.

Mensah, P.; Yeboah-Manu, D.; Owusu-Darko, K.and Ablorde, A. (2002). Street foods in Accra, Ghana: how safe are they?. *Bull. WHO, 80*: 546-54.

Mosupye, F.M. and Van Holy, A. (2000). Microbiological hazard identification and exposure assessment of street food vending inJohannesburg, South Africa. *Int. J. Food Microbiol., 61*: 137-45.

Mwangi, A.M.; den Hartog, A.P.; Mwadime, R.K.; van Staveren, W.A. and Foeken, D.W. (2002). Do street food vendors sell a sufficient variety of foods for a healthful diet? The case of Nairobi. *Food Nutr. Bull., 23*:48-56.

Nguyen-the, C. and Carlin, F. (1994). The microbiology of minimally processed fresh fruits and vegetables. *Crit Rev Food Sci Nutr, 34*: 371-401.

Nicand, E. and Teyssou, R. and Buisson, Y. (1998). Le risque fécal viral en 1998. *Virologie, 2*: 103-116.

Nichols, L.G. (2005). Fly transmission of Campylobacter. *Emerg. Infect Dis., 11*: 361-364.

Nissen, E.; Konig, P.; Feinstone, S.M. and Pauli, G. (1996). Inactivation of hepatitis A and other enteroviruses during heat treatment (pasteurization). *Biologicals, 24*: 339-341.

Ohiokpehai O. Nutritionnal Aspects of street foods in Botswana. *Pakistan J. Nutr.* 2003; 2: 76-81.

Parashar, U.D.; Bresee, J.S.; Gentsch, J.R. and Glass, R.I. (1998). Rotavirus. *Emerg. Infect. Dis., 4* : 561-570.

Parashar, U.D.; Hummelman, E.G.; Bresee, J.S.; Miller, M.A. and Glass, R.I. (2003). Global illness and deaths caused by rotavirus disease in children. *Emerg. Infect. Dis.*, 9:565-572.

Pirtle, E.C. and Beran, G.W. (1991). Virus survival in the environment. *Rev. Sci. Tech.*, 10:733-748.

Powell, S.C. and Attwell, R. (1999). The use of epidemiological data in the control of foodborne viruses. *Rev. Environ. Health*, 14: 31-37.

Reij, M.W. and Van Schothorst, M. (2000). Critical notes on microbiological risk assessment of food. *Brazilian J. Microbiol.*, 31: 1-8.

Richards, G.P. (2001). Enteric virus contamination of foods through industrial practices: a primer on intervention strategies. *J. Ind. Microbiol. Biotechnol.*, 27: 117-125.

Rutjes, S.A.; Lodder-Verschoor, F.; van der Poel, W.H.; van Duijnhoven, Y.T. and Husmani, A.M. (2006). Detection of noroviruses in foods: a study on virus extraction procedures in foods implicated in outbreaks of human gastroenteritis. *J. Food Prot.*, 69: 1949-1956.

Rzezutka, A. and Cook, N. (2004). Survival of human enteric viruses in the environment and food. *FEMS Microbiol. Rev.*, 28: 441-453.

Schwartzbrod, L. (1992). Virus, eaux et coquillages. *In*: *Coquillages et santé publique du risque à la prévention* (Lesne J NSP ed) Renne, pp 35-49.

Steele, M. and Odumeru, J.J. (2004). Irrigation water as source of foodborne pathogens on fruit and vegetables. *J. Food Prot.*, 67: 2839-2849.

Theron, J. and Cloete, T.E. (2002). Emerging waterborne infections: contributing factors, agents, and detection tools. *Crit. Rev. Microbiol.*, 28: 1-26.

Tjoa, W.S.; Dupont, H.L.; Sullivan, P.; Pickering, L.K.; Holguin, A.; Olate, T.; Evans, D.G. and Evans, D.J.Jr. (1977). Location of food consumption and travelers diarrhea. *American. J. Epidemiol.*, 106: 61-66.

Umoh, V.J.; Dagana, A. and Umoh, J.U. (1984). Isolation of *Yersinia enterocolitica* from milk and milk products in Zaria. *Nigeria Inter. J. Zoonoses*, 11: 223-228.

van der Poel, W.; Vinjé, J.; van der Heide, R.; Herrera, I.; Vivo, A. and Koopmans, M. (2000). Norwalk-like calicivirus genes in farm animals. *Emerg. Infect Dis.*, 6: 36-41.

van't Riet, H.; den Hartog, A.P.; Hooftman, D.A.P.; Foeken, D.W.; Mwangi, A.M.; van Staveren, W.A. (2003). Determinant of non-homme prepared food consumption in two low income areas in Nairobi. *Nutr.*, 19: 1006-1012.

Vidal, R.; Solari, V.; Mamani, N.; Jiang, X.; Vollaire, J.; Roessler, P.; Prado, V.; Matson, D.O. and O'Ryan, M.L. (2005). Calicivirus and foodborne gastroenteritis, Chile. *Emerg. Infect. Dis.*, 11: 1134-1137.

Vollaard, A.M.; Ali, S.; van Asten, H.A.; Ismid, I.S.; Widjaja, S.; Visser, L.G; Surjadi, C.H. and van Dissel, J.T. (2004). Risk factors for transmission of foodborne illness in restaurants and street vendors in Jakarta, Indonesia. *Epidemiol. Infect.*, 132: 863-872.

Vose, D.J. (1998). The application of quantative risk assessment to microbial food Safety. *J. Food Prot.*, 61: 640-648.

Ward, B.K. and Irving, L.G. (1987). Virus survival on vegetables spray-irrigated with wastewater. *Water Res.*, 21: 57-63.

WHO (Worl health Organization) (1992). *Essential safety requirements for street-vended foods*. Provisonal edition, Genva, WHO/HPP/FOS 92.3.

WHO (Worl health Organization) (2002a). WHO global strategy for food safety safer food for better health. World Health Organization, Geneva Sitzerland ISBN 924 154574 7. http://www.who.int/foodsafety/publications/genarl/en/strategy-en.pdf.

WHO (Worl health Organization) (2002b). *Foof safety and foodborne illness.* Fact Sheet, n°237, 7p.

WHO (World Health Organization). (2006). Food safety: Avian influenza: food safety issues, http://www.who.int/foodsafety/micro/avian/en/index.html.

Wihelmi, I.; Roman, E. and Sanchez-Fauquier, A. (2003). Virus causing gastroenteritis. *Clin. Microbiol. Infect,* 9: 247-262.

Wilkinson, N.; Kurdziel, A.S.; Langton, S.; Needs, E. and Cook, N. (2001). Resistance of poliovirus to inactivation by high hydrostatic pressures. *Innovative Food Sci. Emerging Technol,* 2: 95-98.

Winarno, F.G. (1991). Allain A. Street food in developing countries: lessons from Asia. *Food, Nutr. Agric,* 1: 11-15.

Woteki, C.E.; Facinoli, S.L. and Schor, D. (2001). Keep food safe to eat: healthfull food must be safe as well as nutritious. *J. Nutr.,* 131: 502-509.

Yang, S.; Angulo, F.J. and Altekruse, S.F. (2000). Evaluation of safe food-handling instructions on raw meat and poultry products. *J. Food Prot.,* 63: 1321-1235.

Yang, S.; Leff, M.G.; McTague, D.; Horvath, K.A.; Jackson-Thompson, J.; Murayi, T.; Boeselager, G.K.; Melnik, T.A.; Gildemaster, M.C.; Ridings, D.L.; Altekruse, S.F. and Angulo, F.J. (1998). Multistate surveillance for food-handling, preparation, and consumption behaviors associated with foodborne diseases: 1995 and 1996 BRFSS food-safety questions. *MMWR CDC Surveill Summ.,* 47: 33-57.

In: Hygiene and Its Role in Health
Editors: P. L. Anderson and J. P. Lachan

ISBN 978-1-60456-195-1
© 2008 Nova Science Publishers, Inc.

Chapter 5

Current Status on the Etiology, Epidemiology, Food Safety Implications and Control Measures in *Escherichia coli* O157:H7 Infections

G. Normanno[*]

Department of Health and Animal Welfare, Faculty of Veterinary Medicine
Str. Prov. per Casamassima Km 3, 70010 Valenzano (Ba), Italy

Abstract

Escherichia coli O157:H7 is an important foodborne pathogen. It was recognized as a cause of severe human illness only in the early 1980's. Since then it has been implicated in foodborne disease outbreaks in many countries throughout the world. Cattle are the main reservoir of this microrganism, and transmission of the infection to humans occurs primarily through the consumption of contaminated food. The pathogenicity of *E. coli* O157:H7 is associated to genes encoding for a number of virulence factors, especially the verotoxin-encoding genes. The infective dose is extremely low - in the order of a few bacterial units. *E. coli* O157:H7 is acid-tolerant and survives in acidic environments such as the gastric barrier and acidic foods. The most severe illnesses induced by *E. coli* O157:H7 are Hemorrhagic Colitis and Hemolytic Uremic Syndrome. Both these clinical forms are characterized by severe morbidity and might sometimes be lethal. Children are the most commonly affected age group and they are affected by the highest death rate. *E. coli* O157:H7 is one of the main food safety hazards having important implications for human health worldwide, since outbreaks lead sometimes to cases of mortality. This review examines the etiological and epidemiological aspects of *E. coli* O157:H7 infection and focuses on the food safety concerns raised by *E. coli* O157:H7 and on control methods for the prevention of food poisoning.

Keywords: Escherichia coli O157:H7, food safety.

[*]Correspondence. Tel:+39 080 4679895; fax:+39 0804679854; E-mail address: g.normanno@veterinaria.uniba.it

1. Introduction

Escherichia coli was firstly described by Theodor Escherich in 1885 and it is considered a typical inhabitant of the intestinal tract of humans and warm-blooded animals. *E. coli* colonizes the intestine during the first few hours after birth and stays on indefinitely as a commensal (Drasar and Hill, 1974). It was used as an indicator of faecal contamination of food and water as early as 1890.

A few clones causing human disease developed within the species. Most of them induce variably severe gastrointestinal symptoms while others cause serious systemic diseases with a high mortality rate. The main pathogenic variants of *E. coli* are categorized according to the virulence factors they produce or based on their pathogenetic mechanisms during infection. Enterotoxigenic strains (Enterotoxigenic *E. coli*, ETEC) synthesize heat-labile and heat-stable (LT and ST) enterotoxins; enteropathogenic strains (Enteropathogenic *E. coli*, EPEC) synthesize adherence factors that generate lesions in the enterocytes; enteroaggregative strains have either diffuse or aggregate patterns of adherence (Enteroaggregative *E. coli*, DAEC, EAggEC, or EAEC) and form microcolonies on the enterocytes; enteroinvasive strains (Enteroinvasive *E. coli*, EIEC) penetrate the enterocytes; cytolethal distending toxin producing *E. coli* (CDTEC) and, finally, enterohemorrhagic strains (Enterohemorrhagic *E. coli* EHEC) produce Verotoxins (VTs) or Shiga toxins (Stx) and are thus also called verotoxin producing-*E. coli* (VTEC or STEC) (Doyle and Padhye, 1989; Batt, 2000; Clarke, 2001). *E. coli* O157:H7 is considered to be the prototype of the EHEC strains (Nataro and Kaper, 1998) and is a genuine emerging foodborne pathogen that probably evolved from the Enteropathogenic *E. coli* O55:H7 (Feng et al., 1998). It is the predominant VTEC serotype in many parts of the world and it has been most commonly associated with large outbreaks (Karmali, 1989). *E. coli* O157:H7 was firstly isolated in 1975 in a woman with grossly bloody diarrhea and recognized as a major foodborne pathogen in 1983 after Riley reported two outbreaks of Hemorrhagic Colitis (HC) associated with the consumption of contaminated hamburgers from a fast food chain in Michigan and Oregon (Riley et al., 1983). In both places the *E. coli* serotype isolated from the patients and the food was O157:H7. Since then, *E. coli* O157:H7 has been considered a serious public health concern.

1.1. Metabolic and Growth Characteristics

E. coli O157:H7 presents many biochemical reactions typical of other strains of *E. coli* although there are some important differences. First, most *E. coli* O157:H7 isolates are slow- or non-fermenters of sorbitol and this feature distinguishes this serotype from the other *E. coli* strains that ferment sorbitol within 24h (Doyle and Schoeni, 1984). Second, *E. coli* O157:H7 is negative with the MUG assay and thus lacks β-glucuronidase activity (Tortorello, 2000). Both features are helpful in the isolation and presumptive identification of the microorganism although sorbitol-fermenting and β-glucuronidase-producing strains of *E. coli* O157:H7 have been isolated from patients with HUS (Gunzer et al., 1992; Karch and Bielaszewsca, 2001). Other important biochemical and metabolic characteristics of *E. coli* and *E. coli* O157:H7 are summarized in Table 1.

Table 1. Main biochemical differential parameters, parameters of development and of survival of *E. coli* and *E. coli* O157

	E. coli	*E. coli* O157
Gram	-	-
Cytochrome Oxidase	-	-
Indole Production	+	+
Citrate and Urease	-	-
β-Glucuronidase	+	-
Enterohemolysin	-	+
Lactose Fermentation	+	+
Sorbitol Fermentation (24h)	+	- (+)
Grow 44°-44.5°C	Well	Poorly
Min. Grow T°C	5	5
Chilling Survival	Yes	Yes
Minimum pH Value	4-4.5	2.5
a_w	0.97	0.97
Max [NaCl]	6.5	6.5
Milk Pasteurization Survival	No	No
Inactivation T°		>63.3 (160°F)

2. Virulence Factors

The following steps are required for an active *E. coli* O157:H7 infection to develop: colonization of the intestine, *in situ* replication of the microrganism, evasion of the host immune response, and production of toxins. *E. coli* O157:H7 is considered to be one of the most formidable biological agents that induce disease in humans because of its considerable range of virulence factors, which has been extensively reviewed elsewhere (Law, 2000b; Caprioli et al., 2005). *E. coli* O157:H7 exerts its pathogenic action through the synthesis of adherence factors, haemolytic factors, iron subtraction factors, host immune response evasion factors, and verocytotoxins (VTs). The most important virulent factor of *E. coli* O157:H7 is the synthesis of VTs and the adhesin *intimin*. Virulence factors are encoded on phage, plasmid, or chromosomal genes, but novel or unknown virulence factors may also exist. These pathogenicity determinants have been acquired by *E. coli* O157:H7 via other organisms which are *E. coli* and non- *E. coli* species (Law, 2000a). In the chromosome genes encoding for the VTs are present together with a pathogenicity island called Locus of Enterocyte Effacing (LEE) that contains the information encoding the set of proteins needed for adherence and for the *attaching and effacing lesions* to occur (A/E lesions) (McDaniel and Kaper, 1997). The information required to synthesize enterohemolysin and the fimbriae potentially involved in the colonization of the mucosal gut is present in the characteristic 60 MDa plasmid of *E. coli* O157:H7, designated as the pO157 plasmid (Karch et al., 1987; Schmidt et al., 1995).

2.1. Adherence Factors

Several adherence factors have been shown to exist in *E. coli* O157:H7, but the main pathogenetic role is played by an outer membrane protein (OMP) called *intimin*. This is a 94-97-kDa OMP, made up of 939 aminoacids, encoded by the *eae* gene (*E. coli* attaching and effacing). Besides the gene coding for intimin, LEE contains several genes, such as *EspA*, *EspB*, and *EspD*, and a type III secretion apparatus. All these encode for a few secretory proteins needed for A/E activity, as well as the *Tir* gene that codes for the intimin receptor (Tir: translocated intimin receptor) (Kenny et al., 1997; Sinclair et al., 2006). Intimin produces a characteristic, close adherence of the microorganism to the enterocyte surface known as "attaching and effacing adherence". This mechanism is also typical of EPEC strains in their action on the enterocytes of the small intestine whereas *E. coli* O157:H7 targets the large intestine (Yu and Kaper, 1992). The bacterium/host cell interaction leads to an exchange of biochemical signals resulting in the localized destruction of microvilli (Mead and Griffin, 1998) and the formation of a cup-like structure on the enterocyte surface. The cup-like structure is the result of a rearrangement of the cytoskeletal components of the cytoskeleton and is the place where *E. coli* becomes anchored and causes the A/E lesions (Knutton et al., 1989; Donnenberg et al., 1997; Paton and Paton, 1998). The *E. coli* O157:H7 strains carrying the *eae* gene isolated in HC and HUS cases were more numerous than the *eae* negative strains isolated during these diseases (Paton, and Paton, 1998). It appears that the presence of *eae* is not essential to cause human disease and that *eae* strains may synthesize other yet non-identified virulence factors (Barret et al., 1992), such as fimbriae, other OMPs, and lipopolysaccharides (LPS), which may be involved in enteric cell adhesion (Karch et al., 1987; Fratamico et al., 1993; McKee and O'Brien, 1995). Further studies are needed to shed light on the role of the fimbriae, LPSs, and other structures that may be involved in the complex bacterial cell/enterocyte interaction, especially in the *eae* negative strains.

2.2. Verotoxins (VTs)

The most potent virulence factor of *E. coli* O157:H7 is associated with the synthesis of VTs or Shiga-like toxins (STXs). Although VTs alone cannot induce disease, they are responsible for the severe symptoms of HC and HUS (Mead and Griffin, 1998). Verotoxins are one of the most potent bacterial cytotoxins known and their name comes from the irreversible cytopathic effect they have on monolayers of VERO (African green monkey kidney) cells (Konowalchuk et al., 1977). Verotoxins are also referred to as *Shiga-like toxins* because of the similarity between VT1 and the Shiga toxin produced by Type 1 *Shigella dysenteriae*. The only difference between the two proteins is in one amino acid of the A subunit (Weeratna and Doyle, 1991). VTs are exoproteins with a molecular weight of about 70,000. Antigenically they are distinguished as VT1 and VT2 and are encoded by genes, namely *stx1* and *stx2,* of temperate bacteriophages inserted into the microorganism chromosome (O'Brien and Holmes, 1987). The compositions of VT1 and VT2 are extremely different since VT2 presents only 56% amino acid homology with VT1. VT1 is a relatively homogeneous protein (5 genetic variants have been described so far), while 12 variants of

VT2 have been observed - VT2c, VT2d, VT2e, VT2f, etc. (Ramachandran et al., 2001; Scheutz et al., 2001). Not all the variants of VT2 are produced by *E. coli* O157 or are associated to disease in humans. VT2e has been found in strains of *E. coli* O138, O139, and O140, the agents of piglet edema disease (Konowalchuk et al., 1977), and VT2f is produced by pigeon-adapted *E. coli* strains (Schmidt et al., 2000). VTs have a common structure, made up of the two subunits, A and B. The B subunit has a pentameric structure (MW of each monomer is 5,000-7,000) and it is involved in the binding between the toxin and the cell receptor. The A subunit (MW of 29,000-31,000) is the active part of the toxin. After being proteolytically nicked and reduced to the A_1 fragment, the A subunit inhibits protein synthesis through catalytic interaction with the 60S ribosomal subunit and the inhibition of the peptide chain elongation step of protein synthesis causes cell death (Sandving and van Deurs, 1996). VTs interact with eukaryotic cells through binding of B subunit with its specific receptor, globotryaosilceramide (Gb_3). This receptor is commonly present on the surface of colonic cells, on the surface of the endothelium of renal microvessels, and in VERO cells (Nataro and Kaper, 1998). VT2c is a particular VT subgroup, since it presents poor affinity with Gb_3 and has a smaller effect on the VERO cell line (Lindgren et al., 1994). The VT2e subgroup, instead, binds to the cell receptor, Gb_4 (Nataro and Kaper, 1998).

The biological effects of VTs on laboratory animals vary depending on the species and amount of toxin used. The most sensitive species are rabbits that present with pooling of fluid in the ileal loop, followed by paralysis and death (Keusch et al., 1972). Besides the VERO cells, other cell lines sensitive to the cytopathic effect of VTs are HeLa, Daubi, KB, human liver cells, and human foreskin fibroblasts. By contrast WI-38, Henle 407, CHO, L, BHK, and several other cells of human neoplastic origin are resistant to the action of VTs (Karmali, 1989).

VTEC strains are able in producing one or both VTs simultaneously. While most of the *E. coli* O157:H7 strains produce both VT1 and VT2, having a cytotoxic action on the renal microvessels, only few strains produce VT1. VT2 is known to be about 1000 times more effective than VT1 (Law, 2000b).

To date, few studies have been carried out on the impact food containing preformed VTs may have on human health. VT1 is known to be a relatively heat-stable toxin, hence VT1 produced by VTEC strains may remain active if the food undergoes mild heat treatment, such as pasteurization. VT1 heated at 45-70°C for up to 60 min has been shown to maintain its toxicity while it becomes completely inactivated when heated at 80°C for 60 min or at 85°C for 5 min (Kittel et al., 1991; Weeratna and Doyle, 1991). This issue requires further investigations.

2.3. Enterohemolysin

Most *E. coli* O157:H7 strains synthesize a particular hemolysin called *enterohemolysin* (Ehx). Ehx is encoded by the *hlyA* gene present in the 60-Mda virulence plasmid pO157 which is highly conserved in EHEC strains (Beutin et al., 1989). Unlike *E. coli* alpha-hemolysin, which produces large clear zones of haemolysis on blood agar after few hours of incubation, Ehx produces a small turbid haemolytic zone on washed sheep's blood agar after an incubation of 24 hours. The specific role of enterohaemolysin in the pathogenesis of HUS is still unclear. Enterohaemolysin has been found in most *E. coli* O157:H7 strains isolated from clinical cases but other experiments have shown that this factor is not essential for the development of HC and HUS (Law, 2000b). Ehx may be involved in *E. coli*'s ability to survive in the host organism since it lyses erythrocytes leading to a release of haemoglobin which provides a source of iron for the microorganism to grow in the gut (Law and Kelly, 1995).

2.4. Acid Resistance

The acid resistance of *E. coli* O157:H7 has very important effects both on human disease and food safety. By virtue of its acid tolerance *E. coli* O157:H7 can easily pass the acid barrier of the stomach and reach areas of the intestine where it can bind to the sites of enteric adherence: this biological feature of the microorganism is associated with the extraordinarily low infective dose required to produce illness in humans which ranges from tens to a few hundreds of bacterial cells (Tuttle et al., 1999). Three induction mechanisms of acid resistance have been reported to exist in strains of enterohemorrhagic *E. coli*: oxidative, arginine-dependent, and glutamine-dependent (Lin et al., 1996). Due to these mechanisms the microorganism can survive at pH 2.5 for 2-7 h at 37°C (Buchanan and Doyle, 1997). Nevertheless, the ability of *E. coli* O157:H7 to survive in an acid environment depends on the other growth parameters, the type of acid it is exposed to, temperature and on the growth phase of the microbial population (cells in the stationary phase are more than 1000 times more acid resistant than cells in the exponential phase). The possible contamination of foods with acid resistant bacteria calls for more careful surveillance of foodstuffs. Foods considered to be microbiologically safe because of their low pH value, such as mayonnaise, yoghurt, cured meats, and apple juice can be vehicles of *E. coli* O157:H7 infection (Meng and Doyle, 1998). Tests have shown that *E. coli* O157:H7 can survive for 5-7 weeks in mayonnaise (pH 3.6-3.9), for weeks in yoghurt kept at 4°C, and for 10-31 days in unpasteurized apple juice (pH 3.6-4.0) kept at 8°C (Caprioli et al., 2001).

2.5. Other Virulence Factors

Several other protein factors have been considered to be putative virulence factors synthesized by *E. coli* O157:H7. They include Extracellular Serin Protease (EspP), the *Clostridium-difficile*-like toxin, the enteroaggregative heat-stable toxin (EAST1) the production of Catalase/Peroxidase and the Cytolethal Distending Toxin (Law, 2000b; Janka et al., 2003). The involvement of these factors in the pathogenesis of *E. coli* O157:H7 infection is still to be clarified.

3. Epidemiology

The epidemiology of *E. coli* O157:H7 infections is very complex and still obscure. It is still unclear whether certain animal species are involved in spreading the microrganism. Transmission is known to occur mainly through contaminated foods but, several other routes of infection have been acknowledged. Victims may become infected after swimming in lakes and other recreational waters, and animal-to-person infection via the faecal-oral route may occur especially with school children during farm visits (Table 2). Since reporting the infection is not obligatory in many countries, the data available are an underestimation of the real incidence of *E. coli* illnesses. The epidemiological picture of the infection is far from being complete because no exhaustive information is available about the presence of *E. coli* O157:H7 in animal reservoirs or in foods of animal origin, nor is there any data on the ability of the microrganism to survive in several foodstuffs. Since 1982, when the first outbreak of HC and HUS ascribable to *E. coli* O157:H7 infection was reported (Riley et al., 1983), several outbreaks have been described (Remis et al., 1984). The most significant of these are reported in Table 2.

3.1. Reservoirs

The association between *E. coli* O157:H7 infection and the consumption of bovine meat was evident from the first epidemic outbreak. Several studies subsequently established that cattle are the main reservoir of *E. coli* O157:H7 (Montenegro et al., 1990; Armstrong et al., 1996). Carriers are usually young animals with no clinical signs that intermittently shed *E. coli* O157:H7 into the environment through their faeces, at about 6.8×10^5 CFU/g (Fegan et al., 2004) with a peak during the spring-summer months (Hancock et al., 1997). This seasonality in shedding the germ is consistently reflected in disease presenting in humans during the same months, probably because of an increase in the consumption of barbecued meat during outdoor activities (Chapman, 1995). The absence of clinical signs and symptoms in carriers is another factor enhancing the risk of meat contamination. Since they have no visible signs of infection these animals are regularly slaughtered. Their meat may become contaminated at the slaughterhouse due to spillage from the intestine or because of contact between carcass surface and hide and may thus become the gateway through which the microrganism enters the human food chain. A number of surveys have been carried out to assess the prevalence of cattle carrying and shedding *E. coli* O157:H7 and the percentage of contaminated carcasses. These studies were carried out in many countries and the results were extremely variable. In the US the percentage of bovine carriers ranged from 2 to 45% (Karch et al., 1987; Faith et al., 1998; Elder et al., 2000); in the United Kingdom the prevalence of the microrganism in animals was 15.7% (Chapman et al., 1997), while in other European countries the percentage of animal carriers and contaminated carcasses was 1% to about 37% (Wells et al., 1991; Blanco et al., 1996; Albihn et al., 1997; Heuvelink et al., 1999; Bonardi et al., 1999; Chapman et al., 2001; Bonardi et al., 2001; Guyon et al., 2001). This variability may be due to the differences in sampling criteria, geographic origin, the number of samples analyzed and survey protocols used in the surveys. *E. coli* O157:H7 has

Table 2. Listing of prior *E. coli* O157 outbreaks occurs from 1982 to 2006

Year	Country	Persons Affected	Age	Cases of Hus	Hospital-izations	Deaths	Serotype	Implicated Food; Source of Infection (confirmed by laboratory or by epidemiological evidences)
1985	Canada	73	/	12	19	19	*E. coli* O157:H7	Sandwich meal
1988	Wisconsin	61	/	/	/	/	*E. coli* O157:H7	Roast Beef
1989/90	Missouri (U.S.)	243	/	2	32	4	*E. coli* O157:H7	Municipal water
1991	Massachusett	18	/	/	/	/	*E. coli* O157:H7	Unpasteurized Apple juice
1992/93	California	34	/	/	/	4	*E. coli* O157:H7	Hamburger
1992/93	Washington (U.S.)	501	/	45	151	3	*E. coli* O157:H7	Hamburger
1993	Nevada	58	/	/	/	/	*E. coli* O157:H7	Hamburger
1992/96	England and Wales (U.K.)	381	/	59	120	14	*E. coli* O157	Cold cooked meat; Milk; Raw vegetables; Cooked minced beef dishes
1994	Virginia (U.S.)	156	9/22 years	1	3	0	*E. coli* O157:H7	Raw (red or pink) minced beef
1994	Washington, California (U.S.)	23	23 months/ 77 years	1	6	0	*E. coli* O157:H7	Dry cured salami
1994	Wisconsin	193	Young to middle-aged adults	0	2	0	*E. coli* O157:H7	Undercooked roast beef and salad cross-contaminated
1995	Illinois (U.S.)	12	2/12 years	3	3	0	*E. coli* O157:H7	Lake water
1995	Ontario (Canada)	21	/	0	21	0	*E. coli* O157:H7	Green salad
1995	Bohemia (Czech Republic)	4	Children	4	4	0	*E. coli* O157	Raw goat's milk
1995	Montana (U.S)	92	/	/	/	/	*E. coli* O157	Leaf Lettuce
1995	Oregon (U.S)	11	/	/	/	/	*E. coli* O157	Jan Deer Jerky
1996	Scotland (U.K.)	496	/	/	151	21	*E. coli* O157	Cold cooked meat; Steak pie
1996	Connecticut	14	2/73 years	3	7	0	*E. coli* O157:H7	Unpasteurized apple juice

Year	Country	Persons Affected	Age	Cases of Hus	Hospital-izations	Deaths	Serotype	Implicated Food: Source of Infection (confirmed by laboratory or by epidemiological evidences)
1996	British Columbia, California, Colorado, Washington (U.S.)	45	1/41 years	12	/	0	E. coli O157:H7	Unpasteurized apple juice
1996	Connecticut and Illinois (U.S.)	/	/	/	/	/	E. coli O157:H7	Mesclun mix lettuce
1996	Sakai City (Japan)	9000	/	0	/	/	E. coli O157:H7	White radish sprouts
1997	Michigan (U.S.)	60	2/79 years	2	25	0	E. coli O157:H7	Alfalfa sprouts
1997	Virginia (U.S.)	48	6/67 years	0	11	0	E. coli O157:H7	Alfalfa sprouts
1997	Colorado (U.S.)	15	/	/	/	/	E. coli O157:H7	Hamburger
1997	Finland	14	3/8 years	0	5	0	E. coli O157:H7	Lake water
1997	Fuerteventura (Spain)	14	/	3	/	0	E. coli O157:H7	Raw vegetables
1998	England (U.K.)	7	/	/	4	0	E. coli O157:H7	Unpasteurized cream
1998	Wyoming (U.S.)	157	9/60 years	4	4	0	E. coli O157:H7	Municipal water
1998	Georgia (U.S.)	32	/	/	/	/	E. coli O157:H7	Swimming pool
1998	Ontario (Canada)	39	18 months/ 69 years	2	14	0	E. coli O157:H7	Genoa salami
1998	Washington (U.S.)	12	Children	/	/	/	E. coli O157:H7	School lunch
1999	Ohio (U.S.)	/	/	/	/	/	E. coli O157:H7	Coleslaw
1999	Oklahoma (U.S.)	7	/	/	/	/	E. coli O157:H7	Apple Cider
2000	Barcelona (Spain)	158	Children <5 years old	6	/	0	E. coli O157:H7	Sausages made with pork
2000	New York (U.S.)	1000	/	2	/	2	E. coli O157:H7	Water well located on the fairgrounds
2000	Oregon (U.S.)	171	/	/	/	/	E. coli O157:H7	Fast food
2000	Pennsylvania and Washington (U.S.)	75	1/52 years	9	19	0	E. coli O157:H7	Direct contact with farm animals

Table 2. (Continued)

Year	Country	Persons Affected	Age	Cases of Hus	Hospital-izations	Deaths	Serotype	Implicated Food; Source of Infection (confirmed by laboratory or by epidemiological evidences)
2001	British Columbia (U.S.)	5	1/7 years	2	3	0	*E. coli* O157:H7	Non-pasteurized goat's milk
2002	Connecticut (U.S.)	45	10/90 years	7	24	1	*E. coli* O157:H7; *E. coli* O157:NM	Not identified
2002	Japan	43	1/77 years	0	/	0	*E. coli* O157:H7	Grilled beef
2002	Texas (U.S.)	45	/	0	/	0	*E. coli* O157:H7	Cajun potatoes; Gravy; Rice; Chili.
2002	Colorado California; Iowa; Michigan; South Dakota; Washington; Wyoming (U.S.)	28	1/72 years	5	7	0	*E. coli* O157:H7	Minced beef
2004	Denmark	25	18 children and 7 adults	0	/	0	*E. coli* O157	Milk
2005	Wales (U.K.)	160	Children	/	/	/	*E. coli* O157	Cooked meat at School meals service
2005	Sweden	120	Adults	7	/	7	*E. coli* O157	Iceberg lettuce
2005	Scotland	15	Adults	/	/	/	*E. coli* O157	Not identified
2005	France	26	/	13	20	0	*E. coli* O157:H7	Beefburgers
2006	Norway	7	2/8 years	7	7	0	*E. coli* O157	Minced beef
2006	Scotland	13	4 children and 9 adults	4	4	0	*E. coli* O157	/
2006	Scotland	3	/	0	3	0	*E. coli* O157	/

also been isolated from carcasses in Australia, Canada and Japan (Sekiya, 1997; Power et al., 2000; Philips et al., 2001). Cattle are not the only source of *E. coli* O157:H7 infection for humans since the microorganism has also been isolated from bison, water-buffalo, sheep, goats, pigs, deer, horses, dogs, birds, flies, and other animals (Griffin and Tauxe, 1991; Caprioli et al., 1993; Chapman et al., 2001; Johnsen et al., 2001; Bouvet et al., 2002; Bonardi et al., 2003; Li et al., 2004; Kaufmann et al., 2006). Non-ruminant species are believed to be transient carriers of *E. coli* O157:H7 (Caprioli et al., 2005).

Whether chicken is a potential reservoir of *E. coli* O157:H7 is still unclear. *E. coli* O157:H7 has been shown to colonize the intestine of chickens rapidly as a result of experimental infection, but investigations carried out in order to isolate the microorganism from farm animals provided negative results (Chapman et al., 1997; Heuvelink et al., 1999). Nevertheless, the results of a survey conducted in Slovakia showed that, out of 216 cloacal swabs analyzed, 20 (9.2%) were positive at the *E. coli* O157 detection, but all the isolates tested negative for H7 antigen (Pilipčinec et al., 1999). *E. coli* O157:H7 was isolated from chicken carcasses on the retail market (Doyle and Schoeni, 1987) suggesting that cross-contamination may occur during storage and marketing. Pathogenic strains of *E. coli* O157:H7 have been isolated from specimens of turkey faeces (Heuvelink et al., 1999).

The environment is a continuous source of contamination along the beef chain. *E. coli* O157:H7 can survive and replicate in animal feeds and in sedimented water on farms. It remains infective in water for at least six months and may thus survive and spread on farms during periods when it cannot be detected in cattle, especially during cold months (Hancock et al., 2001). *E. coli* O157:H7 has been frequently isolated from surfaces (walls, floors, ceilings, etc.) on the farm (24%), from the surfaces of the animal transport vehicles (7.3%), and from surfaces at slaughterhouses (7.8%) (Buncic et al., 2004). Finally, humans may also potentially spread *E. coli* O157:H7 since person-to-person infection and asymptomatic carriers have been identified in nursing home, hospitals daycares and among abattoir workers and others working in close contact with cattle and beef carcasses. When proper personal hygiene is not maintained, these individuals may be a source of food contamination and may cause secondary person-to-person spread.

3.2. Foods

Various foods have been implicated as potential vehicles in incidents or outbreaks of *E. coli* O157:H7 infections: burgers, minced beef, sausages, wurstels, turkey rolls, unpasteurized cow, sheep, and goat milk, cheese made from raw milk, vegetables, unchlorinated drinking water and others (Tab. 2). The fact that *E. coli* O157:H7 may be present in foods of animal origin and in the environment is predictable. Carcasses are mainly contaminated during slaughtering (skinning, evisceration, equipment tools), while meat products (ground meat, etc.) may be cross-contaminated during storage, processing, and marketing. Similarly, milk may become contaminated on the farm or cross-contaminated at processing facilities (McKee et al., 2003). Vegetables, such as coleslaw, alfalfa sprouts, and lettuce have been associated with outbreaks of *E. coli* O157:H7 infections (Sanz et al., 2003), and may become contaminated by manure from infected animals or by contaminated irrigation water. Sea foods may probably become contaminated by *E. coli* O157:H7 present in water from human or animal waste. Food safety issues are raised by the ability of *E. coli* O157:H7 to survive in ready-to-eat foods that have been processed to become microbiologically safe for their low pH (yoghurt, mayonnaise, and dry fermented salami) and have however caused infection outbreaks. After an important outbreak involving 20 laboratory-confirmed cases of *E. coli* O157:H7 diarrhoea associated with commercially distributed dry-cured salami in Washington and California (Centers for Diseases Control and Prevention, 1995), several studies have been carried out on the ability of *E. coli* O157:H7 to survive and produce toxins after maturation. These studies showed that the microbial load of *E. coli* O157:H7 gradually decreases by about a logarithm a week during maturation of cured meats (Normanno et al., 2002). Hence, the safety of these foods depends on the bacterial load contaminating the raw material at the time of sausage making and on the diameter of the salami as larger diameters require longer curing.

Many surveys have been performed to assess the presence of *E. coli* O157:H7 in several foodstuffs such as ground meat, cured meat, milk, cheese, and vegetables (Pradel et al., 2000; Coia et al., 2001; Normanno et al., 2002; Stampi et al., 2004; Normanno et al., 2004). Hussein and Bollinger (2005) reported a global prevalence rates of *E. coli* O157:H7 in beef (whole carcasses, ground, sausage, etc.) ranges from 0.01 to 54.2%.

The results differed greatly with values ranging from very low to very high detection rates probably because the sampling methods used, foodstuffs considered and detection protocols were broadly different.

3.3. Prevalence and Economic Burden

The incidence of *E. coli* O157:H7 infections is substantially low compared to other foodborne pathogens. In 2000, the incidence of human *E. coli* O157:H7 infection per 100,000 persons was 4.10 for Scotland and 2.36 for Northern Ireland (McKee et al., 2003).

It is estimated that in the US there are annually over 73,000 infections and about 60 deaths annually due to *E. coli* O157:H7 infections (Mead et al., 1999). However, the data for 2003 showed that the incidence of *E. coli* O157 infections was 42% lower in the US than in previous years, with 443 laboratory-diagnosed cases (Center For Diseases Control and Prevention, 2004). In 2002 more than 2500 human infections or HUS were reported in the European Union (Kasbohrer, 2004).

The target risk groups are children and the elderly. The highest isolation rate is in the 0-4 year-old group followed by the 5-14 year-old group and the group over 65 (Simmons, 1997).

In a recent study it has been estimated that the yearly cost due to the illnesses caused by O157 infections is about $405 millions of which $370 millions for premature deaths, $30 millions for medical treatments, and $5 millions in productivity losses (Frenzen et al., 2005).

4. Pathology

E. coli O157:H7 infections present a wide spectrum of clinical manifestations ranging from asymptomatic carriage and uncomplicated non-bloody diarrhea to severe illness, including bloody diarrhea and renal failure. Papers of clinical interest present an extensive overview of the pathological features of the infection (Riley, 1987; Karmali, 1989; Nataro and Kaper, 1998; Tkalcic et al., 2003), while this review outlines the main pathogenetic and clinical aspects of the most important diseases associated with the infection: Hemorrhagic Colitis (HC) and the Hemolytic Uraemic Syndrome (HUS). After oral ingestion of *E. coli* O157:H7 and its passage through the acid barrier of the stomach, the microrganism adheres to enterocytes causing A/E lesions and non-bloody diarrhea. The average incubation period is 3 days ranging from 1 to 8 days. At this stage the infection may resolve or continue through replication of *E. coli* O157:H7 and VT production with toxemia. Infection progress to HUS is about 2 to 15% of cases (Dundas et al., 2001) and some risk factors for HUS have been individuated in sex (i.e. females), age (i.e. <5 years), elevated leukocyte count (> 13,000/μL), vomiting, fever, >3 days diarrhea and proteinuria (Rowe et al., 1991; Tserenpuntsag, 2005). The VTs induce microangiopathic lesions in the microvessels of the bowel (HC) and kidneys (HUS), with fibrin/platelet thrombi, capillary occlusion and swelling of the endothelial cells (Karmali, 1989). HC is characterized by severe bloody diarrhea and abdominal pains. In most cases the symptoms will resolve without sequelae. However, in about 10% of young patients (≤ 10 years) the illness will progress to HUS, a syndrome characterized by microangiopathic haemolytic anaemia, thrombocytopenia, renal failure, and central nervous system symptoms. The mortality rate is 3-5% (Nataro and Kaper, 1998). Many survivors (12 to 30%) present severe life-threatening sequelae, including chronic renal failure, hypertension, and neurological symptoms (headache, lethargy, and convulsions). Antibiotic therapy for the management of acute illness may lead to further complications. The case fatality rate ranges from 3 to 7% (Griffin and Tauxe, 1991). The most important clinical features of *E. coli* O157:H7 infection are summarized in Table 3 (Todd and Dundas, 2001).

Table 3. Clinical features of *E. coli* O157 infection (Todd and Dundas, 2001 modified)

Clinical features	Percentage incidence
Vomiting	30-60
Fever	< 30
Abdominal pain	70-80
Diarrhea	95
Diarrhea with blood	>70
Complication rate (HUS)	2-15 in sporadic, 20 in some outbreaks
Asymptomatic infection	10-15
Fatality rate	3-7

5. Detection from Foods

Over the course of time, comprehensive reviews on the methods used for detecting *E. coli* O157:H7 in foods and clinical samples have appeared in the literature (Remis et al., 1984; Padhye and Doyle, 1992; Meng et al., 1994; Phillips, 1999; Chapman, 2000; Bettelheim and Beutin, 2003). Traditional procedures for detecting *E. coli* in foods are unlikely to detect *E. coli* O157:H7 because of specific physiological characteristics of this serotype (Tab. 1). Since the infective dose of *E. coli* O157:H7 is low, sensitive and specific techniques for its detection in food are needed. Rapid and sensitive detection of viable *E. coli* O157 cells, in food is a critical step in the development of effective strategies for the control of the infections. Several methods have been developed for the detection of *E. coli* O157:H7 in food and clinical samples, but to date no universally accepted protocol or "gold standard" method exists for the detection, isolation, and characterization of these bacteria. One obstacle to establishing a method for the detection of *E. coli* O157:H7 in foods is that the indigenous microflora in samples is generally present in greater amounts than few bacterial units of the germ sought for. Another constraint is represented by the correct identification and characterization of isolates, which require serological, biological, and molecular investigations. In terms of risk analysis, the isolation of the strain is not enough and the presence of virulence factors needs to be determined because they might be absent in some *E. coli* O157:H7 strains. Moreover many selective isolation media are based on *E. coli* O157's inability to ferment sorbitol in 24 hours while infections from sorbitol-fermenting strains are becoming more frequent, especially in Europe (Karch and Bielaszewsca, 2001). The method providing the most comprehensive results is based on a selective culture of *E. coli* O157:H7 from which the isolated strains can be typed. One protocol is commonly used in several laboratories and requires neither specialized personnel nor particularly sophisticated equipment while providing satisfactory results. It includes a phase of selective enrichment in modified Tryptone Soy Broth or EC broth added with novobiocin (20mg/l) and incubated at 41±0.5°C for 6-18h, followed by immunomagnetic separation (IMS) and isolation on a selective and differential solid medium, such as Cefixime (0.05mg/l)- Potassium Tellurite (2.5mg/l) (CT)-SMAC, or in a chromogenic medium (ISO 16654, 2001). IMS may be used to capture the target bacteria cells from interfering foodstuffs and concentrate them in a small volume. This step remarkably improves the sensitivity of detection by cultural methods and reduces total analysis time (Wright et al., 1994, Islam et al., 2006). Suspect colonies can be screened for O157 LPS using serological methods (ELISA, latex reagents, etc.) and then identified by biochemical reactions. Once the strain is identified, the presence of virulence factors can be assessed using molecular methods, such as PCR or hybridization with DNA probes for the detection of *eae*, *stx*1 and *stx*2 genes. Biological or serological methods (VERO cell assay, ELISA, RPLA, etc) are useful tools for the evaluation of VT production.

Another approach to detect *E. coli* O157:H7 in foods consists in the screening of the samples (generally after a selective enrichment step) using specific markers for *E. coli* O157 and isolating the microorganism by a selective plating. In fact, molecular techniques (such as PCR, Multiplex-PCR, Real Time-PCR, IMS-PCR, Quantitative Competitive-PCR, etc.) for the detection of genetic markers of virulence, immunoassays for the detection of the O157 antigen, as well as biological assays such as the VERO cell test, are usually employed to directly detect *E. coli* O157:H7 from foods. Nonetheless, each of these methods may have limitations and the results they provide should always be confirmed by isolation and characterization of the strain.

6. Preventing and Control Measures

E. coli O157:H7 infections are a serious public health issue since they can cause epidemic outbreaks affecting many persons with cases of mortality. The epidemiology and control of the infection are rather complex. Since several animals may act as reservoirs, many foods of animal origin (meat and milk) may be contaminated. Faecal contamination of the environment may lead to the contamination of vegetables and water. Moreover, because of its high acid resistance, *E. coli* O157:H7 may persist in processed foods such as cheeses and cured meat. Nevertheless, the infection may be controlled by acting at three levels: the farm, the slaughterhouse (with proper sanitary practices), and the public at large (with information about the safe use of foods).

6.1. Farm

Eradication of the infection on farms where cattle are reared is difficult. The strategies proposed include immunization with different types of vaccines, the administration of probiotics, competitive exclusion treatment or phage therapy (Zhao et al., 1998; Kudva et al., 1999; Tkalcic et al., 2003). These approaches cannot fully ensure eradication of the infection on a farm, and require further investigations. Proper sanitary practices and good hygiene are much more effective as infection control measures. They include changing beverage water frequently, cleaning troughs, reducing faecal contamination of feeds, and the frequent removal and correct disposal of manure (storage and spreading as a soil amendment). Manure is an important source of infection on the farm and for the contamination of fertilized vegetable products, since it has been demonstrated that *E. coli* O157:H7 can survive in bovine faeces from 1 to 18 weeks and for 231 days at 21°C in manure-amended autoclaved soil (Fukushima et al., 1999; Jiang et al., 2002). Furthermore, cattle drinking water represents a source of *E. coli* O157:H7 in farms (Zhao et al., 2006). In addition, in a recent study conducted in order to determine the survival timing of the pathogen in different biological matters, it has been showed that the microorganism survives 97 and 109 days in bovine faeces and water respectively (Scott et al., 2006).

Precautions to be taken during school visits to livestock farms are extremely important. Several cases of infection in school-age children have been ascribed to contact with animals or tasting raw milk on these occasions (Tozzi et al., 2001).

6.2. Slaughterhouse

In abattoirs, a critical point in the meat production chain, the consistent use of Good Hygienic Practices at slaughtering, especially during skinning and evisceration, may considerably reduce the percentages of contaminated carcasses. Particular care should be taken to ensure cleanliness of the hide and sanitation of the stunning box. Recent studies have pointed out that stunning boxes may be an important source of contamination for the hide given that the on-hide median prevalence of positive cattle at slaughter units is 23.6% (Buncic et al., 2004; Small et al., 2005). Pre-skinning decontamination, proper removal of the gastrointestinal tract, avoidance of direct carcass-carcass contact, and frequent disinfection of utensils and surfaces can reduce the percentages of contaminated carcasses at slaughterhouses. Finally, several methods have been proposed to decontaminate carcasses at the end of the processing cycle (washing with hot water, the use of steam, organic acids, gamma radiation, ozone, etc.) (Castillo et al., 2003). Each has limits in terms of applicability and efficiency, at times for technical and/or prescriptive reasons.

6.3. Food Industry and Home

Health education and information on safe food handling and preparation practices may effectively reduce the infection rates. Cooking ground beef to the point that typical strains of salmonellae are killed will also kill *E. coli* O157:H7. Pasteurization of milk (72°C for 16.2 s) will kill more than 10^4 *E. coli* O157:H7 per ml (Doyle, 1991). *E. coli* O157 is more heat-sensitive than salmonellae and is killed by heating to an internal temperature of 68.3°C. Cooking raw meats to an internal temperature of 70°C for two minutes (until there are no pink areas left inside) or an equivalent treatment will provide effective means of preventing infection (Advisory Committee on the microbiological Safety of Food, 1995).

Special care should be taken in the production of ready-to-eat foods such as fermented salami, especially in countries where manufacturing regulations do not prescribe a technological procedure for the reduction of the bacterial load contaminating the mixture before sausage making. It would be appropriate to constantly check the microbiological quality of the raw materials used and perform challenge tests by experimentally inoculating the mixtures to check whether the processing procedure used reduces the load of *E. coli* O157:H7 in the finished product by at least 5 log (Faith, 1998).

Strict observance of hygienic and sanitary practices during food preparation is very important, especially in mass catering services. Accurate washing of vegetables, cleansing of work surfaces, uninterrupted refrigeration of stored foods (4°C), and especially care taken to avoid cross-contamination of raw, cooked and ready-to-eat foods can dramatically reduce the risk of infection.

7. Conclusion

The microbiological safety of food needs to be carefully assessed. The evaluation of potential risks derived from the presence of *E. coli* O157:H7 in foods is an important aspect of assessment of food safety that has not received much attention in the past. To provide the scientific basis for decisions regarding human health, new methods and policies to assess such food safety need to be developed and agreed upon internationally. A this proposal, since 1st January 2006, in European Community is come into force a new body of legislation on the hygiene, safety and control of foods. This regulation includes several Regulations (European Regulation n. 178/2002, 852/2004, 853/2004, 854/2004, 2073/2005, 2074/2005 and others) and aimed to guarantee a high level of safety of foodstuff produced and marketed in EC. Surprisingly, the Reg. (CE) 2073/2005, dealing with the microbiological criteria applicable on foods, considers that the application of microbiological criteria for *E. coli* O157 for the control of the microbiological safety of foods is unlikely to reduce significantly the infection risks for consumers. Nevertheless, it underlines that the application of Good Manufacturing Practices in order to reduce the fecal contamination of foods during the producing chain may constitute a helpful tool for reducing the number of infections due to *E. coli* O157.

In conclusion, an efficient risk analysis for preventing *E. coli* O157:H7 infection requires further investigations. Investigations are needed to shed light on the actual prevalence of *E. coli* O157:H7 in animals acting as reservoirs and in foods of animal origin (using standardized protocols), on its ability to survive in several types of processed foods, and on the likelihood of intoxications due to the presence of preformed VTs in food. Reduction and control of this dangerous infection are predicated on the realization of effective surveillance systems, infection case-studies, and proper health education of food industry personnel handling products "from farm to fork". Finally, efficient food labelling can ensure the provision of adequate information to consumers on safe food preparation practices.

In this perspective, further efforts are needed to integrate medical and veterinary expertise in order to improve competencies and scientific knowledge about the epidemiology of the disease, the ecology of the pathogen along with its behaviour both in the food chain and in complex foods (i.e. fermented and ready to eat foods) and detection methods of the microrganism from foods.

Finally, clear communication of the basis for safety assessment in this area is generally lacking at national and international levels. For this reason, governments all over the world should intensify their efforts to improve food safety in response to an increasing number of food safety problems and rising consumer concerns.

Acknowledgments

The author is grateful to Dr. N.C. Quaglia for her assistance, suggestions, criticism and for her invaluable help in consulting literature cited and table draft.

References

Advisory Committee on the microbiological Safety of Food. 1995. Report on Vero Cytotoxin-producing *Escherichia coli*. *HMSO*, London.

Albihn, A., Zimmernan, U., Rehbinder, V., Jansson, V., Tysén, E., Engvall, A., 1997. Enterohemorrhagic *E. coli* (EHEC)- a nation wide Swedish survey of bovine faeces. *Epidémiol.* Santé Anim. 4, 31-32.

Armstrong, G.L., Hollingsworth, J., Morris, J.G. Jr, 1996. Emerging foodborne pathogens: *Escherichia coli* O157:H7 as a model of entry of a new pathogen into the food supply of the developed countries. *Epidemiol. Rev.* 18, 29-51.

Barret, T.J., Kaper, J.B., Jerse, A.E., Wachsmut, I.K., 1992. Virulence factors in Shiga Toxin-producing *Escherichia coli* isolated from humans and cattle. *J. Infect. Dis*. 165, 979-980.

Batt, C.A., 2000. *Escherichia coli*. In: Robinson, R., Batt, C., and Patel, P. (Ed.), *Encyclopedia of Food Microbiology*, vol. 1. Academic Press, New York, pp. 633-640.

Bettelheim, K.A., and Beutin, L., 2003. Rapid laboratory identification and characterization of verocytotoxigenic (Shiga toxin producing) *Escherichia coli* (VTEC/STEC). *J. Appl. Microbiol.* 95, 205-217.

Beutin, L., Montenegro, M.A., Orskov, I., Prada, J., Zimmermann, S., Stephan, R., 1989. Close association of verotoxin (Shiga-like toxin) production with enterohemolysin production in strains of *Escherichia coli*. *J. Clin. Microbiol.* 27, 2559-2564.

Blanco, M., Blanco, J.E., Blanco, J., Gonzales, E.A., Mora, A., Prado, C., Fernandez, L., Rio, M., Ramos, J., Alonso, M.P., 1996. Prevalence and characteristics of *Escherichia coli* serotypes O157:H7 and other verocytotoxin-producing *Escherichia coli* in healthy cattle. *Epidemiol. Infect.* 117, 251-257.

Bonardi, S., Brindani, V., Pizzin, G., Lucidi, L., D'Incau, M., Liebana, E., Morabito, S., 2003. Detection of *Salmonella* spp., *Yersinia enterocolitica* and verocytotoxin-producing *E. coli* O157 in pigs at slaughter in Italy. *Int. J. Food Microbiol.* 85, 101-110.

Bonardi, S., Maggi, E., Bottarelli, A., Pacciarini, M.L., Ansuini, A., Vellini, G., Morabito, S., Caprioli, A., 1999. Isolation of Verocytotoxin-producing *Escherichia coli* O157:H7 from cattle at slaughter in Italy. *Vet. Microbiol.* 67, 203-211.

Bonardi, S., Maggi, E., Pizzin, G., Morabito, S., Caprioli, A., 2001. Faecal carriage of verocytotoxin-producing *Escherichia coli* O157 and carcass contamination in cattle at slaughter in northern Italy. *Int. J. Food Microbiol.* 66, 47-53.

Bouvet, J., Montet, M.P., Rossel, R., Le Roux, A., Bavai, C., Ray-Gueniot, S., Mazuy, C., Atrache, V., Vernozy-Rozand, C., 2002. Prevalence of verocytotoxin producing *Escherichia coli* (VTEC) and *E. coli* O157 in French pork. *J. Appl. Microbiol.* 93, 7-14.

Buchanan, R.L., and Doyle, M.P., 1997. Foodborne significance of *Escherichia coli* O157:H7 and other enterohemorrhagic *E. coli*. *Food Technology* 51, 69-76.

Buncic, S., Avery, S.M., and De Zutter, L., 2004. Epidemiology of *Escherichia coli* O157 in cattle from farm to fork. pp. 67-84. *Proceedings of International EU-RAIN Conference*, Padua, Italy, 2-3 Dec.

Caprioli, A., Lucangeli, C., Severini, M., 2001. *Escherichia coli* O157. In: De Felip, G. (Ed.), Recenti sviluppi di igiene e microbiologia degli alimenti. *Tecniche nuove*, Italy, pp. 625-641.

Caprioli, A., Morabito, S., Brugère, H., Oswald, E., 2005. Enterohaemorragic *Escherichia coli*: emerging issues on virulence and modes of transmission. *Vet. Res.* 36, 289-311.

Caprioli, A., Nigrelli, A., Gatti, R., Zavanella, M., Blando, A.M., Minelli, F., and Donelli, G., 1993. Characterization of verocytotoxin- producing *Escherichia coli* isolated from pigs and cattle in northern Italy. *Vet. Rec.* 133, 323-324.

Castillo, A., McKenzie, K.S., Lucia, L.M., Acuff, G.R., 2003. Ozone treatment for reduction of *Escherichia coli* O157:H7 and *Salmonella* serotype *Typhimurium* on beef carcasses surfaces. *J. Food Prot.* 66, 775-779.

Center For Diseases Control and Prevention. 2004. Preliminary FoodNet data on the incidence of infection with pathogens transmitted commonly through food- Selected sites, US, 2003. *Morbidity and Mortality Weekly Report* 2004, 53, 338-342.

Centers for Diseases Control and Prevention. 1995. *Escherichia coli* O157:H7 outbreak linked to commercially distributed dry-cured salami- Washington and California, 1994. *Morbidity and Mortality Weekly Report*, 44.

Chapman, P.A., 1995. Verocytotoxin-producing *Escherichia coli*: an overview with emphasis on the epidemiology and prospects for control of *E. coli* O157. *Food Control* 4, 187-193.

Chapman, P.A., 2000. Methods available for the detection of *Escherichia coli* O157 in clinical, food and environmental samples. *W. J. Microbiol. Biotechnol.* 16, 733-740.

Chapman, P.A., Cerdàn Malo, A.T., Ellin, M., Ashton, R., Harkin, M.A., 2001. *Escherichia coli* O157 in cattle and sheep at slaughter, on beef and lamb carcasses, and in raw beef and lamb products in South Yorkshire, UK. *Int. J. Food Microbiol.* 64, 139-150.

Chapman, P.A., Siddons, C.A., Malo, A.T.C., Harkin, M.A., 1997. A one year study of *Escherichia coli* O157 in cattle, sheep, pigs, and poultry. Epidemol. Infect. 119, 245-250.

Clarke, S.C., 2001. Diarrhoegenic *Escherichia coli* – an emerging problem? *Diagn. Microbiol. Infect. Dis.* 41, 93-98.

Coia, J.E., Jhonston, Y., Steers, N.J., Halson, M.F., 2001. A survey of *Escherichia coli* O157 in raw meats, raw cow's milk and raw milk cheeses in south-east Scotland. *Int. J. Food Microbiol.* 66, 63-69.

Commission Regulation (EC) No 2073/2005 of 15 November 2005 on microbiological criteria for foodstuffs. *Official Journal of the European Union L.* 338 of 22 December 2005.

Donnenberg, M.S., Kaper, J.B., Finlay, B.B., 1997. Interactions between enteropathogenic *Escherichia coli* and host epithelial cells. *Trends Microbiol.* 5, 109-114.

Doyle, M.P., 1991. *Escherichia coli* O157:H7 and its significance in foods. *Int. J. Food Microbiol.* 12, 289-302.

Doyle, M.P., and Schoeni, J.L., 1984. Survival and growth characteristics of *Escherichia coli* associated with hemorrhagic colitis. *Appl. Environ. Microbiol.* 48, 855-856.

Doyle, M.P., and Schoeni, J.L., 1987. Isolation of *Escherichia coli* O157:H7 in meats and poultry. *Appl. Environ. Microbiol.* 53, 2394-2396.

Doyle, M.P., Padhye, V.V., 1989. *Escherichia coli*. p. In: Doyle, M.P. (Ed.), *Foodborne Bacterial Pathogens*. Marcel Dekker, New York, pp. 235-271.

Drasar, B.S., and Hill, M.J., 1974. *Human intestinal flora*. Academic Press, Ltd., London, UK.

Dundas, S., Todd W.T., Stewart, A.I., Murdoc, P.S., Chaudhuri, A.K.R., Hutchinson, S.J. 2001. The central Scotland *Escherichia coli* O157:H7 outbreak: risk factor for hemolytic uremic syndrome and death among hospitalized patients. *Clin. Infect. Dis*. 33, 923-931.

Elder, R.O., Keen, J.E., Siragusa, G.R., Barkocy-Gallagher, G.A., Koohmaraie, M., Laegreid, W., 2000. Correlation of enterohemorrhagic *Escherichia coli* O157 prevalence in faeces, hides, and carcasses of beef cattle during processing. *Proc. Natl. Acad. Sci. USA* 97, 2999-3003.

Faith, N.G., Parniere, N., Larson, T., Lorang, T.D., Kaspar, C.W., Luchansky, J.B., 1998. Viability of *Escherichia coli* O157:H7 in salami following conditioning of batter, fermentation, and drying of sticks, and storage of slices. *J. Food Prot*. 61, 377-382.

Fegan, N., Higgs, G., Vanderlinde, P., and Desmarchelier, P., 2004. Enumeration of *Escherichia coli* O157 in cattle faeces using the most probable number technique and automated immunomagnetic separation. *Lett. Appl. Microbiol*. 38, 56-59.

Feng, P., Lampel, K.A., Karch, H., and Whittam, T.S., 1998. Genotypic and phenotypic changes in the emergence of *Escherichia coli* O157:H7. *J. Infect. Dis*. 177, 1750-1753.

Fratamico, P.M., Bhaduri, S., Buchanan, R.L., 1993. Studies on *E. coli* serotype O157:H7 strains containing a 60-Mda plasmid and on 60-Mda plasmid-cured derivatives. *J. Med. Microbiol*. 39, 371-381.

Frenzen, P.D., Drake, A., Angulo, F.J., 2005. Emerging Infections Program FoodNet Working Group. Economic cost of illness due to *Escherichia coli* O157 infection in the United States. *J. Food Prot*. 68, 2623-2630.

Fukushima, H., Hoshina, K., Gomyoda, M., 1999. Long-term survival of Shiga toxin-producing *Escherichia coli* O26, O111, and O157 in bovine faeces. *Appl. Environ. Microbiol*. 65, 5177-5181.

Griffin, P.M., Tauxe, R.V., 1991. The epidemiology of infections caused by *Escherichia coli* O157:H7, other enterohemorrhagic *E. coli*, and the associated hemolytic uraemic syndrome. *Epidemiol. Rev*. 13, 60-98.

Gunzer, F., Bohm, H., Russman, H., Bitzan, M., Aleksic, S., Karch, H., 1992. Molecular detection of sorbitol fermenting *Escherichia coli* O157 in patients with hemolytic-uraemic syndrome. *J. Clin. Microbiol*. 30, 1807-1810.

Guyon, R., Dorey, F., Malas, J.P., Grimont, F., Foret, J., Rouviere, B., Collobert, J.F., 2001. Superficial contamination of bovine carcasses by *Escherichia coli* O157:H7 in a slaughterhouse in Normandy (France). *Meat Sci*. 58, 329-331.

Hancock D.D., Besser, T.E., Rice, D.H., Herriott, D.E., Tar, P.I., 1997. A longitudinal study of *Escherichia coli* O157 in fourteen cattle herds. *Epidemiol. Infect*. 118, 193-195.

Hancock, D., Besser, T., Lejeune, J., Davis, M., Rice, D., 2001. The control of VTEC in animal reservoir. *Int. J. Food Microb*. 66, 71-78.

Heuvelink, A.E., Zwartkruis, J.T.M., van den Biggelaar, F.L.A.M., van Leeuwen, W.J., de Boer, E., 1999. Isolation and characterization of verocytotox-producing *Escherichia coli* O157 from slaughter pigs and poultry. *Int. J. Food Microbiol*. 52, 67-75.

Hussein H.S., Bollinger, L.M., 2005. Prevalence of shiga toxin-producing *Escherichia coli* in beef. *J. Food Prot*. 68, 2224-2241.

Islam, A.M., Heuvelink, A.E., Talukder, K.A., de Boer, E., 2006. Immunoconcentration of Shiga toxin-producing *Escherichia coli* O157 from animal faeces and raw meats by using

Dynabeads anti-*E. coli* O157 and the VIDAS system. *Int. J. Food Microbiol.* 109,151-156.

ISO 16654, 2001. Microbiology of food and animal feeding stuffs. Horizontal method for the detection of *Escherichia coli* O157.

Janka, A., Bielaszewsca, M., Dobrindt, U., Greune, L., Schimdt, M.A., and Karch, H., 2003. Cytolethal distending toxin gene cluster in enterohemorragic *Escherichia coli* O157:H⁻ and *Escherichia coli* O157:H7: characterization and evolutionary considerations. *Infect. Immun.* 71, 3634-3638.

Jiang, X., Morgan, J., Doyle, M.P., 2002. Fate of *Escherichia coli* O157:H7 in manure-amended soil. *Appl. Environ. Microbiol.* 68, 2605-2609.

Johnsen, G., Wasteson, Y., Heir, E., I. Berget, O., Herikstad, H., 2001. *Escherichia coli* O157:H7 in faeces from cattle, sheep and pigs in the southwest part of Norway during 1998 and 1999. *Int. J. Food Microbiol.* 65, 193-200.

Karch, H., and Bielaszewsca, M., 2001. Sorbitol-fermenting Shiga toxin producing *Escherichia coli* O157:H⁻ strains: epidemiology, phenotypic and molecular characteristics, and microbiological diagnosis. *J. Clin. Microbiol.* 39, 2043-2049.

Karch, H., Heesemann, J., Lauls, R., O'Brien, A.D., Tacket, C.O., Levine, M.M., 1987. A plasmid of enterohemorrhagic *Escherichia coli* O157:H7 is required for expression of a new fimbrial antigen and for adhesion to epithelial cells. *Infect. Immun.* 55, 455-461.

Karmali, M.A., 1989. Infection by verotoxin-producing *Escherichia coli*. *Clin. Microbiol. Rev.* 2, 15-38.

Kasbohrer, A., 2004. Current European trends in foodborne zoonoses. 1-3. *Proceedings of International EU-RAIN Conference*, Padua, Italy, 2-3 Dec.

Kaufmann, M., Zweifel, C., Blanco, M., Blanco, J.E., Blanco, J., Beutin, L., Stephan, R. 2006. *Escherichia coli* O157 and non-O157 Shiga toxin-producing *Escherichia coli* in fecal samples of finished pigs at slaughter in Switzerland. *J. Food Prot.* 69, 260-266.

Kenny, B., DeVinney, R., Stein, M., Reinscheid, D.J., Frey, E.A., Finlay, B.B., 1997. Enteropathogenic *E. coli* (EPEC) transfers its receptor for intimate adherence into mammalian cells. *Cell* 91, 511-520.

Keusch, G.T., Grady, G.F., Mata, L.J., McIver, J., 1972. The pathogenesis of *Shigella diarrhea* 1. Enterotoxin production of *Shigella dysenteriae* 1. *J. Clin. Invest.* 51, 1212-1218.

Kittel, F.B., Padhey, N.V., and Doyle, M.P., 1991. Characterization and inactivation of verotoxin-1 produced by *Escherichia coli* O157:H7. *J. Agr. Food Chem.* 39, 141-145.

Knutton, S., Baldwin, T., Williams, P.H., McNeisch, A. S., 1989. Actin accumulation at sites of bacterial adhesion to tissue culture cells: basis of a new diagnostic test for enteropathogenic and enterohemorrhagic *Escherichia coli*. *Infect. Immun.* 57, 1290-1298.

Konowalchuk, J., Speirs, J.I., Stavric, S., 1977. Vero response to a cytotoxin of *Escherichia coli*. *Infect. Immun.* 18, 775-779.

Kudva, I.T., Jelacic, S., Tarr, P.I., Youderian, P., Hovde, C., 1999. Biocontrol of *Escherichia coli* O157 with O157-specific bacteriophages. Appl. Environ. Microbiol. 65, 3767-3773.

Law, D., 2000a. The history and evolution of *Escherichia coli* O157 and other shiga toxin-producing *E. coli*. *World J. Microbiol. Biotechnol.* 16, 701-709.

Law, D., 2000b. Virulence factors of *Escherichia coli* O157 and other shiga toxin-producing *E. coli. J. Appl. Microbiol.* 88, 729-745.

Law, D., Kelly, J., 1995. Use of heme and hemoglobin by *Escherichia coli* O157 and other Shiga-like-toxin-producing *Escherichia coli* serogroups. *Infect. Immun.* 63, 700-702.

Li, Q., Sherwood, S.J., Logue, C.M., 2004. The prevalence of *Listeria, Salmonella, Escherichia coli* and *E. coli* O157 on bison carcasses during processing. *Food Microbiol.* 21, 791-799.

Lin, J., Smith, M.P., Chapin, K.C., Baik, H.S., Bennet, G.N., Foster, J.W., 1996. Mechanism of acid resistance in enterohemorragic *Escherichia coli. Appl. Environ. Microbiol.* 62, 3094-3100.

Lindgren, S.W., Samuel, J.E., Schmitt, C.K., O'Brien, A.D., 1994. The specific activities of Shiga toxin type (SLT-II) and SLT-II related toxins of enterohemorragic *Escherichia coli* differ when measured by Vero cell cytotoxicity but not by mouse lethality. *Infect. Immun.* 62, 623-631.

McDaniel, T.K., Kaper, J.B., 1997. A cloned pathogenicity island from enteropathogenic *E. coli* confers the attaching and effacing phenotype on *E. coli* K-12. *Mol. Microbiol.* 23, 399-407.

McKee, M.L., O'Brien, A.D., 1995. Investigation of enterohemorragic *E. coli* O157:H7 adherence characteristics and invasion potential reveals new attachment pattern shared by intestinal *E. coli. Infect. Immun.* 63, 2070-2074.

McKee, R., Madden, R.H., Gilmur, A., 2003. Occurrence of verocytotoxin producing *Escherichia coli* in dairy and meat processing environments. *J. Food Protect.* 66, 1576-1580.

Mead, P.S., and Griffin, P.M., 1998. *Escherichia coli* O157. *Lancet* 352, 1207-1212.

Mead, P.S., Slutscker, L., Dietz, V., McCaig, L.F., Bresee, J.S., Shapiro, C., Griffin, M.P., Tauxe, R.V., 1999. Food-related ilnesses in the United States. *Emerg. Infect. Dis.* 5, 607-625.

Meng, J., and Doyle, M.P., 1998. Microbiology of Shiga toxin-producing *Escherichia coli* in foods. In: Kaper, J.B., and O'Brien, A.D. (Ed.), *Escherichia coli* O157:H7 and other Shiga toxin-producing *E. coli* strains. *American Society for Microbiology*, Washington, D.C., pp. 92-108.

Meng, J., Doyle, M.P., Zhao, T., and Zhao, S., 1994. Detection and control of *Escherichia coli* O157:H7 in foods. *Trends F. Sci. Technol.* 5, 179-185.

Montenegro, M.A., Bulte, M., Trumpf, T., Aleksic, S., Rauter, G., Helmut, R., 1990. Detection and characterization of faecal vero-toxin-producing *Escherichia coli* O157 from healthy cattle. *J. Clin. Microbiol.* 28, 1417-1421.

Nataro, J.P., and Kaper, J.B., 1998. Diarrhagenic *Escherichia coli. Clin. Microbiol. Rev.* 11, 142-201.

Normanno, G., Dambrosio, A., Parisi, A., Quaglia, N.C., La Porta, L., Celano, G.V., 2002. Survival of *Escherichia coli* O157:H7 in a short ripened fermented sausage. *Ital. J. Food Sci.* 14, 181-185.

Normanno, G., Parisi, A., Dambrosio, A., Quaglia, N.C., Montagna, C.O., Chiocco, D., and Celano, G.V., 2004. Typing of *Escherichia coli* O157:H7 isolated from fresh sausage. *Food Microbiol.* 21, 79-82.

O'Brien, A.D., Holmes, R.K., 1987. Shiga and Shiga-like toxins. *Microbiol. Rev.* 51, 206-220.

Padhye, N.V., and Doyle, M.P., 1992. *Escherichia coli* O157:H7: epidemiology, pathogenesis, and methods for detection in food. *J. Food Protect.* 55, 555-565.

Paton, J.C., and Paton, A.W., 1998. Pathogenesis and diagnosis of Shiga toxin-producing *Escherichia coli* infection. *Clin. Microbiol. Rev.* 11, 450-479.

Philips, D., Summer, J., Alexander, J.F., Dutton, K.M., 2001. Microbiological quality of Australian beef. *J. Food Prot.* 64, 692-696.

Phillips, C.A., 1999. The epidemiology, detection and control of *Escherichia coli* O157. *J. Sci. Food Agric.* 79, 1367-1381.

Pilipčinec, E., Tkáčiková, L., Naas, H.T., Cabadaj, R., Mikula, I., 1999. Isolation of verotoxigenic *Escherichia coli* O157 from poultry. *Folia Microbiol.* 44, 455-456.

Power, C.A., Johnson, R.P., McEwen, S.A., McNab, W.B., Griffiths, M.W., Usborne, W.R., De Grandis, S.A., 2000. Evaluation of the Reveal and SafePath rapid *Escherichia coli* O157 detection tests for use on bovine faeces and carcasses. *J. Food Prot.* 63, 860-866.

Pradel, N., Livrelli, V., De Champs, C., Palcoux, J.B., Reynaud, A., Scheutz, F., Sirot, J., Joly, B., and Forestier, C., 2000. Prevalence and characterization of Shiga-toxin producing *Escherichia coli* isolated from cattle, food, and children during one year prospective study in France. *J. Clin. Microbiol.* 38, 1023-1031.

Ramachandran, V., Hornitzky, M.A., Bettelheim, K.A., Walker, M.J., Djordjevic, S.P., 2001. The common ovine shiga toxin 2- containing *Escherichia coli* serotypes and human isolates of the same serotypes possess a Stx2d toxin type. *J. Clin. Microbiol.* 39, 1932-1937.

Regulation (EC) No 178/2002 of the European Parliament and of the Council of 28 January 2002 laying down the general principles and requirements of food law, establishing the European Food Safety Authority and laying down procedures in matters of food safety. *Official Journal of the European Communities L.* 31/1 of 1February 2002.

Regulation (EC) No 852/2004 of The European Parliament and of the Council of 29 April 2004 on the hygiene of foodstuffs. *Official Journal of the European Union L.* 139, vol. 47 of 30 april 2004.

Regulation (EC) No 853/2004 of The European Parliament and of the Council of 29 April 2004 laying down specific hygiene rules for on the hygiene of foodstuffs. *Official Journal of the European Union L.* 139, vol. 47 of 30 april 2004.

Regulation (EC) No 854/2004 of The European Parliament and of the Council of 29 April 2004 laying down specific rules for the organization of official controls on products of animal origin intended for human consumption. *Official Journal of the European Union L.* 139, vol. 47 of 30 April 2004.

Remis, R.S., McDonald, K.L., Riley, L.W., Puhr, N.D., Wells, J.G., Davis, B.R., Blake, P.A., Cohen, M.L., 1984. Sporadic cases of hemorrhagic colitis associated with *Escherichia coli* O157:H7. *Ann. Intern. Med.* 101, 738-742.

Riley, L.W., 1987. The epidemiologic, clinical, and microbiologic features of hemorrhagic colitis. *Ann. Rev. Microbiol.* 41, 383-407.

Riley, L.W., Remis, R.S., Helgerson, S.D., McGee, H.B., Wells, J.G., Davis, B.R., Hebert, R.J., Olcott, H.M., Johnson, L.M., Hargrett, N.T., Blake, P.A., and Cohen, M.L., 1983.

Hemorrhagic colitis associated with a rare *Escherichia coli* serotype. *N. Engl. J. Med.* 308, 681-685.

Rowe, P.C., Walop, W., Lior, H., Mackenzie, A.M., 1991. Hemolytic anemia after childhood *Escherichia coli* O157:H7 infection: are females at increased risk? *Epidemiol. Infect.* 106, 523-530.

Sandving, K., van Deurs, B., 1996. Endocytosis, intracellular transport, and cytotoxic action of Shiga toxin and ricin. *Physiol. Rev.* 76, 949-966.

Sanz, S., Giménez, M., and Olarte, C., 2003. Survival and growth of *Listeria monocytogenes* and *E. coli* O157:H7 in minimally processed artichokes. *J. Food Prot.* 66, 2203-2209.

Scheutz, F., Beutin, L., Pierard, D., and Smith, H., 2001. Nomenclature of verocytotoxins. In: Duffy, G., Garvey, P., and McDowell, D. (Ed.), Verocytotoxigenic *E. coli*. *Food and Nutrition* Press Inc., Trumbull, CT, USA, pp. 447-452.

Schmidt, H., Beutin, L., Karch, H., 1995. Molecular analysis of the plasmid-coded hemolysin of *Escherichia coli* O157:H7 strain EDL 933. *Infect. Immun.* 63, 1055-1061.

Schmidt, H., Scheef, J., Morabito, S., Caprioli, A., Wieler, L., Karch, H., 2000. A new shiga toxin variant (Stx2f) from *Escherichia coli* isolated from pigeons. *Appl. Environ. Microbiol.* 66, 1205-1208.

Scott L., McGee, P., Sheridan, J.J., Earley, B., Leonard, N., 2006. A comparison of the survival of *Escherichia coli* O157:H7 grown under laboratory condition or obtained from cattle faeces. *J. Food Prot.* 69, 6-11.

Sekiya, J., 1997. *Escherichia coli* O157:H7 in livestock in Japan. *Rev. Sci. Tech. Off. Int. Epiz.* 16, 391-394.

Simmons, N.A., 1997. Global perspectives on *Escherichia coli* O157:H7 and other verocytotoxic *E. coli* spp.: UK views. *J. Food Prot.* 60, 1463-1465.

Sinclair J.F., Dean-Nystrom, E.A., O'Brien, A.D., 2006. The established intimin receptor Tir and the putative eucaryotic intimin receptors nucleolin and beta1 integrin localize at or near the site of enterohemorrhagic *Escherichia coli* O157:H7 adherence to enterocytes in vivo. *Infect Immun.* 74, 1255-1265.

Small, A., Wells-Burr, B., Buncic, S., 2005. An evaluation of selected methods for the decontamination of cattle hides prior to skinning. *Meat Science* 69, 263-268.

Stampi, S., Caprioli, A., De Luca, G., Quaglio, P., Sacchetti, R., Zanetti, F., 2004. Detection of *Escherichia coli* O157 in bovine meat products in northern Italy. *Int. J. Food Microbiol.* 90, 257-262.

Tkalcic, S., Zhao, T., Harmon, B.G., Doyle, M.P., Brown, C.A., Zaho, P., 2003. Faecal shedding of enterohemorragic *Escherichia coli* in weaned calves following treatment with probiotic *Escherichia coli*. *J. Food Prot.* 66, 1184-1189.

Todd, W.T.A., and Dundas, S., 2001. The management of VTEC O157 infection. *Int. J. Food Microbiol.* 66, 103-110.

Tortorello, M.L., 2000. *Escherichia coli* O157:H7. In: Robinson, R., Batt, C., and Patel, P. (Ed.), *Encyclopedia of Food Microbiology*. Academic Press, New York, vol. 1 pp. 646-652.

Tozzi, A.E., Gorietti, S., Caprioli, A., 2001. Epidemiology of human infections by *Escherichia coli* O157 and other verocytotoxin-producing *Escherichia coli*. In: Duffy,

G., Garvey, P., McDowell, D. (Ed.), Verocytotoxigenic *Escherichia coli. Food and Nutrition* Press Inc., Trumbull, pp. 161-179.

Tserenpuntsag, B., Chang, H.G., Smith, P.F., Morse, D.L., 2005. Hemolytic uremic syndrome risk and *Escherichia coli* O157:H7. *Emerg. Infect. Dis.* vol.11 No 12.

Tuttle, J., Gomez, T., Doyle, M.P., Wells, J.G., Zhao, T., Tauxe, R.V., and Griffin, P.M., 1999. Lessons from a large outbreak of *Escherichia coli* O157:H7 infections: insights into the infective dose and method of widespread contamination of hamburger patties. *Epidemiol. Infect.* 122, 185-192.

Weeratna, R.D., Doyle, M.P., 1991. Detection and production of verotoxin 1 of *Escherichia coli* O157:H7 in food. *Appl. Environ. Microbiol.* 57, 2951-2955.

Wells, J.G., Shipman, L.D., Greene, K.D., Sowers, E.G., Green, J.H., Cameron, D.N., Downes, F.P., Martin, M.L., Griffin, P.M., Ostroff, S.M., Potter, M.E., Tauxe, R.V., and Wachsmuth, I.K., 1991. Isolation of *Escherichia coli* serotype O157:H7 and other Shiga-like-toxin producing *Escherichia coli* from dairy cattle. *J. Clin. Microbiol.* 29, 985-989.

Wright, D.J., Chapman, P.A., and Siddons, C.A., 1994. Immunomagnetic separation as a sensitive method for isolating *Escherichia coli* O157 from food samples. *Epidemiol. Infect.* 113, 31-39.

Yu, J., and Kaper, J.B., 1992. Cloning and characterization of the *eae* gene of enterohemorrhagic *E. coli* O157:H7. *Mol. Microbiol.* 6, 411-417.

Zhao, T., Doyle, M.P., Harmon, B.G., Brown, C.A., Mueller, P.O.E., Parks, A.H., 1998. Reduction of carriage of enterohaemorragic *Escherichia coli* O157 in cattle by inoculation with probiotic bacteria. *J. Clin. Microbiol.* 36, 641-647.

Zhao, T., Zhao, P., West, J.W., Bernard, J.K., Cross, H.G., Doyle, M.P., 2006. Inactivation of enterohemorrhagic *Escherichia coli* in rumen content- or faeces-contaminated drinking water for cattle. *Appl. Environ. Microbiol.* 72, 3268-3273.

In: Hygiene and Its Role in Health
Editors: P. L. Anderson and J. P. Lachan

ISBN 978-1-60456-195-1
© 2008 Nova Science Publishers, Inc.

Chapter 7

Is Hand Hygiene Linked to Health Benefits in the Community in Developed Countries?

Thea F. van de Mortel[*]
School of Health and Human Sciences
Southern Cross University,
PO Box 157, Lismore, 2480 NSW
Australia

Abstract

Mortality rates from infectious diseases have declined dramatically in developed countries over the last century, largely due to improvements in nutrition, sanitation, and vaccination, and to the development of effective antimicrobials. Research has demonstrated that hands can be contaminated by pathogens, and that washing hands or using a waterless hand sanitizer can reduce that microbial contamination. Increased frequency of hand hygiene in homes, child care facilities, schools, and workplaces is therefore hypothesized to reduce infectious illness in the community, thus reducing morbidity and mortality and improving productivity as well as providing both a health and a cost benefit to the community. There is some evidence to support this hypothesis in the developing world, where infectious illnesses are very common and a major source of morbidity and mortality for the population, particularly for children. However, in a modern society that has proper sanitation, clean water, plentiful food and access to good health care, does increased hand hygiene frequency or the use of antimicrobial hand hygiene solutions significantly improve health and reduce costs in the community outside of the hospital setting? Various studies have examined infectious illness and/or illness absenteeism outcomes in response to hand hygiene programs in first world homes, child care facilities, elementary schools, colleges and some workplaces, with effects ranging from a lack of significant improvement to reductions in illness and illness absenteeism of up to 50%. However, the studies are often confounded by poor research design, including

[*] Email: tvandemo@scu.edu.au

lack of randomisation and blinding, failure to calculate sample sizes and power, failure to analyse on the basis of intention to treat, and failure to take clustering into account when calculating sample sizes and analysing data, most of which have a tendency to increase the chance of spurious positive findings. Reductions in mild infectious illnesses, such as colds, must also be offset against possible adverse effects of frequent hand hygiene such as skin damage and the increased risk of atopy in children exposed to a very hygienic environment in early life. This chapter will discuss the relative benefits and costs of hand hygiene programs in developed countries in the community setting and make some suggestions on the design and analysis of future programs.

Introduction

Mortality rates from infectious diseases have declined dramatically in developed countries over the last century. In 1900, the mortality rate from infectious diseases in the United States was 797 deaths per 100,000 persons; by 1996 it had plummeted to 59 deaths per 100,000 [1]. Similar patterns have been found across the developed world. This change in infectious diseases mortality is thought to be largely due to improvements in housing, nutrition, water quality, sanitation, and vaccination, and to the development of effective antimicrobials. For example, deaths due to tuberculosis, one of the main causes of infectious diseases mortality in 1900, declined by around 4-5% per annum in developed countries before the introduction of effective chemotherapy. This was due in part to housing programs that reduce overcrowding and other public health measures, such as isolation of infected persons, and pasteurisation of milk to reduce the incidence of bovine tuberculosis [2-4]. Tuberculosis mortality declined by a further 12-13% per annum in developed countries after 1945 following the development of effective antimicrobials such as Streptomycin and Isoniazid [1, 4], although the onset of the Human Immunodeficiency Virus (HIV) pandemic in the 1980s saw a bounce in the incidence and mortality of tuberculosis.

Vaccination programs are another major contributor to the reduction in incidence of, and mortality related to, other previously common infectious diseases. Such programs have substantially reduced the incidence, morbidity, and mortality associated with measles, mumps and rubella, have virtually eliminated diphtheria, tetanus and poliomyelitis, and completely eliminated smallpox [3].

Improvements in nutrition in first world countries over the last century have also contributed to a reduction in infectious diseases' mortality and morbidity, as underweight status and nutritional deficiency decrease the effectiveness of the body's specific and non-specific immune defences [5]. For example, in squatter settlements in Karachi, Luby et al. [6] found that children who were severely malnourished were 40% more likely to develop pneumonia than children who were not malnourished. Additionally, an analysis of 10 studies of children under the age of five years, found that the fraction of infectious disease attributable to being underweight was between 45% and 61% for diarrhoea, measles, malaria, and pneumonia, and 53% for other infectious diseases [5, 7]. Likewise, certain micronutrient deficiencies are estimated to increase the mortality related to diarrhoea, measles, pneumonia, and malaria by 13% - 24% [5, 8, 9].

Water quality and sanitation have also made important contributions to the reduction in infectious diseases incidence and mortality. A review of 35 years (1950-1985) of research on the effects of improved water quality and sanitation on health in developing countries, concluded such improvements reduced childhood morbidity and mortality related to infectious diseases in those countries [10]. A more recent review of 144 studies on the effect of improved water quality and sanitation on the incidence of diarrhoea and a range of parasite infections, found substantial reductions in infectious diseases morbidity ranging from 26% - 78%, and mortality reductions of up to 65% related to diarrhoeal illness [11].

Research has demonstrated that hands can be contaminated by pathogens, and hand hygiene - washing hands or using a waterless hand sanitizer – can reduce the degree of microbial contamination (see a review in [12]). Increased frequency of hand hygiene in homes, child care facilities, schools, and workplaces is, therefore, hypothesized to reduce infectious illness in the community, thus reducing infectious disease morbidity and mortality, improving productivity, and providing both a health and a cost benefit to the community.

There is some evidence to support this hypothesis in the developing world, where infectious illnesses are very common and a major source of morbidity and mortality for the population, particularly for children. For example, in squatter settlements in Karachi, where diarrhoea and acute respiratory infections such as pneumonia are leading causes of death, a program that provided soap and instruction in handwashing and bathing significantly reduced the incidence of diarrhoea, pneumonia and impetigo [6]. Curtis and Cairncross [13] conducted a meta-analysis of studies that related handwashing to the risk of infectious intestinal or diarrhoeal diseases in the community. They found 17 studies that met their review criteria, 15 of which were conducted in developing countries in Asia, Africa and South America including Bangladesh, Malawi, India, Brazil, Indonesia and Burundi. They found that interventions that promoted handwashing reduced the risk of diarrhoeal disease by 47%, however, they also concluded that all of the studies had methodological flaws, most were of poor quality, and the range of results was considerable, so the strength of the effect was in some doubt. In a modern society that has proper sanitation, clean water, plentiful food and access to good health care including vaccines and antimicrobials, do programs aimed at increasing hand hygiene frequency significantly improve health and reduce costs in the community outside of the hospital setting?

The effects of hand hygiene programs on infectious diseases incidence have been studied in various community settings in the developed world including the home, child-care centres, schools, universities, and workplaces.

Hand Hygiene in the Home

Larson et al. [14] studied the effects of introducing antimicrobial products for hand hygiene, general cleaning and laundry into the home in a randomised, placebo controlled, double-blinded trial. Two hundred and thirty-eight mostly Hispanic New York households were randomly allocated to control or intervention groups. Sample size calculations were used to ensure sufficient power (80%) to detect a significant difference. The intervention group was given antimicrobial products to use over a period of 48 weeks, and the incidence of infectious disease symptoms and hygiene practices of the treatment and control groups were monitored by self-report via weekly telephone calls, monthly home visits and quarterly interviews. Physicians validated a sub-sample of reports of symptoms via personal checks. The data were analysed on the basis of intention to treat. Logistic regression analysis was used to adjust for potential confounders. The authors found no significant difference in the incidence of infectious symptoms or the number of symptoms between the control and intervention groups. Adverse effects of the intervention were not reported.

The authors outlined three limitations. The study was conducted primarily on large Hispanic families in crowded suburban conditions, which would tend to make it more likely to find a significant intervention effect, as the bioburden would be larger under these conditions. Conversely, frequent contact with researchers plus provision of free product may have encouraged greater cleanliness in both treatment and control groups leading to fewer infectious disease symptoms in both groups. Additionally, as participants were not observed using the products, the products may not have been used as directed.

Sandora et al. [15] examined whether hand hygiene education and introduction of alcohol-based hand sanitizer in the home reduced the secondary spread of infections in families with children in child-care. Two hundred and ninety-two families with at least one child in day care for at least 10 hours per week in one of 26 child-care centres that consented to be involved were included in the study. Child-care centre was used as the unit of randomisation due to the possible correlation between child-care centre and clustering of illnesses in families with children attending the same centre. Over a five-month period, intervention households were given a supply of alcohol-based hand sanitizer and biweekly written information supporting hand hygiene. Control families were given written information on nutrition during the same period. Families recorded the timing and duration of illnesses in a symptom diary and reported symptoms of infectious illness and amount of hand hygiene product used to data collectors by telephone interview biweekly. The main outcome measure was the overall rate of secondary respiratory and gastrointestinal illness. The data were analysed on the basis of intent to treat, and were adjusted for number of children in a household, income, race, primary caregiver occupation and education level, and previous experience using hand sanitizer. After adjustment for the variables described above, there was a significant reduction (59%) in secondary gastrointestinal illness in intervention families when compared with control families, although there was no difference in the incidence of upper respiratory tract infection (URTI) between groups. Eisenberg et al. [16] suggest that there are usually multiple transmission pathways for infectious diseases, and if each pathway is sufficient to maintain transmission on its own, then an intervention that only deals with a single pathway may be ineffective. The incidence of adverse events was a secondary outcome measure. Participants reported 112 adverse events related to hand sanitizer use including dry skin, skin irritation, dislike of the product, allergy and stinging.

The study by Sandora et al. [15] has several limitations. Firstly, neither the families nor the data collectors were blinded to treatment allocation, which tends to increase the chance of finding a statistically significant intervention effect [17]. Secondly, while the researchers calculated the sample size that would be needed to detect a 20% difference with 80% power, they were unable to recruit the full sample that they needed, which reduced the power to find a significant difference to 75%. Thirdly, illness incidence and use of hand sanitizer were collected by self-report, which may be subject to socially desirable responding, where participants 'fake good' to obtain approval or avoid censure [18]. Fourthly, the sample had limited socio-economic diversity and socio-economic status was comparatively high. There is some evidence to suggest that socio-economic status can influence uptake of health promoting behaviours [19, 20]. A large proportion of families also declined to participate, which would dilute the effectiveness of the intervention in the general population.

Why did Larson et al. [14] find no significant benefit from their interventions when Sandora et al. [15] found a significant reduction in the incidence of secondary gastrointestinal illness in families using an alcohol-based hand sanitizer? The studies differed somewhat in focus and that may be one contributing factor, however, the latter study was not blinded, which tends to increase the likelihood of obtaining a spurious significant intervention effect, and the participants were of high socio-economic status which tends to increase the effectiveness of a health promotion intervention.

Hand Hygiene in Child-Care Settings and Elementary Schools

Preschools/Child Care Centres

Infectious diseases in pre-school children have an associated cost. Carabin et al. [21] followed 273 toddlers in 52 day-care centres for up to six months to determine the incidence of illness absenteeism due to colds, vomiting and diarrhoea and the associated direct and indirect costs. The average adjusted direct cost of illness per child over a six-month period included approximately $100 dollars (Canadian) for medications and doctors' consultations. The authors also estimated indirect costs ranging from $11.51 to $117.12 due to lost wages when parents had to take time off work, or pay family members or babysitters to care for sick children. This raises the question: Do hand hygiene programs reduce the incidence of infectious illness in child-care centres, and is this translated into a significant decline in illness absenteeism and related direct and indirect costs?

A number of studies have examined the effect of hand hygiene interventions (within a suite of other infection control interventions) on infectious illness frequency and/or illness absenteeism in child-care centres (Table 1). The reductions in illness frequency/illness absenteeism ranged from no significant effect to significant reductions in particular types of infections such as upper respiratory tract infections and diarrhoea in particular age groups. For example, Kotch et al. [22] found their infection control interventions (which included hand hygiene education) translated into a moderate significant reduction in severe diarrhoea in children under 24 months, however, they did not measure illness absenteeism or cost their program, so it is not possible to determine if it increased parental productivity or reduced costs (Table 1).

Carabin et al. [23] conducted a cluster-randomised trial of the effectiveness of a one-day training program on hygiene in reducing the incidence of respiratory and diarrhoeal illness in toddlers attending day care centres. The hygiene program included multiple infection control interventions including the encouragement of frequent hand hygiene (Table 1).

Table 1. Research studies examining the effects of hand hygiene (HH) interventions on infectious illness incidence or infectious illness absenteeism in child-care centres

Author/s (year)/ study location	Design	Interventions	Outcomes	Limitations
Kotch et al. (1994) [22] North Carolina, USA	Cluster randomised controlled trial (CRCT) Sample: 371 children in 24 day care centres 31 intervention classrooms and 36 control classrooms Control and intervention centres were paired by enrolment size Duration: seven months	Handwashing by staff and children emphasized; staff required to demonstrate correct technique Disinfection of toilet and diapering areas Daily disinfection of toys, sinks and kitchens Separation of diapering areas from food preparation areas Hygienic preparation of food Daily laundering of linen and dress ups Biweekly information collected from parents on diarrhoea and respiratory symptoms	Handwashing improved significantly in intervention classrooms Moderate significant improvement in rates of severe diarrhoea in children <24 months of age when potential confounding variables were controlled for Adjusted incidence of severe diarrhoea in children <24 months was 0.58 episodes per year in intervention centres and 1.12 episodes per year in control centres	Effect on illness absenteeism not measured Cost effectiveness of the intervention not described Multiple interventions make it impossible to quantify the role of HH in diarrhoea reduction Data on compliance obtained by covert observation which is subject to problems with interrater reliability and observer bias Data not analysed on the basis of intent to treat Adverse effects not reported Data collectors were not blinded to treatment allocation, although parents, who provided illness reports were blinded to the intervention status of their centre

Author/s (year)/ study location	Design	Interventions	Outcomes	Limitations
Carabin et al. (1998) [23] Quebec, Canada	CRCT Stratified by median incidence of URTI in pre-intervention period Block randomised by geo-graphical region Sample: 1,729 children in 47 day care centres 43 intervention classrooms in 24 day care centres, 40 control classrooms in 23 day care centres Duration: 15 months	Clean toys bi-daily with bleach Wash hands upon arrival, after playing outside, after using the bathroom, and before lunch Reminder cues for handwashing Open window for 30 minutes per day Clean sand in sand-box bi-weekly with bleach	The interventions significantly reduced the incidence risk of upper respiratory tract infection in the short term (25% reduction); no significant long-term effect The intervention did not significantly reduce the incidence of diarrhoea; monitoring of diarrhoea rates did significantly reduce diarrhoea rates and faecal contamination of children's and educators' hands	Data collectors not blinded to treatment allocation Effect of intervention on HH rates not measured Costs and illness absenteeism not reported Effects of HH can't be separated from those of the other infection control interventions Analysis partially conducted on the basis of intent to treat, however children who did not attend for five days during the study period were excluded from the analysis and centres that dropped out due to closure or failure to provide data were also excluded Adverse effects not reported

Table 1. (Continued)

Author/s (year)/ study location	Design	Interventions	Outcomes	Limitations
Roberts et al. (2000) [24], [25] ACT, Australia	CRCT Sample: 558 children in 23 child-care centres 11 intervention, 12 control centres Duration: nine months	Carers and children educated on HH importance and methods Carers used a plastic sandwich bag to protect fingers when blowing children's noses Daily washing of toys encouraged but not measured	A significant reduction in colds in children under 24 months of age. A non-significant reduction in illness absences due to URTI, i.e. six absences per child year in the intervention group versus seven absences per child year in the control group Diarrheal episodes significantly reduced (48%) in children over 24 months of age from 2.1 episodes per child year to 1.2. Absenteeism related to diarrheal episodes not significantly reduced	Not possible to separate out effects of HH from those of daily toy washing, and gloving to wipe noses Cost effectiveness of intervention not described Parents may have become aware of treatment allocation Data on compliance collected by observation which is subject to observer bias Adverse effects not reported
Pönkä et al (2003) [27]	Controlled, non-randomised, open cluster trial	One training session with supporting reference documents on infection control measures	A statistically significant reduction in diarrhoea in children under three years of age (-50 absences per month per 1000 children)	Non-randomised, non-blinded Relative cost benefits not reported

Author/s (year)/ study location	Design	Interventions	Outcomes	Limitations
Helsinki, Finland	Sample: 17, 388 children in 288 day care centres 60 intervention and 228 control centres Duration: two months baseline; three months intervention phase	Encouraged HH on arrival, after being outside, sneezing, toileting or changing diapers, and before eating Improved diaper changing practices and environmental cleaning Weekly washing of toys, daily washing of teething rings and dummies Regulation of air exchanges Isolation of children with infectious disease symptoms	When absences for URTI, diarrhoea, otitis media and conjunctivitis were pooled, there was a 26% reduction in absences in the intervention group in children aged < three Non-significant trend demonstrating reductions in illness absenteeism in children under three No significant difference in illness absenteeism in children over three Non-significant trend for increased infectious illness in the intervention group (+14%)	Effects of HH can't be separated from those of the other infection control interventions Adverse effects not reported Some dropouts of centres that did not comply with reporting absences Not analysed on the basis of intent to treat Short duration: long-term effectiveness?
Rosen et al (2006) [26]	CRCT	Educational training of carers on hand hygiene and other interventions	There was a threefold statistically significant increase in hand washing in the intervention centres over the period of the study (RR ranged from 2.77 to 3.30)	Only illness absenteeism recorded

Table 1. (Continued)

Author/s (year)/ study location	Design	Interventions	Outcomes	Limitations
Jerusalem, Israel	Stratified by sector: religious and secular Sample: 1029 children in 40 preschools 20 intervention, 20 control preschools Duration: 4.5 months Analysed on the basis of intent to treat	An educational program for children Installation of liquid soap dispensers Paper towels and individual cups Home video of intervention	There was no significant relationship between HH and either illness absenteeism or absenteeism in general (RR = 1.0)	Frequency of infectious illness unknown Although originally blinded to the treatment allocations, observers became aware of allocations during the study Cost effectiveness of interventions not described Compliance data collected by observers, subject to issues with interrater reliability and observer bias Adverse effects not reported

Table 2. Research studies examining the effects of hand hygiene interventions on infectious illness incidence or infectious illness absenteeism in elementary schools

Author (year) Location	Design	Hand hygiene interventions	Outcomes	Limitations
Courtney (1996) [41] South Dakota, USA	CRCT Sample: 1140 grade 3-6 students in six schools Three experimental and three control schools Duration: 2.5 months during winter and early spring	HH education provided by teachers to each class Dirty and clean fingers plated on agar plates Alcohol wipes provided to be used three times daily after morning and afternoon recess and before lunch Attitudes to HH assessed pre and post intervention	Attitudes towards HH improved significantly in experimental schools compared to controls No significant difference in illness absenteeism between controls and experimental schools No correlation between percent HH compliance of classes and illness absenteeism	Method of randomisation not described Participants and data collectors not blinded Sample size calculations not reported Inadequate number of clusters in each arm of the study Limited study duration: ? Seasonality and long term maintenance of effect Clustering not accounted for in data analysis Cost effectiveness not calculated Adverse effects not reported

Table 2. (Continued)

Author (year) Location	Design	Hand hygiene interventions	Outcomes	Limitations
Kimel (1996) [42] Chicago, USA	Cluster controlled trial (non-randomised) Sample: 199 students in 9 kindergarten and first grade classes in one school Duration: two months baseline data; three months intervention data (during peak flu season)	30 minute hand washing education program Demonstrations of germ transmission and handwashing techniques Raise teachers awareness of the importance of handwashing via a survey of teachers Absentee rates compared between control and intervention groups	A significant difference in flu-like absenteeism between control (3.8%) and intervention (1.8%) groups during December/January No significant difference between the two groups in February: control group 5.1%, intervention group 5.4%	Not randomised or blinded Clustering not accounted for in analysis Insufficient number of clusters per arm Sample size not calculated Confounding variables not assessed or controlled for Medium to high SES Limited study duration: long term maintenance of effect? Intervention evaluated during peak illness season Cost effectiveness not calculated Adverse effects not reported

Author (year) Location	Design	Hand hygiene interventions	Outcomes	Limitations
Master et al 1997 [43] Michigan, USA	Cluster Controlled trial (non-randomised) Sample: 143 intervention students (six classrooms) and 162 control students (eight classrooms) in one school Duration: 37 school days in winter	Demonstration of correct handwashing technique Discussion of germ theory Mandatory handwashing for intervention group, scheduled after arrival at school, before and after eating lunch, and prior to going home Illness absenteeism recorded	Children in intervention group had 25% less absences, and 57% less gastrointestinal symptoms. There was no significant difference in absences related to respiratory symptoms	Not randomised or blinded Clustering not accounted for in analysis Insufficient number of clusters per arm Sample size not calculated Limited study duration: long-term maintenance of effect? Intervention evaluated during peak illness season Cost effectiveness not calculated Adverse effects not reported
Hammond et al. (2000) [40]	Cluster Controlled trial (non-randomised)	Scheduled hand hygiene with alcohol-based hand sanitizer on entering and leaving the classroom, before and after lunch, after using the toilet, prior to going home, and after coughing and sneezing	There was a statistically significant 19.8% reduction in illness absenteeism in the intervention group compared to the control group when the school groups were evaluated cumulatively	Not randomised or blinded Analysis was not conducted on the basis of intention to treat Clustering not accounted for in analysis

Table 2. (Continued)

Author (year) Location	Design	Hand hygiene interventions	Outcomes	Limitations
Delaware, Ohio, Tennessee, California, USA	Sample size: ~6,000 students in 16 schools in five districts Number of experimental and control schools/ classes unclear Duration: 10 months	Three reinforcing visits by study coordinators Recorded illness absenteeism	When each school district was analysed separately, three of the five districts had a significant reduction in absenteeism in the intervention group, one had a non-significant reduction, and one had a non-significant increase in absenteeism	Direct and indirect costs of illness and absenteeism not assessed Sample size calculations not reported Parental consent not sought Ethics review not mentioned Adverse effects not reported
Dyer et al. (2000) [39]	Crossover study Sample: 420 students in one private school; seven intervention classes and seven control classes	Hand hygiene education program Students advised to use a benzalkonium hand sanitizer upon entering the classroom, before eating, after sneezing and coughing, and after using the toilet	41% reduction in illness absenteeism, 28.9% drop in gastro-intestinal illness and 49.7% drop in respiratory illness in first intervention group	Not randomised or blinded Clustering not accounted for in analysis

Author (year) Location	Design	Hand hygiene interventions	Outcomes	Limitations
California, USA	Duration: four weeks first group, two weeks washout, four weeks second group	Teachers recorded absences	Upon crossover, there was a 31.7% decrease in illness absenteeism, a 44.2% drop in gastro-intestinal illness and 50.2% drop in respiratory illness Monitored for adverse effects, however none reported	Insufficient number of clusters per arm Sample size not calculated No ethics approval sought Parental consent not sought Limited study duration: ? Seasonality and long term maintenance of effect Cost benefit not calculated No diversity of SES Handwashing frequency not monitored
White et al. (2001) [38]	CRCT Placebo controlled, double-blinded	Hand hygiene eduction program included handwashing technique, prevention of illness transmission, and the relationship between germs and illness	33.8% reduction in incidence of illness absenteeism in intervention group Gastrointestinal and respiratory absence-incidence were reduced in the intervention group by 38.6% and 31.7% respectively	Method of randomisation not reported Clustering not accounted for in analysis Large dropout rate (56% classrooms non-compliant)

Table 2. (Continued)

Author (year) Location	Design	Hand hygiene interventions	Outcomes	Limitations
California, USA	Duration: five weeks Sample size: Initially 1626 students in 72 classes in one private and two public elementary schools; due to dropouts final sample was 769 students in 32 classes	Children taught to cough and sneeze into their cuff, sleeve or elbow Scheduled HH six times daily using a benzalkonium solution Illness absenteeism recorded by administrative staff	Seven students dropped out due to deteriorating skin condition 56% sample non-compliant	Analysis not conducted on the basis of intent to treat Direct and indirect costs of illness and absenteeism not assessed Sample size calculations not reported HH frequency not monitored Limited study duration: ? Seasonality and long term maintenance of effect
Guinan et al. (2002) [37] PA, USA	Cluster Controlled trial (non-randomised) Sample size: 290 children in five independent schools; two test and two control classrooms per school Duration: three months	A 1-hour HH education component that included reminding buddies to wash hands Demonstration of HH using an alcohol-based HS Illness absenteeism recorded by teachers Cost benefit analysis	A significant reduction in illness absenteeism of 50.6% compared to controls Estimated yearly savings of $US24,300 for the five schools	Not randomised or blinded Cost savings largely due to allocation of one hour of casual teaching time for each absent day for remedial teaching (RT). Short absences may not require RT, or RT may be carried out during normal teaching times No description of dropouts or reporting of adverse effects Clustering not accounted for in analysis; insufficient number of

Author (year) Location	Design	Hand hygiene interventions	Outcomes	Limitations
Guinan et al. (2002) [37] PA, USA (Continued)				clusters per arm Sample size not calculated No ethics approval sought Parental consent not sought Limited study duration: ? seasonality and duration of effect No diversity of SES
Morton and Schultz (2004) [35] New England, USA	Crossover trial Sample: 253 students from 17 classes in one school Duration: 46 days first group, seven day washout, 47 days second group	School nurse taught 45 minute germ unit to each class. Glo Germ and UV light used to allow children to visualize areas that harbour germs HH with alcohol-based handrub encouraged on arrival to school, before lunch, before rubbing nose or eyes Illness absences collated by school nurse Weekly hand checks for adverse effects	A significant 43% reduction in illness absenteeism in the intervention group Twenty-two children did not participate due to lack of consent 10 children dropped out due to skin irritation problems	Method of randomisation not reported; not blinded Clustering not accounted for in analysis Sample size not calculated Limited study duration: Seasonality and duration of effect? Cost effectiveness not calculated Analysis not conducted on the basis of intent to treat

Outcome measures included the incidence of colds and diarrhoea, which were recorded by day care educators, and the degree of bacterial contamination of the indoor and outdoor environment, which was measured by faecal coliform counts. The authors used a Bayesian hierarchical model to analyse the effects of intervention while controlling for clustering effects at the level of classroom and day care centre. They controlled for the effect of monitoring/observation (the Hawthorne effect) on infection incidence rates (IR) by calculating the change in IR in the control group from Fall 1996 (pre- intervention period) to Fall 1997 (the post-intervention period) and subtracting that from the change in IR in the intervention group during the same period. When the effect of monitoring was controlled for they found that the effectiveness of the intervention in reducing the illness IR was insignificant, however, monitoring alone significantly reduced the IR of diarrhoea by 37%. When comparing the total pre and post intervention periods, the authors found that the interventions reduced upper respiratory tract illness by 25% when compared with the control. Interestingly, the authors suggested that the lack of a significant reduction in infectious illness IR in the intervention group in the fall-fall comparison, when compared with the significant effect when the whole pre and post intervention period was included in the analysis, demonstrated that the intervention was only effective in the short term. They commented that 50% of the staff taking part in the study had left the centre they worked in or moved on to another class by the second year of the study, and the high turnover would impact on the effectiveness of the intervention. The authors concluded that observing and recording illnesses was a more effective way of improving hand hygiene and environmental cleanliness than the training session on hygiene.

Roberts et al. [24], who studied the influence of hand hygiene education and other infection control initiatives in 23 Australian child care centres over a period of nine months, found that there was a significant link between hand hygiene compliance and URTI in children under 24 month of age, which led to a non-significant decline in illness absenteeism (Table 1). The intervention translated into one less absence per year for URTI and two less colds per year in children under the age of 24 months. Roberts et al. [24] noted that in centres where there was less than 70% compliance with the interventions, there was no effect on URTIs. The interventions consisted of hand hygiene education in conjunction with the use of a plastic sandwich bag glove to wipe children's noses and daily washing of toys.

In parallel, Roberts et al. [25] also examined the frequency of diarrheal episodes and related absenteeism. They found that compliance with the interventions was associated with a 48% reduction in episodes of diarrhoea in children over the age of 24 months, which translated into 1.2 diarrheal episodes per child year for the intervention children compared to 2.1 episodes for the control children of the same age group. The effect was greater (a 66% reduction in diarrhoea) in child-care centres with high compliance when compared to those with low compliance. As with the URTIs, there was no significant difference in absenteeism rates. As more families have both parents working, it is harder for parents to keep children home when they have infectious illnesses. The authors concluded that parents tend to send their children to child-care unless infections were severe. Again, the other infection control measures mentioned above may have impacted on the transmission of infection besides hand hygiene compliance.

Rosen et al. [26] in a study of the effect of a hand hygiene education campaign on illness absenteeism in 40 Jerusalem preschools found that despite an approximately threefold increase in hand hygiene rates in the intervention group, there was no significant influence on illness absenteeism or overall absenteeism in children who received the intervention (Table 1). This study measured only illness absenteeism, and therefore the effect on the frequency of infectious illness and associated costs is unknown.

Four of these five trials demonstrated a reduction in infectious illness rates in subsets of children attending child-care centres in response to hygiene programs *that included hand hygiene as a component*, however the reduction in illness incidence led to a significantly reduced illness absenteeism rate in the under three age group in only one [27] of the trials that measured illness absenteeism, therefore there was probably limited productivity gains for parents overall. None of these studies implemented changes to hand hygiene alone, so it is not possible to quantify the effects of hand hygiene per se as the effects of the other infection control measures confound the results. As none of these studies provided costings for their interventions or examined direct and indirect costs of the reported illnesses for the families involved, it is not possible to tell whether there was any cost benefit from these interventions. It would be interesting to see what the cost-benefit ratio was. Given that colds and diarrhoea are rarely life threatening in the developed world, the costs of introducing a specific hand hygiene campaign may be better recouped in situations where they decrease the risk of infectious illnesses with a substantial morbidity and mortality risk.

While two other studies [28, 29], have examined the effect of infection control programs - including hand hygiene as one of the components - on infectious illness or infectious illness absenteeism in the child care setting, and found effects ranging from none to a 32% reduction in the incidence of colds, they suffered from substantial methodological flaws. These flaws included lack of randomisation and blinding, failure to calculate sample sizes and power, inadequate sample sizes and failure to take clustering into account when calculating sample sizes and analysing data, most of which tend to increase the chance of spurious positive findings [30—33].

Whilst a number of research studies have been conducted on elementary school children to see if introduction of a hand hygiene program could reduce infectious illness absenteeism rates, similar methodological problems to those discussed previously are associated with these studies (Table 2). Meadows and Le Saux [34] conducted a systematic review of the effectiveness of rinse-free hand sanitisers for the prevention of illness-related absenteeism. They screened 141 studies and found six [35-40] that met the inclusion criteria for their review of which one was only available in abstract form [36]. All five published studies found that the introduction of a hand sanitiser significantly decreased illness absenteeism. The reduction in illness absenteeism ranged from 19.8% - 50.6%, however, the studies were characterised by a range of methodological flaws and poor reporting that impacted on the accuracy of the results. Meadows and Le Saux [34] concluded that the strength of the benefit needed to be interpreted cautiously.

Several additional studies [41-43] have examined the effects of hand hygiene education and improved handwashing or hand cleansing with alco-wipes on infectious illness absenteeism (Table 2).

Of the eight controlled trials that examined the effects of hand hygiene programs on infectious illness incidence or infectious illness absenteeism, six found a significant reduction in infectious illness absenteeism ranging from 19.8% to 50.6% in the intervention group, however only two trials were randomised [35, 38], only one was double-blinded [38], and none accounted for clustering in the data analysis.

Children at one school tend to be more alike than children selected at random from the population (different neighbourhoods have different socio-economic status and perhaps different lifestyles), and children within a school may also interact with, and influence one another [33]. One school may be exposed to a highly infectious outbreak during a study period when another school is not. Children within a class are more likely to be exposed to an infectious illness when others in their class have it, and their hand hygiene behaviour is more likely to influence their peers. This is why students in one class or school can't be treated as independent data points when the data are being analysed.

There is also a seasonal influence on the incidence of many infectious illnesses [44]. For example, gastroenteritis caused by rotovirus or norovirus peaks in winter as those viruses survive better in the environment at lower temperatures [45, 46]. Similarly, influenza viruses survive better in the low humidity conditions associated with winter [47, 48]. Timing the intervention in periods of highest infectious illness incidence, as many of the hand hygiene studies did, overestimates the benefits when the authors extrapolate their findings to the whole year.

Despite their flaws it was interesting that the direction, although not the magnitude, of the response was similar in the majority of studies, which provides some evidence to suggest a reduction in infection rates with improved hand hygiene in elementary school-aged children. It is possible, although unproven, that a reduction in infectious illness rates among school aged children can reduce infection rates in the community due to lowered transmission to parents, siblings and other contacts. Only one of the studies attempted to measure the cost benefit of the intervention [37], one measured the effect of the interventions over a whole school year [40], and three studies monitored for adverse effects [35, 38, 39]. Morton and Shultz [35] had 10 dropouts due to skin irritation, while White et al. [38] had seven dropouts due to skin irritation and Dyer et al. [39] had none.

Adverse events associated with hand hygiene programs include exacerbation of eczema, dry and damaged skin and allergic reactions to hand hygiene products [49]. Handwashing can actually increase the number of bacterial colonies on the skin and bacterial dispersal from hands by changing the skin pH, which damages the skin's natural antibacterial action, and by causing skin irritation [49]. Irritated skin is more likely to harbour and shed increased numbers of microorganisms [50]. While antimicrobial products such as rinse-free alcohol-based gels with emollients cause less skin damage than handwashing with soap [51], and are more effective than soap at killing hand flora (see review in [52]), there is also some concern that widespread use of antimicrobials in the community will contribute to antimicrobial resistance [49]. For example, a hospital-based study has demonstrated an increased carriage of antimicrobial resistant organisms in nurses who used an antimicrobial soap for 2 months [53]. Larson [49] recommends that use of antimicrobial agents by the community be restricted to situations where there is physical contact with persons at high risk for infection, or persons who are infected with an organism that is transmissible via direct contact, or in work settings associated with infectious disease transmission such as food handling, or child-care centres.

Another unintended consequence of improved hand hygiene in children may be an increase in atopic illnesses such as asthma and eczema. The 'hygiene hypothesis' suggests that early exposure to infections provides some protection against atopy and that babies/toddlers who are exposed to a very clean environment are therefore at increased risk of developing atopy [54, 55]. Type 1 immune responses occur in response to viral infections and are dominated by the production of gamma interferon [55]. Type 2 responses are dominated by the production of the interleukins 4 and 5, and stimulate IgE production and atopy [55]. Infants are born with strong Type 2 responses (atopic), but their immune systems can be modified towards stronger Type 1 responses (non-atopic) by exposure to common childhood infections [55].

For example, children with multiple siblings tend to have a lower risk of atopy as do children living in homes with a high number of persons per bedroom [54], and both overcrowding and a high number of siblings are associated with increased infection risk. Growing up on a farm with a high degree of contact with farm animals, attending a child-care centre, having childhood measles and orofaecal infections are also protective against atopy [56-58]. Again, attending day care is associated with an increased risk of infections such as colds and diarrhoea, and this is thought to mature children's immune responses and push them in the direction of Type 1 (non-atopic) responses. This is further supported by the results of Illi et al. [59] who demonstrated that children who had two or more simple colds (without wheeze) in the first 12 months of life had a 50% reduction in the risk of developing asthma by the age of seven. This picture is somewhat complicated by the finding that lower respiratory tract infections such as respiratory syncytial virus bronchiolitis, can increase the risk of developing asthma, however, the overall trend is towards increased risk of atopy with decreased infection rates in infancy. Selective vaccination may the key to reducing the incidence of infectious diseases that increase asthma risk without decreasing those that are protective [55].

Hand Hygiene in University Residences

White et al [60, 61] examined the effects of a hand hygiene education campaign and access to alcohol gel hand sanitizer on the incidence of infectious illness in 391 students living in four university dormitories in Boulder, USA over a period of eight weeks during autumn. The hand hygiene education was presented by means of weekly messages on bulletin boards and flier messages in bathroom stalls, and alcohol gel dispensers were installed in the bedrooms, washrooms, and dining halls of the intervention residences. Control students were told they were participating in a wellness study, but were not told the particular focus of the study. Pre-study and post-study assessments of students' health knowledge, attitudes and behaviours, and social support for healthy practices were conducted. Upper respiratory tract infection symptoms, absenteeism and some health practices were assessed via weekly surveys. The authors recorded a significant difference in handwashing frequency per hour in the intervention group (10.4% higher than the control), and a significantly greater use of the hand sanitizer, 0.03 uses per hour in the control group versus 0.26 uses per hour in the intervention group. Illness rates were significantly lower in the intervention group in three of the eight study weeks and there was a 20% decrease in illness symptoms overall. The illness rates for the experimental and control groups were 20.2% and 27.5%, and the percentage of students reporting one or more absent days per group was 5.7% versus 9.5% respectively.

The limitations of this study are similar to those discussed previously. The trial, while controlled, was not blinded, and residences were not allocated to treatment and control randomly. The intervention was carried out on clusters but sample size calculations were not carried out at all, and two clusters per arm are well under the recommended number of clusters for a trial of this type. The Medical Research Council [62] suggests that trials with less than five clusters per arm are inadvisable as parametric tests are unreliable with small numbers, and in order to achieve statistical significance with non-parametric tests at least four to six clusters per arm are needed.

Additionally, statistical analyses did not take clustering into account and the illness and absence data were obtained by self-report surveys, which may be biased problems with recall and by socially desirable responding, particularly when they are eliciting information on behaviours that carry a high social value [18]. These limitations increase the likelihood of false positive results. In the health care setting, researchers sometimes report that compliance following hand hygiene interventions declines over time as the novelty wears off [63-65], and this may also be the case in the community. The lack of long-term follow-up means that there is no way of determining how effectively the behaviour change would be maintained over time. The short study duration of most of these trials also impacts on the accuracy of the study conclusions as seasonality influences the incidence of infectious diseases. The costs associated with the program and possible cost savings to students were not reported, so there is no way of determining if the interventions were cost effective. Adverse effects of the hand sanitizer were not monitored.

Hand Hygiene in the Military Environment

Several studies of the effectiveness of hand hygiene interventions on the health of military personnel have also been carried out. Ryan et al. [66] examined the effect of a handwashing program on the respiratory illness rates and absenteeism of basic recruits at a naval training centre. Baseline rates of respiratory illness and hospitalisations were obtained for 44,797 recruits in 1996 from clinical records at the Great Lakes recruiting centre, USA. In 1997, a handwashing program was implemented, which involved directing recruits to wash their hands five times a day, allowing wet sinks to pass inspection (previously sinks had to be dry to pass inspection which tended to discourage recruits from washing their hands), installation of liquid soap dispensers at all sinks, and monthly education of instructors on the importance of handwashing. Monthly inspections of barracks were also utilized to encourage handwashing and ensure sufficient handwashing supplies. Respiratory illness rates and rates of hospitalisation of 47,300 and 44,128 recruits were then assessed over 1997 and 1998 respectively, via weekly counts in the medical clinic.

There was a statistically significant 45% reduction in the overall rate of infectious illness after the introduction of the hand hygiene program, and no change in the rate of hospitalisation for respiratory illness. A sub-sample of 1,442 recruits was surveyed regarding their handwashing frequency, incidence of respiratory illness, and training days lost to illness. Recruits who reported frequent handwashing had less self-reported illness and less self-reported hospitalisations than those who reported infrequent handwashing, but there was no difference in self-reported absenteeism rates. Respiratory illness rates and hospitalisations were also compared for a group of advanced recruits housed in different barracks, who did not participate in the handwashing program. There were no significant differences in their respiratory illness rates and hospitalisations between 1996, and 1997-1998, although it was interesting to see that the respiratory illness incidence in this group was as low throughout the three years as the lowest post-handwashing intervention rates in the intervention group. It may be that the advanced recruits had developed immunity to a range of pathogens due to high exposure in their basic training period.

There were a number of limitations that may have influenced the results. Firstly, the control group was not a true control, as it was not matched to the intervention group. The intervention group were younger and basic trainees, whereas the controls were a group of advanced trainees with a baseline infection rate half that of the intervention group. This means that temporal changes in the environment, circulating pathogens or susceptibility of the intervention population could have influenced the results. Allocation to treatment and control was not randomised and participants and data collectors were not blinded to the purpose of the study. Participants were allocated to the intervention by cluster but clustering was not accounted for in the data analysis. Adverse effects of the program were not monitored. Secondly, the outcomes were measured differently before and after the intervention: pre-intervention the statistics were collected by a retrospective review of medical records, whereas post-intervention they were collected by weekly monitoring of clinic visits. Thirdly, the survey data relied on self-report of handwashing frequency and illness incidence, which may be influenced by problems with recall and social desirability response bias. The authors noted that the response rate to the surveys was 99% indicating that the participants saw the survey as mandatory. Finally, and most importantly, the authors noted that there was a large outbreak of adenoviral illness in 1997 (the first intervention year), and a mass vaccination campaign was carried out to bring the outbreak under control, which may have confounded the results. Was the significant reduction in respiratory illness a result of the handwashing campaign or was it a result (at least in part) of the adenovirus vaccination campaign? The fact that the rates of respiratory illness were as low in the second intervention year tends to suggest that the major influencing variable was the handwashing intervention, however, the study methodology did not include any measure of whether handwashing in the intervention group was higher in the post intervention phase than the pre-intervention phase, so it is not possible to make a direct connection between the two.

In the second study of hand hygiene and infection rates in military personnel, van Camp and Ortega [67], monitored the effects of introducing hand sanitizing solution to two fighter squadrons' operations buildings in high traffic areas over the winter period, following previous media campaigns to encourage hand hygiene and cough hygiene to all base personnel. Acute infectious illness rates were monitored over a baseline winter period and an intervention winter period via a computerized medical tracking system that recorded when and why personnel were ill, and the amount of lost duty time. The squadrons with access to the hand hygiene solution had a significantly lower rate of illness and illness absenteeism than did the non-squadron personnel (who did not have access to hand hygiene solution). When compared to the previous winter, the intervention personnel had a reduced infectious illness and absenteeism rate, while the control personnel had similar rates of infection and absenteeism to the previous winter. The cost of a recovered duty day was calculated as less than $US0.61. The authors concluded that the hand hygiene education intervention on its own did not change infection rates, but that the use of the hand sanitizer was a cost effective method of reducing illness absenteeism. The study however, was limited by the fact that it was not prospective, randomised or blinded, and the personnel in the intervention and control groups were different in rank, education and work tasks, all of which may have influenced the results. Adverse effects were not monitored.

Methodological Issues in Hand Hygiene Research

This review demonstrates that much of the research on the influence of hand hygiene on infectious illness incidence and absenteeism rates is confounded by methodological deficiencies including lack of randomisation and blinding, lack of adequate controls, insufficient sample size, failure to analyse on the basis of intent to treat, and failure to account for clustering in data analysis. According to Kunz et al. [30] "randomisation is the only means of controlling for unknown and unmeasured differences as well as those that are known and measured" (p. 2). In a systematic review, Kunz and Oxman [17] compared the outcomes of clinical trials that had been randomised versus non-randomised trials of the same intervention. They found eight studies where they were able to compare randomised and non-randomised trials of the same intervention. In five of the eight studies, the intervention effect was overestimated in non-randomised trials. In one study the effect was underestimated, and in one there was no difference in effect between the randomised and non-randomised trials. In a larger and more recent review, Kunz et al. [30] found 35 comparisons of randomised and non-randomised trials of the same interventions. The estimates of effect were larger in the non-randomised trials in 22 of those comparisons, whereas only four comparisons found smaller treatment effects in the non-randomised trials and eight found similar results across both randomised and non-randomised trials. These reviews highlight the fact that lack of randomisation tends to inflate the effect size of an intervention.

Another issue with many of the hand hygiene studies reviewed in this chapter is the lack of blinding to treatment allocation. The term blinding can refer to allocation concealment at the time of randomisation, which means that researchers are not able to predict the treatment allocation of the next individual or cluster enrolled in their trial [68], and the aim of this practice is to prevent selection bias, so that consciously or unconsciously, the researchers don't stack the intervention group with participants that are more likely to deliver a significant intervention effect [69]. Allocation concealment is ensured by using methods of randomisation that don't allow for prediction. For example, randomisation by day or time allows prediction and manipulation of the timing of referral of cases for randomisation, whereas allocation by random number table does not. This is one of the reasons that trials should report their method of randomisation. Kunz and Oxman [17] compared adequacy of allocation concealment in studies of the same intervention. The studies with inadequate concealment overestimated the intervention effects by between 17% and 41%. Shultz et al. [69], in their review of the effect of trail quality on study outcomes, found that inadequate allocation concealment increased the odds ratios by an average of 40% compared to trials where allocation was properly concealed. Keeping participants and data collectors blinded to the treatment allocation throughout the study is another form of blinding, and it is utilised to prevent bias in reporting by participants and data massaging by data collectors.

One of the most persistent methodological problems with studies that examine the effect of hand hygiene programs on hand hygiene rates and infection rates in the community is that sample size calculations and statistical analyses often don't take into consideration that the participants have been randomised on the basis of groups or clusters rather than randomised on an individual basis. When standard methods are used to calculate sample sizes and test hypotheses these are based on the assumption that the observations are statistically independent, however, this is not the case when a class or centre has been selected as the unit of intervention [33]. According to Wear [33] there are two sources of variance in cluster designs: the variability of individuals within a cluster and the variance between clusters. If the data are analysed without accounting for clustering, the risk of a false positive error is increased as confidence intervals are falsely narrow and p-values are falsely low. Cornfield [71] suggests that analysis by individual in cluster-randomised trials is an exercise in self-deception. For example, a review of 21 research papers on public health found nine trials that failed to account for clustering when analysing their data [32]. All of these trials reported significant findings. When the data were reanalysed to take clustering into account, the positive results were found to be spurious in seven of the nine trials.

According to Kerry and Bland [72], 'the ratio of the total number of subjects required using cluster randomisation to the number required using simple randomisation is called the design effect' (p. 550). Wear [33] calls it the 'variance inflation factor'. The larger the number of participants in each cluster, the greater the design effect. This means in practice, that it is better to have more clusters with less participants in each cluster, than it is to have a minimal number of clusters. To illustrate this point, Kerry and Bland [72] discuss a study on a behavioural intervention designed to reduce cholesterol levels, randomised at the level of GP practices. If the researchers could recruit less than 10 patients per practice they would require 558 practices to be involved in the study (a total sample size of 5580 patients) to obtain adequate power. If the number of practices were reduced to 126, then 50 patients would need to be recruited from each practice (total sample size 6300 patients). If only 32 practices were used, then 500 patients would need to be recruited from each practice (total sample size of 16,000 patients) to maintain the same level of power.

In order to ensure sufficient power to detect a significant effect, it is important to take clustering into account when making sample size calculations. The sample size obtained through the normal methods of calculating sample size when the allocation is at the level of individuals can be multiplied by the variance inflation factor to give a more accurate estimate of the required sample size in studies utilizing cluster designs. Wear [33] provides a method to calculate the variance inflation factor and therefore correct sample size for a cluster design. Alternatively, Rosen et al. [73] published an equation that can be used to calculate how many clusters are needed per arm for a CRCT designed to test the effect of a hand hygiene intervention on preschool children. The published equation contains an error. The corrected equation (Pers. com. LJ Rosen, 25th June, 2007) is:

$$N \text{ per arm} = (1/KD) (1+(D-1)BDC) (1+(K-1)ICC) (p_0 (1-p_0) + p_1 (1-p_1)) (z_a +z_b)^2 / (p_0-p_1)^2$$

where D = trial length in days, K = children per cluster, the intraclass correlation (ICC) and between day correlation (BDC) (estimated from a previous trial) are 0.0274 and 0.0548 respectively, and where z_a and z_b are 1.96 and 0.84 respectively for 80% power at the two-sided 0.05 level. The p_0 in the equation is the projected control group daily illness absenteeism rate, and p_1 is the expected treatment group daily absenteeism rate.

Another frequent design flaw is the failure to analyse data on the basis of intention to treat. Analysing data by first excluding non-compliant participants can bias the results because one of the reasons participants may be non-compliant is that the intervention causes adverse effects that would impair the effectiveness of the intervention, or the intervention is too difficult to follow which again would impair its effectiveness in the real world [74]. For example, use of a particular hand sanitizer or frequent hand hygiene may cause reddening, drying, stinging, and exacerbate eczema in susceptible individuals, and they may choose to stop using the product or following the intervention protocol. Therefore excluding cases from the analysis on the basis of non-compliance may cause the clinical effectiveness of the intervention to be overestimated as once the program is rolled out to the wider community, a similar proportion of people prone to adverse effects may also choose not to comply [75]. Analysis on the basis of intention to treat provides a pragmatic estimate of the benefit of a change in policy rather than of potential benefit in participants who receive the intervention exactly as planned [75].

A number of reviews have examined the effects of low quality trials and poor reporting on estimates of effect size. Moher et al. [31], randomly selected 11 meta-analyses that involved 127 studies on various interventions. They assessed the quality of reporting, and examined the effects of reporting on the estimates of benefits. They found that low quality trials overestimated the benefit of the intervention by 34% compared with high quality trials, and that trials with inadequate allocation concealment overestimated the benefit of the intervention by 37%. Kunz et al. [30] review of high versus low quality trials showed that lower quality trials on average increased the effect size by 34%, but that estimates of effect in low quality trials ranged between 55% smaller to 350% larger than those in high quality trials.

When studying hand hygiene interventions, long-term follow-up is an issue, as the effectiveness of an intervention may wane over time due to turnover of personnel and loss of interest by participants. In fact, Ryan et al. [66] in their study of the influence of alcohol-based hand sanitizer on infection rates did not include data after 1998 because of 'inconsistent application of all aspects of the handwashing program at the site after that time' (p. 82). Similarly, the study by Carabin et al. [23] in the child-care setting, found that the infection control intervention resulted in a reduction in infectious illness, however the effect waned within 12 months.

Other methodological problems include the methods of measuring outcomes. Many studies have investigated ways to increase hand hygiene frequency and/or compliance, yet there is still no agreement on the best methods of measuring the research outcomes. Studies relying on self-report can be influenced by problems with recall or socially desirable responding [18]. When data are collected by overt observation, participants may change their behaviour when they know they are being observed (the Hawthorne effect) [76, 77]. Data collected by observation can be influenced by observer bias [78] and if there is more than one observer, interrater reliability can be an issue. Solution audit can be a reliable way to get an objective measure of changes to hand hygiene frequency, however it doesn't allow the researcher to find out about which participants are compliant, or how well or in what situations hand hygiene is being performed [79]. All of these issues need to be considered when deciding how to measure research outcomes.

In the hospital setting there is some disagreement amongst researchers about definitions of infectious disease [80]. As the way in which infectious illness is defined can influence outcomes in hand hygiene studies, it is important that consideration is given to the choice of infectious illness definitions.

Suggested Design for Community Hand Hygiene Studies

A randomised, double-blinded, placebo-controlled trial is the gold standard for a trial of HH efficacy in the community setting. Randomisation helps to control for unknown or unmeasured differences between comparison groups. Randomisation should be carried out using a random numbers table. Double blinding is important to avoid bias that can be introduced when either the participants or the data collectors know the treatment allocation. The use of a control sample allows the researcher to check that the change in outcome has occurred in response to the intervention and not by chance or due to some other unknown variable.

Choice of sample size should be based on sample size calculations to ensure that the study has sufficient power to detect a significant difference in response to an intervention. As the interventions in community trials are almost always allocated on the basis of clusters (families, schools, child-care centres, or squadrons) rather than on an individual basis, a sample size formula that accounts for clustering of the data should be employed. Equally importantly, the statistical methods used to analyse the data must take clustering into account to avoid spurious positive results. Data should also be analysed on the basis of intent to treat, as excluding dropouts from the analysis biases the outcomes in the favour of the intervention.

The trial duration should be at least 12 months to determine if there are seasonal influences on the effectiveness of the intervention, and to determine how well the effects of the intervention are maintained in the long term. If the study duration is limited, the researchers should acknowledge that interventions run during the peak infectious season are likely to overestimate the benefit of the intervention in the real world, especially as the effect of an intervention tends to wash out over time. The sample should include a diverse range of subjects from different socio-economic strata as socio-economic status can influence uptake of health promoting behaviours. As many of the studies that have examined this topic suggest that hand hygiene interventions can reduce the costs and productivity losses associated with infectious diseases, it would be ideal to also measure the direct and indirect costs associated with implementing the intervention, and the cost benefit associated with any reduction in infectious illness or illness absenteeism. An ethics committee should review the study design, and the consent of participants (or their parents) should be sought. Adverse effects and dropouts should be reported. Sufficient detail should be provided in research papers to allow the research to be replicated.

Conclusion

When taken as a whole, the published research on hand hygiene and incidence of infectious illness in the community tends to support the hypothesis that hand hygiene can reduce infectious illness in the community as the majority of studies that have included hand hygiene as at least one component of an infection control intervention have demonstrated a reduction in infectious illness incidence, although the magnitude of the benefit has varied widely. The possible benefits of such programs need to be weighed against the risk of skin damage, allergy and atopy. However, much of the published research on the benefits of hand hygiene programs in the community is plagued by methodological deficiencies, and these tend to increase the chance of spurious positive findings. Infection control researchers need to design robust hand hygiene studies, and work on developing a consensus on the outcomes to measure and how to best measure them, the definitions to use, and the best methods of analyses to answer important infection control questions. Instead of individual researchers conducting studies limited in size and scope due to lack of resources and time, large collaborations across multiple sites may be required to ensure a sufficient number of clusters, total sample size and resources to get unequivocal answers to those questions.

References

[1]   Armstrong, G.L., Conn, L.A. and Pinner, R.W. (1999). Trends in infectious disease mortality in the United States during the 20th century. *JAMA. 281*, 61-66.
[2]   Catalano, R. and Frank, J. (2001). Detecting the effect of medical care on mortality. *Journal of Clinical Epidemiology. 54*, 830-836.
[3]   Centres for Disease Control (1999). Achievements in public health 1900-1999: control of infectious diseases. *Morbidity and Mortality Weekly Report. 48*, 621-9.
[4]   Chadha, V.K. (1997). Global trends of tuberculosis - an epidemiological review. *NTI Bulletin. 33*, 11-18.
[5]   Black, R.E., Morris, S.S., and Bryce, J. (2003). Where and why are 10 million children dying every year? (Child survival I). *Lancet. 361*, 2226-2234.

[6]   Luby, S.P., Agboatwalla, M., Feikin, D.R., Painter, J., Bilhimer, W., Altaf, A. and
       Hoekstra, R.M. (2005). Effect of handwashing on child health: a randomised controlled
       trial. *Lancet. 366*, 225-33.

[7]   Fishman, S., Caulfield, L.E., de Onis, M., Blossner, M., Hyder, A.A., Mullany, L. and
       Black, R.E. (2004). Childhood and maternal underweight. In M. Ezzati, A.D. Lopez, A.
       Rodgers, and C.J.L. Murray (Eds.), *Comparative quantification of health risks: global
       and regional burden of disease attributable to selected major risk factors*. Geneva:
       WHO.

[8]   Rice, A.L., West, K.P. and Black, R.E. (2004). Vitamin A deficiency. In M. Ezzati,
       A.D. Lopez, A. Rodgers, C.J.L. Murray (Eds.), *Comparative quantification of health
       risks: global and regional burden of disease attributable to selected major risk factors*.
       Geneva: WHO.

[9]   Caulfield, L. and Black R.E. (2004). Zinc deficiency. In M. Ezzati, A.D. Lopez, A.
       Rodgers, and C.J.L. Murray (Eds.), *Comparative quantification of health risks: global
       and regional burden of disease attributable to selected major risk factors*. Geneva:
       WHO.

[10]   Esrey, S.A. and Habicht, J.P. (1986). Epidemiologic evidence for health benefits from
       improved water and sanitation in developing countries. *Epidemiologic Reviews. 8*, 177-
       128.

[11]   Esrey, S.A., Potash, J.B., Roberts, L. and Shiff, C. (1991). Effects of improved water
       supply and sanitation on ascariasis, diarrhoea, dracunculiasis, hookworm infection,
       schistosomiasis, and trachoma. *Bulletin of the World Health Organization. 69*, 609-621.

[12]   Boyce, J.M. and Pittet, D. (2002). Guidelines for hand hygiene in health-care settings:
       Recommendations of the Healthcare Infection Control Practices Advisory Committee
       and the HICPAC/SHEA/APIC/IDSA Hand Hygiene Taskforce. *Morbidity and
       Mortality Weekly Report*. 51, 1-48.

[13]   Curtis, V. and Cairncross, S. (2003). Effect of washing hands with soap on diarrhoea
       risk in the community: a systematic review. *The Lancet. 3*, 275-281.

[14]   Larson, E., Lin, S.X., Gomez-Pichardo, C. and Della-Latta, P. (2004). Effect of
       antibacterial home cleaning and handwashing products on infectious disease symptoms.
       Annals of Internal Medicine. 140, 321-9.

[15]   Sandora, T.J., Taveras, E.M., Mei-Chiung, S., Resnick, E.A., Lee, G.M., Ross-Degnan,
       D. and Goldmann, D.A. (2005). A randomised controlled trial of a multifaceted
       intervention including alcohol-based hand sanitizer and hand hygiene education to
       reduce illness transmission in the home. *Pediatrics. 116*, 587-594.

[16]   Eisenberg, J.N.S., Scott, J.C., and Porco, T. (2007). Integrating disease control
       strategies: balancing water sanitation and hygiene interventions to reduce diarrheal
       disease burden. *American Journal of Public Health. 97*, 846-852.

[17]   Kunz, R. and Oxman, A.D. (1998). The unpredictability paradox: review of empirical
       comparisons of randomised and non-randomised clinical trials. *British Medical
       Journal. 317*, 1185-90.

[18]   Huang, C., Liao, H. and Chang, S. (1998). Social desirability and the clinical self-
       report inventory: Methodological reconsideration. *Journal of Clinical Psychology. 54*,
       517-528.

[19] Ettner, S.L. and Grzywacz, J.G. (2003). Socioeconomic status and health among Californians: An examination of multiple pathways. *American Journal of Public Health*. 93, 441-444.

[20] Najman, J.M. (1994). Class inequalities in health and lifestyle. In C. Waddell, and A.R. Petersen (Eds.), *Just health: inequality in illness, care and prevention*. Churchill Livingstone: Melbourne. pp 27-46.

[21] Carabin, H., Gyorkos, T.W., Soto, J.C., Penrod, J., Joseph, L. and Collet, J. (1999). Estimation of direct and indirect costs because of common infections in toddlers attending day care centres. *Pediatrics. 103*, 556-564.

[22] Kotch, J.B., Weigle, K.A., Weber, D.J., Clifford, R.M., Harms, T.O., Loda, F.A., Gallagher, P.N., Edwards, R.W., LaBorde, D. and McMurray, M.P. (1994). Evaluation of an hygienic intervention in child day-care centres. *Pediatrics. 94*, 991-4.

[23] Carabin, H., Gyorkos, T.W., Soto, J.C., Joseph, L., Payment, P. and Collet, J.P. (1999). Effectiveness of a training program in reducing infections in toddlers attending day care centers. *Epidemiology. 10*, 219-27.

[24] Roberts, L., Smith, W., Jorm, L., Patel, M., Douglas, R. and McGilchrist, C. (2000). Effect of infection control measures on the frequency of upper respiratory infection in child care: a randomised, controlled trial. *Paediatrics. 105*, 738-742.

[25] Roberts, L., Jorm, L., Patel, M., Smith, W., Douglas, R. and McGilchrist, C. (2000). Effect of infection control measures on the frequency of diarrheal episodes in child care: a randomised, controlled trial. *Paediatrics. 105*, 742-745.

[26] Rosen, L., Manor, O., Engelhard, D., Brody, D., Rosen, B., Peleg, H., Meir, M. and Zucker, D. (2006). Can a handwashing intervention make a difference? Results from a randomised controlled trial in Jerusalem preschools. *Preventive Medicine. 42*, 27-32.

[27] Pönkä, A., Poussa, T. and Laosmaa, M. (2004). The effect of enhanced hygiene practices on absences due to infectious diseases among children in day care centres in Helsinki. *Infection. 32*, 2-7.

[28] Niffenegger, J.P. (1997). Proper handwashing promotes wellness in child care. *Journal of Paediatric Health Care. 11*, 26-31.

[29] Bartlett, A.V., Jarvis, B., Ross, V., Katz, T., Dalia, M.A., Englender, S.J. and Anderson, L. (1988). Diarrheal illness among infants and toddlers in day care centres: effects of acute surveillance and staff training without subsequent monitoring. *American Journal of Epidemiology. 127*, 808-817.

[30] Kunz, R, Vist, G. and Oxman, A.D. (2007) Randomisation to protect against selection bias in healthcare trials. *Cochrane Database Systematic Reviews. 18*, MR000012.

[31] Moher, D., Pham, B., Jones, A., Cook, D.J., Jadad, A.R., Moher, M., Tugwell, P. and Klassen, T.P. (1998). Does the quality of reports of randomised trials affect estimates of intervention efficacy reported in meta-analyses. *Lancet. 352*, 609-613.

[32] Simpson, J.M., Klar, N. and Donner, A. (1995). Accounting for cluster randomisation: a review of primary prevention trials, 1990 through 1993. *American Journal of Public Health. 85*,1378-1383.

[33] Wear, R.L. (2002). Advanced statistics: statistical methods for analysing cluster and cluster-randomised data. *Academic Emergency Medicine. 9*, 330-341.

[34] Meadows, E. and Le Saux, N. (2004). A systematic review of the effectives of antimicrobial rinse-free hand sanitizers for prevention of illness-related absenteeism in elementary school children. *BMC Public Health. 4*, 50-60.

[35] Morton, J.L. and Schultz, A.A. (2004). Healthy hands: use of alcohol gel as an adjunct to handwashing in elementary school children. *Journal of School Nursing. 20*, 161-167.

[36] Thompson, K. (2004). The effects of alcohol hand sanitizer on elementary school absences. *American Journal of Infection Control. 32*, E127.

[37] Guinan, M., McGuckin, M. and Ali, Y. (2002). The effect of a comprehensive handwashing program on absenteeism in elementary schools. *American Journal of Infection Control. 30*, 217-20.

[38] White, C., Shinder, F., Shinder, A. and Dyer, D. (2001). Reduction in illness absenteeism in elementary schools using an alcohol-free instant hand sanitizer. *Journal of School Nursing. 17*, 258-65.

[39] Dyer, D.L., Shinder, A. and Shinder, F. (2000). Alcohol-free instant hand sanitizer reduces elementary school illness absenteeism. *Family Medicine. 32*, 633-638.

[40] Hammond, B., Ali, Y., Fendler, E., Dolan, M. and Donovan, S. (2000). Effect of hand sanitizer use on elementary school absenteeism. *American Journal of Infection Control. 28*, 340-46.

[41] Courtney, K. (1995). *The effect of a handwashing education program on illness-related absenteeism and attitudes towards handwashing* [dissertation]. UMI Dissertation Service.

[42] Kimel, L.S. (1996). Handwashing education can decrease illness absenteeism. *Journal of School Nursing. 12*, 14-18.

[43] Master, D., Longe, S. and Dickson, H. (1997). Scheduled handwashing in an elementary school population. *Family Medicine. 29*, 336-339.

[44] Grassley, N.C. and Fraser, C. (2006). Seasonal infectious disease epidemiology. *Proceedings of the Royal Society B. 273*, 2541–2550.

[45] Cook, S.M., Glass, R.I., Lebaron, C.W. and Ho, M.S. (1990). Global seasonality of rotavirus infections. *Bulletin of the World Health Organization. 68*, 171–177.

[46] Mounts, A.W., Ando, T., Koopmans, M., Bresee, J.S., Noel, J. and Glass, R.I. (2000). Cold weather seasonality of gastroenteritis associated with Norwalk-like viruses. *Journal of Infectious Diseases. 181*, S284–S287.

[47] Loosli, C.G., Lemon, H.M., Robertson, O.H. and Appel, E. (1943). Experimental airborne influenza infection. I. Influence of humidity on survival of virus in air. *Proceedings of the Society for Experimental Biology and Medicine. 53*, 205–206.

[48] Hemmes, J.H., Winkler, K.C. and Kool, S.M. (1960). Virus survival as a seasonal factor in influenza and poliomyelitis. *Nature. 188*, 430–431.

[49] Larson, E.L. (2001). Hygiene of the skin: when is clean too clean? *Emerging Infectious Diseases. 7*, 225-30.

[50] Larson, E., Aiello, A., Lee, LV., Della-Latta, P., Gomez-Duarte, C. and Lin, S. (2003). Short- and long-term effects of handwashing with antimicrobial or plain soap in the community. *Journal of Community Health. 28*, 139-150.

[51] Graham, M., Nixon, R., Burrell, L.J., Bolger, C., Johnson, P.D.R. and Grayson, M.L. (2005). Low rates of cutaneous adverse reactions to alcohol-based hand hygiene

solution during prolonged use in a large teaching hospital. *Antimicrobial Agents Chemother*, *49*: 4404-4405.

[52]   Piceansathian, W. (2004). A systematic review on the effectiveness of alcohol-based solutions for hand hygiene. *International Journal of Nursing Practice. 10*, 3-9.

[53]   Cook, H.A., Cimiotti, J.P., Della-Latta, P., Saiman, L. and Larson, E.L. (2007). Antimicrobial resistance patterns of colonizing flora on nurses hands in the neonatal intensive care unit. *American Journal of Infection Control. 35,* 231-6.

[54]   da Costa Lima, R., Victoria, C.G., Menezes, M.B. and Barros, F.C. (2003). Do risk factors for childhood infections and malnutrition protect against asthma? A study of Brazilian male adolescents. *American Journal of Public Health. 93*, 1858-1864.

[55]   Johnston, S.L. and Openshaw, P.J.M. (2001). The protective effect of childhood infections. *British Medical Journal. 322*, 376-7.

[56]   Ball, T.M., Castro-Rodriguez, J.A., Griffith, K.A., Holberg, C.J., Martinez, F.D. and Wright, A.L. (2000). Siblings, day-care attendance, and the risk of asthma and wheezing during childhood. *New England Journal of Medicine. 343*, 538-43.

[57]   Matricardi, P.M., Rosmini, F., Riondino, S., Fortini, M., Ferrigno, L., Raicetta, M. and Bonini, S. (2000). Exposure to foodborne and orofaecal microbes versus airborne viruses in relation to atopy and allergic asthma: epidemiological study. *British Medical Journal. 320*, 412-417.

[58]   Shaheen, S.O., Aaby, P., Hall, A.J., Barker, D.J., Hayes, C.B., Shiell, A.W. and Goudiaby, A. (1996). Measles and atopy in Guinea-Bissau. *Lancet. 347*, 1792-6.

[59]   Illi, S., von Mutius, E., Lau, S., Bergmann, R., Niggerman, B., Sommerfeld, C. and Wahn, U. (2001). Early childhood infectious diseases and the development of asthma up to school age: a birth cohort study. *British Medical Journal. 322*, 390-5.

[60]   White, C., Kolble, R., Carlson, R., Lipson, N., Dolan, M., Ali, Y. and Cline, M. (2003). The effect of hand hygiene on illness rate among students in university residence halls. *American Journal of Infection Control. 31*, 364-70.

[61]   White, C., Kolble, R., Carlson, R. and Lipson, N. (2005). The impact of a health campaign on hand hygiene and upper respiratory illness among college students living in residence halls. *Journal of American College Health. 57*, 175-81.

[62]   Medical Research Council (2002). Cluster randomised trials: methodological and ethical considerations. London: MRC.

[63]   Conly, J.M., Hill, S., Ross, J., Leitzman, L and Louise, T.J. (1989). Handwashing practices in an intensive care unit: the efforts of an educational program and its relationship to infection rates. *American Journal of Infection Control. 17*, 330-9.

[64]   Dubbert, P.M., Dolce, J., Richter, W., Miller, M. and Chapman, S.W. (1990). Increasing intensive care unit staff handwashing: effects of handwashing and group feedback. *Infection Control and Hospital Epidemiology. 11*, 191-4.

[65]   Larson, E.L., Bryan, J.L., Adler, L.M. and Blane, C. (1997). A multifaceted approach to changing handwashing behavior. *American Journal of Infection Control. 25*, 3-10.

[66]   Ryan, M.A., Christian, R.S. and Wohlrabe, J. (2001). Hand washing and respiratory illness among young adults in military training. *American Journal of Preventive Medicine. 21*, 79-83.

[67] van Camp, R.O. and Ortega, H.J. (2007). Hand sanitizer and rates of acute illness in military aviation personnel. *Aviation, Space and Environmental Medicine. 78*, 140-142.

[68] Li, P., Mah, D., Lim, K., Sprague, S. and Bhandari, M. (2005). Randomisation and concealment in surgical trials: a comparison between orthopaedic and non-orthopaedic randomised trials. *Archives of Orthopaedic and Trauma Surgery. 125*, 70–7.

[69] Day, S.J. and Altman, D.J. (2000) Statistics notes: blinding in clinical trials and other studies. *BMJ. 321*, 504-5.

[70] Schultz, K.F., Chalmers, I., Hays, R.J. and Altman, D.J. (1995). Empirical evidence of bias. Dimensions of methodological quality associated with estimates of treatment effects in controlled trials. *JAMA. 273*, 408-12.

[71] Cornfield, J. (1978). Randomisation by group: a formal analysis. *American Journal of Epidemiology. 108*, 100-102.

[72] Kerry, S.M. and Bland, M. (1998). Statistics notes: sample size in cluster randomisation. *British Medical Journal. 316*, 459.

[73] Rosen, L., Manor, O., Engelhard, D. and Zucker, D. (2006). Design of the Jerusalem handwashing study: meeting the challenges of a preschool-based public health interventions trial. *Clinical Trials Design. 3*, 376-384.

[74] Ellenberg, J.H. (1996). Intent-to-treat analysis versus as-treated analysis. *Drug Information Journal. 30*, 535-544.

[75] Hollis, S. and Campbell, F. (1999). What is meant by intention to treat analysis? Survey of published randomised controlled trials. *BMJ. 319*, 670-674.

[76] Pedersen, D., Keithly, S. and Brady, K. (1986). Effects of an observer on conformity to handwashing norm. *Perceptual and Motor Skills. 62*, 169-70.

[77] Drankiewicz, D. and Dundas, L. (2003). Handwashing among female college students. *American Journal of Infection Control. 31*, 67-71.

[78] Rosenthal, R. (1969). Interpersonal expectations: effects of the experimenter's hypothesis. In R. Rosenthal and R.L. Rosnow (Eds.), *Artifact in behavioral research.* New York: Academic Press. Pp. 181-277.

[79] van de Mortel, TF. (2006). An examination of covert observation and solution audit as tools to measure the success of hand hygiene interventions. *American Journal of Infection Control. 34,* 95-9.

[80] Silvestri, L., Petros, A.J., Sarginson, R.E., de la Cal, M.A., Murray, A.E. and van Saene, H.K.F. (2005). Handwashing in the intensive care unit: a big measure with modest effects. *Journal of Hospital Infection. 59*, 172-9.

In: Hygiene and Its Role in Health
Editors: P. L. Anderson and J. P. Lachan

Chapter 7

Understanding Sexual Behavior of Adolescents: Contributions to Sexual Health Promotion and HIV/AIDS Prevention

Sónia F. Dias[1]

Institute of Hygiene and Tropical Medicine
New University of Lisbon, Portugal

Abstract

The purpose of this study was to improve the understanding of sexuality and sexual behaviors of adolescents and to identify factors that are relevant for sexual health promotion and HIV/AIDS prevention in adolescents. In order to achieve these goals, two studies, one quantitative, and one qualitative were undertaken. The quantitative study described knowledge, attitudes and sexual behaviors that are important to AIDS prevention and examined the relationship between adolescent sexual behavior and demographic factors, personal characteristics, and social context of young people (family, peers, school and community). Data were collected from the Portuguese sample of Health Behaviour in School-aged Children/WHO study, 2002. The qualitative study was used to identify and understand the dynamics of protective and risk factors relevant to AIDS prevention at individual and contextual level. In this study, 12 focus groups were conducted in six secondary schools from different geographic areas of Portugal. In the quantitative study the percent of adolescents reporting ever had sexual intercourse was 23.7%. With respect to use of condoms, 29.9% of the adolescents reported that they or their partner didn't use a condom last time they had engage in sexual intercourse. The findings put forward differences in gender and age in knowledge, attitudes and sexual behaviors. The logistic regression analysis showed that the variables "have sexual

---

[1] Correspondence to: Instituto de Higiene e Medicina Tropical, Universidade Nova de Lisboa, Rua da Junqueira, 96; 1349-008 Lisboa, Portugal, Tel: 00 351 967058421, Fax: 00 351 213632105, e-mail: smfdias@yahoo.com; sfdias@ihmt.unl.pt

intercourse" and "didn't used condom last time they engage in sexual intercourse" are associated with socio-demographic characteristics, individual, family, peers, school and community variables. The qualitative study results underline that issues related to sexuality are complex and knowledge, attitudes and sexual behaviors are influenced by multiple determinants at different levels: individual, family, peers, school and community. The findings suggest that protective and risk factors interact with each other within a network of possible relations that either reduce or increase the probability of involvement in risk behaviors. The results of the two studies suggest that adolescents can't be seen like a homogeneous group concerning knowledge, attitudes and sexual behaviors and HIV/AIDS. They highlight the significance of early interventions that involve young people, but also agents of socialization in the reduction of risk factors and the promotion of protecting factors. This study confirms that complementary use of different methodologies is an appropriate strategy to increase knowledge and understanding about complex meanings in which sexuality is submersed. This work can be useful to design and implement a comprehensive programme on sexual health promotion and AIDS prevention in young people.

Introduction

Over the past two decades, research about adolescent sexual behavior has been motivated largely by the health and social problems that may result of progressively early sexual initiation and unprotected sexual intercourse (Collins, Robin, Wooley, and al., 2002; United Nations, 2005; WHO, 2004a). Beyond physical and emotional risks that adolescents can experience as resulted of sexual activity, consistent evidence seems to indicate that early sexual activity is associated with lesser educational levels and bigger economic disadvantages, with implications at the individual, social and economic level (UNESCO, 2003).

Adolescents have been a priority focus for research because epidemiological data have demonstrated that they are in particular risk of HIV/AIDS and other Sexually Transmissible Infections, greatly determined by their sexual behavior (United Nations, 2005; WHO, 2004a). Large number of adolescents initiate sexual activity during adolescence, have an inconsistent use of condom, present a high probability to have multiple sexual partners and are involved in an association between consumption of drugs or alcohol and unprotected sexual intercourse (Aggleton, Chase, and Rivers, 2004; Garriguet, 2005; Manlove, Ryan, and Franzetta, 2004; United Nations, 2005).

The study "Health Behaviour in School-aged Children" (Ross, Godeau, and Dias, 2004), indicates that the percentages of 15 year-olds adolescents who report having had sexual intercourse was 28%. The mean age of first intercourse among 15 year-olds who reported ever having sexual intercourse was 14.3 years for girls and 14.0 for boys. The proportion of sexually active young people who report that a condom was used last time they had sexual intercourse ranges from 80.2% for boys and 69.6% for girls. Interestingly, Portuguese boys were the ones that had less answered positively to this question (Ross, Godeau, and Dias, 2004).

Data of the "Youth Risk Behavior Surveillance: 2005" (Eaton, Kann, Kinchen, Ross, Hawkins, Harris, et al., 2005), demonstrate that 46.8% of the students between 9° and 12°

grade already initiated sexual activity, being that 6.2% had the first sexual intercourse before 13 years old. In sexually active adolescents, 70% of boys and 55.9% of girls had reported to have used the condom in the last sexual relation. Of the adolescents that already had initiated the sexual activity, 14.3% affirmed to have had 4 or more sexual partners in its life and 23.3% reported to have consumed drugs or alcohol before having had the last sexual intercourse (Eaton et al., 2005).

These evidence and the results of numerous empirical studies underline the need and relevancy to develop and implement programs for the adolescents that are effective in sexual health promotion and STI's prevention, including HIV/AIDS (Schaalma, Abraham, Gillmore, and Kok, 2004). Nevertheless, there is evidence to suggest that many programs not always have obtained the desirable results (Goold, Bustard, Ferguson, Carlin, Neal, and Bowman, 2006; Robin et al., 2004).

One of the reasons that contribute for this fact is that our understanding of sexuality and sexual behaviors in adolescence, behind the large body of research, is general or sometimes limited. To decrease the health risks associated with having sex, health professionals and educators typically encourage adolescents to postpone engaging in sexual intercourse and to use a condom if they do have sex. To improve upon and increase the effectiveness of risk reduction interventions, it is critical to understand the various factors involved in young adolescents' decisions to engage in sexual activity and to use condoms (United Nations, 2005; WHO, 2004b).

Historically, adolescents' sexual decision-making has been viewed largely as an individual-level phenomenon. Consequently, many intervention efforts target adolescents' individual-level influences, with the goal of eliminating or reducing specific sexual risk behaviors. Unfortunately, these interventions have often been designed without understanding or addressing pervasive contextual influences that directly and indirectly influence sexual behavior of adolescents, and so, may not be sufficient to sustain newly adopted healthy behavioral changes over large periods of time (Fenton et al., 2005; Reininger et al., 2005; Shoveller, Johnson, Langille, and Mitchell, 2004).

Over the past few years, researchers and practitioners in diverse fields of public health have begun to recognize the value of adopting a socio-ecological perspective. Bronfenbrenner's ecological model (1979) assumes that young people's behavior occurs as a joint interaction between the individual and their multiple environments. The ecological model has been applied to several areas of the health, having earn special recognition in prevention of adolescence behavior problems (Jacobson and Crockett, 2000), specifically in sexual risk behaviors (Concoran, 2000; DiClemente, Salazar, Crosby, and Rosenthal, 2005; Kotchick, Shaffer, Forehand, and Miller, 2001).

Kirby (2002a), provided a review of predictors of sexual activity and use of contraception and suggested that individual characteristics, family, peer, school and community have all been associated with adolescent sexual outcomes. In this sense, prevention and health promotion interventions may be enhanced by addressing the complexity of the sexual behavior of adolescents, incorporating the ecological model. Indeed, inter-relations between biological, intra-psychic, affective, social and environment factors which adolescents live influences development outcomes, and teen sexuality (Henrich, Brookmeyer, Shrier, and Shahar, 2006; Grzywacz and Fuqua, 2000; WHO, 2003a, 2004b).

Moreover, numerous studies have examined risk factors of sexual behaviors, while markedly fewer studies have identified protective factors underlying adolescents' sexual health (Garwick, Nerdahl, Banken, Muenzenberger-Bretl, and Sieving, 2004; McManus, 2002; Reininger et al., 2005). Several authors have highlighted that protective factors pertaining to sexual behaviors of adolescents had been underestimated in the research and they had only recently gained relevance, especially in planning strategies of prevention and health promotion of adolescents. (DiIorio, Dudley, Soet, and McCarty, 2004; Fergus and Zimmerman, 2005; Pantin, Schwartz, Sullivan, Meadow, and Szapocznik, 2004; Ross, Godeau, Dias, Vignes, and Gross, 2004).

Numerous studies have demonstrated that preventive interventions cannot only focus in the reduction of risk factors, but also must dress protective factors - personal, social, institutional and environment resources - that reduce risk factors and develop resilience that promote adolescents' healthy development (Kingon and Sullivan, 2001; McManus, 2002; Siqueira and Diaz, 2004; Talashek et al., 2003). In this sense, there is a need to modify the intervention strategies paradigm in order to integrate prevention actions in a large context focusing global health of the adolescents (Biglan, Mrazek, Carnine, and Flay, 2003; Caskey and Rosenthal, 2005; Fergus and Zimmerman, 2005; Weissberg, Kumpfer, and Seligman, 2003).

As already pointed, much of previous research has concentrated on the phenomenon of sexuality at individual level assuming that sexual behavior is the result of rational decision-making. Several authors have argued that sexuality is too complex to be conceptualized in terms of individual behaviors indicators that have been measured through the use of quantitative methods and epidemiologic KAP studies (Crawford and Popp, 2003). Quantitative methods gives only a partial picture of the complex factors shaping sexuality and does not enable researchers and developers of intervention programmes to consider the contexts in which knowledge, attitudes and norms are gained and sexuality negotiated (Jackson and Cram, 2003; Power, 2002).

In reality, the complex nature of sexuality needs a more contextualized definition of the phenomenon and a wider view of other levels of influence (Frith, 2000). Therefore, there is a recognition about the need to complementary such data with qualitative methods (Lipovsek, Karim, Gutiérrez, Magnani, and Gomez, 2002). This complementary is useful to enrich a depth understanding of the different dimensions of object in study, namely factors and specificities of political, cultural, social, and personal context.

Much research into adolescent sexuality and risk behaviors are usually understood with health professionals' viewpoint (DiCenso, et al., 2001). Several authors argue that little is know about adolescents' perspective about risk and protective factors of sexual behaviors (Hoppe et al., 2004; Zwane, Mngadi, and Nxumalo, 2004). These analyses are essential to future research and development of effective interventions that incorporate participatory methods in order to promote adolescent sexual health (Crawford and Popp, 2003; Deren et al., 2003; Morgan, 1998).

The fact that recent data indicate that more youths initiate sexual activity during their adolescence, it becomes a priority examine factors related with sexual initiation, but also increase knowledge and understanding about factors that can help sexually active youths to take sexual healthy decisions (Hopkins, Tanner, and Raymond, 2004). Evidence had supported that when youths have information, competences, support and services they make responsible choices and adopt healthy sexual behaviors (WHO, 2004b).

This study involves examining sexual behaviors of adolescents within the context of their environment. The purpose of this study was to improve our understanding of sexuality and sexual behaviors of adolescents and to identify factors that are relevant for sexual health promotion and HIV/AIDS prevention in adolescents. In order to achieve these goals, two studies, one quantitative, and one qualitative were undertaken. The quantitative study described sexual behaviors and examined the relationship between adolescent sexual behavior and demographic factors, personal characteristics, and social context of young people (family, peers, school and community). The qualitative study was used to understand adolescents' perception of the dynamics of protective and risk factors relevant to sexual behavior at individual and contextual level.

Quantitative Study

Method

Data were collected from the Portuguese sample of Health Behaviour in School-aged Children- a collaborative WHO study (Currie et al., 2004). This study included pupils in the 8th and 10th grade of high school from 135 randomly chosen Portuguese schools, representing the entire country as stratified by Education Regional Divisions: North: 42.9%, Centre: 17.7%, Lisbon: 30.7%, Alentejo: 4.1%, and Algarve: 4.5%. The sample included 3762 students, 52% (1956) girls and 48% (1806) males whose mean age was 15.12 (standard deviation=1.35).

Data were collected through the questionnaire used in HBSC study (Currie et al., 2004). The questionnaire had two parts: 1) the mandatory questions of HBSC survey that included questions on socio-demographics characteristics (age, sex, socioeconomic status and nationality), family and school ethos, social relations and social support, physical activity and leisure, nutrition, safety, aspects of psychosocial health, general health symptoms, tobacco and alcohol use, and sexual behavior; 2) an additional national questionnaire included questions on knowledge, attitudes and behaviors about AIDS and sexual behavior. The questionnaire required approximately 55 minutes to complete.

This survey is based on a self-administered questionnaire conducted in schools. The sampling unit used in this survey was the class. The schools in the sample were randomly selected from a national list of schools, stratified by region (5 Education Regional Divisions). In each school classes were randomly selected in order to meet the required number of students for each grade according to international research protocol, which was proportional to the number of same grade mates for each specific region according to the numbers provided by Ministry of Education. Teachers administered the questionnaires in the classroom. Adolescents' participation in the survey was voluntary, however, no instances of refusal were reported. Adolescents who were absent from school on the day of survey were not included. The process of distribution and collection of questionnaires, in the entire country, by mail, was co-ordinated by the national team. Pupils completed the questionnaires on their own and teachers were only allowed to help with administrative procedures. Pupils left their anonymous questionnaires in an envelope; the last pupil was requested to seal the envelope. A 93% response rate was reached considering schools, and 87% considering pupils.

Data Analyses

First, data were analyzed using descriptive analysis of the variables related with sexual behaviors. χ^2 test was used to assess the significance of comparisons. Second, logistic regression analyses were conducted, considering "had sexual intercourse" and "use of condom last sexual intercourse" as dependent variables and a set of demographic, personal, family, peers, school and community variables used as independent variables. The results are express in "odds ratios" with 95% confidence interval. These Logistic regression models included only independent variables that were significantly associated with dependent variables in the bivariate analysis.

Results

The percent of adolescents reporting had ever had sexual intercourse was 23.7%, although 53.9% perceived that adolescents of their age had already had sexual relations. The results indicated gender differences in sexual behaviors: only 15% of girls compared to 33% of boys reported sexual intercourse ($\chi^2(1) = 167.28$, p<.001). First sexual experience occurred between 12-14 years-old for 48% of adolescents, before 11 years for 17.3 % and 15 years or older for 34.5%. Boys were more likely to report first experience earlier than girls.

Nearly half (44.2%) of non-Portuguese adolescents contrasting with 21.4% Portuguese adolescents reported that they had ever had sex ($\chi^2(1)= 72.15$, p<.001).

With respect to use of condoms, 29.9% of the adolescents reported that they or their partner didn't use a condom last time they had engage in sexual intercourse. Gender differences weren't found. While 43.6 % of Portuguese adolescents reported used of condom last sexual relation, only 27.4% of non-Portuguese adolescents had safe sex (χ^2 (1) =12.53, p<.001).

As shown in table 1, logistic regression analysis indicated that compared to sexually inexperienced adolescents, adolescents who had initiated sexual relations were more likely to be older (OR=1.30; 95%CI:1.18-1.42), be male (OR=2.13; 95%CI:1.65-2.75), be non-Portuguese nationality, (OR=2.06; 95%CI:1.34-3.15). Risk-taking behaviors were also significantly related to sexual activity: smoke cigarettes (occasionally, OR=1.54; 95%CI:1.12-2.14 and frequently, OR=2.72; 95%CI:1.89-3.91), drunkenness (occasionally, OR=1.43; 95%CI:1.09-1.87 and frequently, OR=2.29; 95%CI:1.48-3.51), fights (occasionally, OR=1.34;95%CI:1.01-1.76 and frequently, OR=2.01; 95%CI:1.24-3.23). Regarding family variables, sexually active adolescents are significantly more likely to report lower parental monitoring (OR=.90; 95%CI:.84-.98) and sexually inexperienced adolescents had higher levels of mothers' education (OR=.41; 95%CI:.18-.94). The results showed that perceiving that friends had sexual relations (OR=2.80; 95%CI:2.12-3.69), higher number of nights going out with friends (OR=1.20; 95%CI:1.11-1.28), and higher frequency of discos (occasionally, OR=1.53; 95%CI:1.16-2.02 and frequently, OR=2.02; 95%CI: 1.43-2.85) were significantly related to sexual experience. Adolescents who reported be dissatisfied with school are significantly more likely to report had ever had sexual intercourse (OR=1.35; 95%CI:1.05-1.74).

Table 1. Associations with sexual intercourse: results of logistic regression

		OR	95% CI	p-value
Age		1.295	(1.178-1.424)	<.001
Sex	Female	1.0		*<.001*
	Male	2.127	(1.649-2.745)	
Nationality	Portuguese	1.0		.001
	Not Portuguese	2.056	(1.341-3.154)	
*Satisfaction with the life**		1,043	(.975-1.115)	.218
Refuse to have	Easy	1.0		.303
unwanted sexual	Difficult or unable	1.092	(.767-1.557)	.625
relations	Don't know	.696	(.408-1.189)	.185
Refuse to have	Easy	1.0		.079
unprotected sexual	Difficult or unable	.995	(.728-1.359)	.975
relations	Don't know	.549	(.322-.937)	.028
Frequency of smoke	Never	1.0		.001
cigarettes (last	Occasionally	1.544	(1.115-2.138)	.009
month)	Frequently	2.717	(1.889-3.907)	<.001
Frequency of	Never	1.0		<.001
drunkenness	Occasionally	1.426	(1.089-1.867)	.010
(last month)	Frequently	2.285	(1.488-3.510)	<.001
Frequency of	Never	1.0		.336
consumption illegal	Occasionally	.729	(.474-1.119)	.149
drugs (last month)	Frequently	.763	(.334-1.741)	.521
Frequency of getting	Never	1.0		.007
involve in a fight	Occasionally	1.336	(1.014-1.758)	.039
(last 12 months)	Frequently	2.006	(1.246-3.229)	.004
Perceived risk of HIV	Vulnerable	1.0		.489
infection	Invulnerable	.951	(.705-1.282)	.741
	Don't know	.836	(.608-1.149)	.270
Talk with peers about	Easy	1.0		.382
Aids	Difficult or don't talk	.818	(.521-1.284)	
Talk with parents	Easy	*1.0*		.359
about Aids	Difficult or don't talk	1.132	(.869-1.475)	
Family structure	Nuclear	1.0		.237
	Single parent	1.288	(.885-1.875)	.185
	Reconstructed	1.455	(.914-2.315)	.114
	Other	1.269	(.758-2.126)	.365
Mother's Educational	Not educated	1.0		.90
Level	Primary	.580	(.269-1.254)	.166
	Secundary (9th grade)	.560	(.257-1.219)	.144
	Secundary (12th grade)	.479	(.214-1.071)	.073

Table 1. (Continued)

		OR	95% CI	p-value
	College degree	.410	(.179-.938)	.035
*Parental monitoring***		.903	(.835-.976)	.010
Number of nights going out with friends (week)		1.195	(.113-1.283)	<.001
Frequency of going to a disco	Never	1.0		<.001
	Occasionally	1.531	(1.161-2.020)	.003
	Frequently	2.019	(1.432-2.846)	<.001
Adolescents' perceptions of peer sexual debut	Hadn't sexual intercourse	1.0		<.001
	Had sexual intercourse	2.800	(2.123-3.695)	
School satisfaction	Satisfied	1.0		.021
	Dissatisfied	1.348	(1.047-1.736)	
School achievement	Good	1.0		.824
	Average or lower	.971	(.753-1.253)	
Community perception ***		1.104	(.896-1.359)	.352

* Scale range between 0 (minimum) to 10 (maximum).
** Parental monitoring (5 items; α=.71) assessed by perceived parental awareness of child's peers and activities. Higher score reflect higher parental supervision.
*** Community perception (5 items, α=.56) assessed by perceived community organization and neighborhood attachment. Higher score reflect higher negative community perceptions.

Logistic regression analysis based in the variable "use of condom last sexual relation" identified several associations (table 2). The results suggested that first sexual experience at 11 years-old or early (12-14 years-old: OR=.31; 95%CI:.18-.52, and 15-16 years-old: OR=.37; 95%CI:.21-.63), frequency of drunkenness (frequently, OR=2.11; 95%CI:.663-1.212) and be difficult or do not talk with parents about AIDS (OR=1.43; 95%CI:.95-2.16) tend to increased the probability of nonuse of condoms. Adolescents who reported lower number of nights going out with friends found to be less likely to use condoms during last sexual relation, higher number of nights, OR=.847; 95%CI:.95-2.16).

Table 2. Associations with use of condom last sexual relation: results of logistic regression

.		OR	95% CI	p-value
Nationality	Portuguese	1.0		.104
	Not Portuguese	1.591	(.909 - 2.787)	
Satisfaction with the life		.968	(.875 - 1.070)	.521
Refuse to have unprotected sexual relations	Easy	1.0		.762
	Difficult or unable	1.165	(.730 - 1.858)	.522
	Don't know	.877	(.352 - 2.185)	.778
Talk with partner about condom	Easy	1.0		.486
	Difficult or unable	1.300	(.645 - 2.621)	.463
	Don't know	2.277	(.472 - 10.999)	.306
Negotiate use of condom in a sexual relation	Easy	1.0		.665
	Difficult or unable	1.313	(.678 - 2.544)	.419
	Don't know	1.364	(.366 - 5.088)	.644

		OR	95% CI	p-value
Frequency of drunkenness (last month)	Never	1.0		.012
	Occasionally	1.023	(.654 - 1.600)	.922
	Frequently	2.107	(1.212 - 3.663)	.008
Frequency of consumption illegal drugs (last month)	Never	1.0		.451
	Occasionally	1.057	(.610 - 1.831)	.843
	Frequently	1.697	(.745 - 3.868)	.208
Age of first sexual intercourse	11 years old	1.0		<.001
	12-14 years old	.308	(.184 - .515)	<.001
	15 years old	.365	(.213 - .625)	<.001
Perceived risk of HIV infection	Vulnerable	1.0		.812
	Invulnerable	.858	(.538 - 1.368)	.519
	Don't know	.909	(.555 - 1.489)	.705
Talk with parents about Aids	Easy	1.0		.045
	Difficult or don't talk	1.434	(.951 - 2.162)	
Number of nights going out with friends (week)		.847	(.763 - .941)	.002
Frequency of going to a disco	Never	1.0		.667
	Occasionally	.895	(.565 - 1.418)	.637
	Frequently	.785	(.464 - 1.330)	.368

Qualitative Study

Method

The option for focus group as research method was determined by our interest in concept of 'sexuality' as a socially negotiated phenomenon, strongly influenced by contextual factors in favor of the conceptualization of 'sexual behavior' as product of individual decisions (Frith, 2000; Hollander, 2004; Parker, Easton, and Klein, 2000; Warr, 2005). Several authors argue that focus groups reveal the way in which particular individuals' opinions are accommodated or assimilated within an evolving group process (Barbour and Kitzinger, 1999; Green and Thorogood, 2004; Hollander, 2004). This method provides insights into not only individual behavior but also social, cultural and political factors that influence it (Goldman and Schmalz, 2001; Krueger and Casey, 2000; Peterson-Sweeney, 2005). Our choice of focus groups was also determined because focus groups are particularly appropriate for facilitating discussion of taboo topics, like sexuality (Hyde et al., 2005).

Twelve focus groups were conducted, a purposive sample of 72 adolescents, half males and half females. The participants were selected from 10th grade in order to increase the possibility to have adolescents that were more involved in romantic or sexual relationships. The focus groups were carried out in six public schools situated in different regions of the country, in order to include a bigger diversity in terms of social-demographic characteristics of the participants. In each school two single sex focus groups were conducted with six participants in each group.

It was develop a guide for focus groups with of the topics and questions to be explored in discussion. This guide didn't have the purpose of impose a strict structure, but constitute a form to consider the diversity of aspects that intended to discuss, and organize the information to collect.

In the first contact with each group it was presented the moderator and general objective of the study, obtained voluntary consent of the adolescents, and guaranteed anonymity and confidentiality of the data. The focus groups was preceded of an introduction where were discussed some important aspects for the organization of focus groups discussion and participation of each element of the group. It was asked authorization for record focus groups. The focus groups were carried out in the schools in places that permitted privacy. Each focus group had around 90 minutes of duration and all the discussions were tape-recorded and later transcribed.

Data Analysis

For focus groups discussions analysis, it was develop a model, integrating the contribution of several models, as ecological models, and several socio-cognitive models of behavior change apply to the study of the sexual behaviors and HIV/AIDS. This proposed comprehension model presumes that adolescents are exposed to several protective and risk factors distributed by different aspects of their ecological context. This analysis intend to understand protective and risk factors at individual, family, peers, school and community level that contribute to the adoption of healthy or risky sexual behaviors.

Data were analyzed by thematic decomposition analysis (Krueger and Casey, 2000; Morgan, 2001). The first stage of the data analysis involved organization the focus group transcripts into broad content categories complementing with theoretical questions previously defined. After an initial sorting process, the second stage of data analysis was to adjusted categories and proceeding to encoding while continued the re-reading of the discussions. In the analysis, first we establish broad areas of consensus amongst focus group participants on various topics, and second, we draw attention to areas of controversy or debate.

Results

The results presented are going to translate risk and protective factors to sexual behaviors identified in study at individual and contextual level (family, peers, school and community). The results of focus groups discussions cannot be generalized beyond this context, rather they are illustrative of the opinions of a select group on the topics discussed. In each category will be presented excerpts of conversation from transcribed text in order to illustrate adolescents´ meanings.

Individual Factors

Risk Factors

Deficit of Skills

Participants stated that adolescents who don't have the necessary ability to negotiate and refuse sex and don't think in the consequences of the behaviors present a higher risk because these characteristics can work as risk factors. One girl stated, *"There are girls that don't know how to say no. The boyfriend say: oh if you don't want is because you don't like me enough... and the girls end for doing it."* One male respondent said, *"There are some guys that do what others say and don't think for their head. Sometimes they suffer great deceptions, just to do it because the others did."*

Positive Attitudes toward Sexual Risk-Behavior and Expectation of Positive Consequences

Adolescents highlighted positive effects when became sexually active, as acquisition of a status and perception of a better auto-image (associated to the traditional ideology of masculinity). Some boys explained, *"Is more to affirm as a man. We fell more grown up... we feel better with ourselves.";* *"Sometimes it because the desire of wanting to try what the others have already done and to be equal to them."* On the other hand, girls indicated that their male partners expect them to have sex with them to prove that they (the girls) love them (the boys), so frequently they have sex to express theirs love and make sure that they are going to maintain theirs relationships.

Negative Believes about Condoms

The adolescents presented more negative than positive believes about condoms. Loss of physical sensations, pleasure and sensibility, cutting the spontaneity of the relationship, fear in using condoms because it can hurt and little effectiveness of condoms were given as the dominant reasons for not using condoms. One female argued, *"There are some guys that feel that with condoms are not real sexual relationships. They feel that with condoms they don't have pleasure and so they don't like using it."*

Intention of Not Using Condoms

While almost participants highlighted the importance of using condoms, many in their general discussion indicated, in several situations, intention of not using it. One boy said, *"Almost everyone knows that it is necessary to use condoms, but they are taken by the atmosphere... it happens and we won't say no only because we don't have condoms..."*

Adolescents view condom as an effective prevention measure and believe that it is important to avoid sexually transmitted disease, but very few reported always using condoms. One boy reported, *"We know that we should use condoms but when we are in the situation we forget it, we stop thinking and we forget everything..."*

Perception of Low Self-Efficacy in the Adoption of Protective Strategies

The adolescents believe that lack of self-control is a risk factor. A large group of boys acknowledged fears or difficulties in using the condoms. They claimed that condoms were a threat to their self-image and in those who sensed that their erectile performance would be out of their control if condoms were imposed on them. One male stated, *"It is natural that everyone is afraid the girl thinks that he is an inexperienced and in that situation boys are afraid and prefer not using."*

Lack of Knowledge on HIV/AIDS

Most of the adolescents, although they consider that they are informed, affirmed to have doubts. One girl said, *"But there are a lot of doubts. People can be informed of the essential, but all have doubts... it is necessary to explain and tall with adolescents."*

Inaccurate Perception of the Vulnerability to HIV Infection

The majority of participants did not mention personal vulnerability. Adolescents used a wide range of invalid strategies to rationalize low personal risk of becoming infected: first time, adhering to romantic notions about the long-term and monogamous nature of serial relationships. Some adolescents stated, *"Some teenagers don't see any HIV risk because it is their first time having sex. They believe they don't have any disease or nothing."; "If we have sexual relationships with a person that is not known... there we took risk. With our girlfriend we don't take risks we trust...and I'm not going to do with someone that I don't know."; "I only have sex with my boyfriend, I don't have sex with A, B, or C..."*

Although most of adolescents believe that they are immune to risk, some expressed a sense of fatalism that mitigates against planning for the future. One boy argued, *"We never know... we can get AIDS with some needles that are lost in the ground... we live in a neighborhood that is so bad and with lots of drugs users that we never know..."*

Students who considered that is possible for any person becoming HIV infected attribute to a blood transfusion the principal cause of infection. One girl explained, *"We can help someone who has an accident with blood and the person can have AIDS and because we don't know, we can be infected."*

Preventive Strategies That Represent Risk of Infection

The dominant strategies mentioned to reduce the infection risk are good knowledge and trust of the sexual partner. One boy said, *"If we know the person before doing it the risks are minimums". We can't do with the first girl that we see."* They believed that abstinence from casual sex is sufficient to protect against HIV infection, while protected sex with regular partners is safe. One boy stated, *"One way to protect ourselves is not having sex with someone strange."*

Some adolescents believe that infected people can be detected and avoided: *"I think that I'm not in risk of being HIV infected because when a person has AIDS we know ... the person have an anemic aspect".*

Pregnancy Prevention

Unwanted pregnancy was the main concern to participants and it seems to have implications in the preventive strategies that adolescents adopted when they have sexual relationships. Protection to HIV/AIDS goes to second plan. One girl explained, *"If the boy is afraid that the girl becomes pregnant he uses condom, but if he doesn't worry and he is only interested in doing it maybe he will not use anything."* One boy said, *"I know a case that they didn't use condom because she used the pill."*

Protective Factors

Skills
Adolescents argued to enable to impose their will and to know how to avoid pressures is extremely important. One male stated, *"No matter how much pressure you are suffering, you should only do what you want,... we should not force ourselves to do anything that we don't want.".* One girl said, *"If she doesn't want, she has to explain to her boyfriend that she is not prepared and say that she decided not to do it."*

Negative Attitudes towards Unprotected Sex and Expectation of Negative Consequences
A small group of participants presented negative attitudes towards unprotected sex, highlighting the existence of negative consequences. One boy stated, *"Nowadays, nobody even think not to take precautions, the youths have the notion of the future and they worry in protecting themselves, only a foolish one takes risks."*

Positive Attitudes about Condoms
A minority of participants indicated more positive attitudes about condoms than negative. The arguments used are associated with the naturalness and easiness of using it, and the need of protection. One boy said, *"That is prepared to be simple. It is the form of having safe sexual relationships."*

Intention to Adopt Protective Behaviors and Use Condoms
A small number of adolescents strongly believed that they will use the condom when they have sexual intercourse. One boy declared *"I don't even put in hypothesis not to use it because I couldn't manage to do it without using it, I won't feel well."*

Perception of Self-Efficacy
About a quarter of the participants presented a perception of self-efficacy in the adoption of healthy sexual behaviors. One female affirmed, *"I think I can persuade my boyfriend to use it. I would say: you do like I want or I don't do it."* One male explained, *"Everyone knows how to put a condom before having sexual relationships. I think in first time, boys can feel a little anxious, but then we don't think about that and we use it."*

High Levels of Accurate Knowledge about HIV/AIDS
The participants believed high levels of accurate knowledge about modes of prevention can be a protective factor. Some considered that they are already quite informed. One female stated, *"Before doing it they have to think, they have to be aware of what can happen and know how it can be avoided."*

Accuracy Perception of the Vulnerability to HIV/AIDS

A small group of participants stated that everyone who practices sexual risk behaviors is at risk of HIV infection. Unprotected sexual relationships and multiplicity of partners are the dominant reasons to be at risk. One boy admitted, *"Who doesn't take precautions, can be caught."*

Preventive Protective Strategies

When asked for strategies that they can adopt to reduce infection risk, although they refer trust in the sexual partner they seem to be aware that the use of condoms is the only strategy that confers full protection. One girl said, *"I think that I can say that I trust in my boyfriend and I don't think there is any problem, but it is never 100% safe. It is better always to protect ourselves with condoms."*

Some participants in the discussions described a strategy to make sure that they have a condom when they need one. One boy affirmed, *"I also think that the best thing is to always have condoms in your pocket because you don't know what time you are going to have sex".*

Family Factors

Risk Factors

Negative and Hostile Family Environment

According to adolescents' opinions a negative family environment with a high level of family conflict can increased risk for sexual debut and other sexual risk behaviors. One boy explained, *"Girls who don't have the love of their parents, tend to do other things, that's why they become sexually active."* Males, on the other hand, linked lack of parental love to problem behavior, *"...teenagers need to feel loved by their parents because if not, they will stay away and may end up doing wrong things like drugs and sex with the first girl that appears."*

Lack of Parent-Child Communication about Sexual Issues

The majority of adolescents stated that lack of communication and information can be risk factors. One boy said, *"Because they don't talk with parents, adolescents do what friends say. And girls are more influenced by boyfriends."*

Many felt that sexual education by parents was an ideal but not always realistic goal. Both male and female adolescents reported that it was difficult to talk to their parents about sexual issues. Some adolescents said that talking about sexuality in the family is taboo. Not only embarrassment, but also anxiety about how to talk about it, as well as the respect for their parents plays an important role in parent-child communication. A group of adolescents affirmed there is a lack of sexual health knowledge among parents and that is a barrier to a sexual health communication.

In general, adolescents wanted more open discussions with their parents about sex, though most felt parents were uncomfortable, afraid or unsure how to broach the subject. They also believed parents treated boys and girls differently: *"Parents believe they don't need* to talk with a daughter because it is too early for her. But sometimes fathers talk about sex with sons."; "They would give condoms to a son but not to a daughter. They expect boys ... to be a little on the wild side, but they don't expect the girls to be that way." Girls spontaneously said that their mothers' communications about sex often seemed to assume the form of warnings: "She told me that I can get a baby and that it isn't nice...and them with boys parents don't care about it."

It was clear that even in the context of a rather open conversation about sex, there was no emphasis on the feelings, experiences and pleasures of sexual intercourse. Girls tend to perceive parental discussions about sex as restrictive and with and emphasis in the risk of sexual activity. It seemed that one of the consequences of this "discourse of danger", some times dominant in the conversations between mothers and daughters, was that daughters did not openly discuss their sexuality or their sexual behavior with their parents: sexual desire, sexual feelings and sexual behavior became a secret. One girl explained, "I'm afraid that my mom and the rest of family will find out, because my father said that if he finds out about it then my bag is already packed. So I'm afraid because if my parents find out then I must leave house."

Authoritarian Parenting Style

The majority of participants highlighted the adverse effect of being given too little autonomy or trust by parents. One girl explained, "The world forbidden, don't do it just because, increased the desire and curiosity of doing it. Then when we are alone, without parents, we do all without thinking and without responsibility because we have to take advantage of a moment of liberty".

Lack of Parental Supervision

Adolescents indicated that the lack of parental supervision can be a risk factor. One boy said, "Some parents don't care about what their children do. Sometimes they don't go to school and they don't care. This is very bad."

Protective Factors

Family Connectedness

When asked to discuss the role of family in the sexual behavior of adolescents, participants said that the influence of parents in adolescent sexual behaviors depends on quality of the parent-son relation. The majority focused on the impact of parental love and family relationships and expressed the view that a stable and loving family was an important part of an adolescent's life, including the decision to engage in sexual intercourse.

Positive Parent-Child Communication

A positive and open parent-child communication was related with an influence in how teenagers make their sexual decisions as well with a reduction in sexual risk-taking behavior. One girl said, "If we can talk with our parents, and we felt supported when we talk with them about all kind of issues, they can help us a lot. They have more experience so they will help us to protect to futures situations."

Authoritative Parenting Style

An authoritative parenting style, where parents don't forbid, but are vigilant about what happen in theirs children's life and explain the risks promotes responsibility, competence and the development of skills to avoid risk behaviors. One boy affirmed, *"If parents give some liberty to their children they will become more responsible. They should say: be careful about this and this, but you have to decide what is better for you."*

Parental Monitoring

Parent monitoring, like awareness where children are, what they are doing after school, know their friends, was stated as a protective factor. One boy said, "Parents should be aware of our life. It's important for us. Then they should tell us what is wrong and what is correct. It is for us own good".

Peer Factors

Risk Factors

Peer Norms

The normative expectations of others and the motivation to comply with these expectations generated responses that highlight the influence of peers on the sexual behavior of the adolescents. High levels of sexual activity were perceived as normative for both sexes. One difference that did emerge was that sexual activity for young boys was socially accepted, whereas attitudes toward girls' sexual activity were more variable. The majority of young women made no mention of peer norms pressured them to have sex. Participants indicated if adolescents perceive that their friends are having unprotected sex and engaging in other types of risky sex, they may be more likely to adopt their friends' behaviors.

Consistent with traditional gender roles, males were expected to have frequent sex, taking place at the earliest possible opportunity after meeting a potential partner. Boys admitted, *"Males are concerned with being viewed as not masculine enough or "immature" by girls.";* *"Talking about experience, girls don't want a virgin boy, they want someone with experience."*

Adolescents view sexual behavior and condom use as elements within a complex script that rules heterosexual interactions. While many of girls participants highlighted the importance of using condoms and their intention to use them in relationships, their general discussion indicated the manner in which negative peer norms encroach on consistent use of condoms. Social norms limit the extent to which young women can negotiate the use of condom in relationships and are prepared to carry condoms with them. Participants mentioned that girls who carry condoms risked being labeled a promiscuous. One girl explained, *"It will worry a guy if a girl carries lots of condoms. He will worry and start thinking that maybe she will have sex with other boys."*

Some female participants were aware of importance of protecting themselves in terms of pregnancy and diseases. Indeed, some said that they ignore social norms about carrying condoms and replace them with their own norms, *"If she's carrying a condom in her bag, everyone will say that she likes sex. I think that girl is taking care of herself because she doesn't want to be affected by pregnancy or AIDS."*

Among male and female participants there was the notion that condoms are generally unnecessary in steady relationships but that they should be used in casual sex. Some indicated that they would make use of condoms to prevent pregnancy with regular partners but that condom use is most important for preventing getting a disease in casual relationships. One boy affirmed, *"You don't need to use a condom with your girlfriend but you have to use one with your casual partner because you don't know if she has a disease".*

Perceived Peers and Partners' Pressure to Sexual Risk-Behaviors

In all groups, peer pressure to have sexual relationships was the main risk factor given. Adolescents are often influenced by others to engage in behaviors they would otherwise not engage in. Some participants felt that they are outcast from group if they are not doing what their peers are doing. These adolescents exhibited a degree of awareness of the way in which peer and gender pressures placed their health at risk. The results suggest that peer pressure on boys strongly encourage intercourse. It was described that oftentimes, those who tried to resist to conforming to peers norms by avoiding sex are also subjected to taunting and teasing. In an attempt to avoid being called names, adolescents find their self conforming to group behavior. Boys admitted, *"Guys were asking me how I could not have sex with my girlfriend. They said I didn't know anything about sex and she didn't like me enough. That's why many boys have to have sex with theirs girlfriends."; "Some friends encourage you to have sex. They tease you and accused you of being stupid for not having sex and sometimes they try to convince that sex without condoms are better."*

Although some girls chose to abstain from sexual intercourse and reported that peers respected their choice, others reported a great deal of partners' pressure to become sexually active, *"The problem is that some guys want so much to have sex that they do it forcefully. And girls are afraid of losing their partner so they didn't deny sex."*

However, there were participants in the discussions who had chosen not to adhere to peers norms. One Boy said: *"I don't care about what others say, I will only have sex when I decide".* One girl affirmed: *"I refuse. I don't want to be doing that without a condom. I can say no, thanks."*

Lack of Power in Heterosexual Relationships

The pressure on boys may translate into some degree of force or coercion on young women in sexual encounters. Many girls reported that young women experience partners' pressure to become sexually active. The imbalance in power between male and female partners in heterosexual relationships limits the ability of girls to either refuse sex or negotiate use of condoms. Several themes related to condom used emerged and they included personal sense of powerlessness and male dominance, condom beliefs that may be barriers to use, and lack of skills in negotiating the use of condoms. One girl said: *"Boys don't like to use condoms, and they try to convince the girlfriend saying: we don't need to use condoms, you are my princess and I'm going to stay with you for all my life... you trust me and I believe in you and only without condoms is a full relation... and so many girls don't use it".* Males agreed that females "break down" quicker than males when pressured to have sex or to have unprotected sex.

Association between Alcohol and Sexual Risk Behaviors

Most participants mentioned that the intake of large amounts of alcohol was a determining factor in their risk-taking sexual behavior. Boys reported that while intoxicated they feel an intense physiological excitement to have sex which overruled the threat of HIV infection, *"In a bar or disco, and when you were drinking a lot, you don't even think about the risks. You are so excited to have sex that you don't care about with whom you are going to have sex or if you are going to use a condom".*

For young women drinking allows them to forget about social rules of having a clean reputation. Participants reported that alcohol consumption reduced girls' capacity for refuse sex or negotiate use of condoms. One girl explained, *"You've got no more inhibitions, you're not shy anymore, you have no worry about anything and you can't say no."* One boy affirmed, *"When a girl drinks a lot, she behaves like a guy and for us it is easier because she always wants to have sex."* Boys believed it is easier to have sex and don't use condom under the influence of alcohol. One male participant admitted, *"Sometimes boys offer drinks to get her drunk and she will accept to have sex."*

Protective Factors

Positive Communication, Support and Understanding

All groups of participants agreed that talking about sexuality with peers is very important because they can hear advices, clarify doubts and talk without fear of consequences. Adolescents considered that friends support, help and understand them very well. Girls said, *"Friends are the easiest form to obtain information about sexuality and that kind of things...talking with my friends I have learned lots of things that not even knew.";* *"If our friend is more experienced she will say you not to break down to boyfriends' pressures and thus she can help us with this situation and we aren't so alone..."*

Perceived Positive Peers' Norms and Positive Attitudes from Partners to Use Condoms

A group of adolescents mentioned that the majority of their friends didn't have sexual relations yet and pointed out that this fact decrease pressure to have sexual relations because they feel that they are act according peers' norms. One girl explained, *"By example, in my group of friends I know there aren't many that already had, there are cases but they are not the majority. Then we don't feel so much pressure."*

Some participants considered that most of adolescents used condoms in theirs sexual relations. One boy affirmed, *"I think that my friends us. And it is very easy to carry condoms with us and always have a condom when we need one."* The majority of participants have the perception that girls have a positive attitude to condoms use and this is pointed as a protective factor.

Interpersonal Positive Consequences

Some participants identified positive interpersonal consequences of use of condoms. The argument presented is that improves the relationships. Boys argued that using condom in sexual relation reduce conflict and disagreement *"The use of condom reduce conflict between girls and boys because there are no disagreement";* and girls whose partners want to use condoms feel more respected because boyfriend worries about her, *"If it is a well-mannered boy he will use condom. If a boy loves his girlfriend he will use it because he thinks about her and respect her."*

How Parents' Factors Interact with Peers Influence

Participants indicated that peers and family have the most influence on the sexual behavior of adolescents. The absence of open communication about sex let adolescents very alone with their sexuality with little support and guidance from their parents. On the other hand, seemed also to contribute to adolescents be even more dependent on their friends' perception of sexuality and sexual behaviors.

School Factors

Risk Factors

Poor School Achievement, Low Academic Aspirations and School Abandonment

In agreement with some adolescents, poor school achievement, low academic aspirations or school abandonment can constitute risk factors, *"Who doesn't have the objective of studying, of thinking about the future or doesn't have responsibilities is more susceptible.";* *"The youths that don't go to school have less support and are more isolated. They don't have anything to do all day and then they take more risks."*

Lack of Sexual Education in Schools

They stated that lack of information about sexuality in school can constitute a risk factor for sexual behaviors. One girl said, *"They didn't speak anything about that in school and I think it is wrong. It is very important that schools can transmit information about sexual issues because there are many adolescents that have difficulties in speaking with their parents and they are alone with doubts..."*

Critics to the Sexual Education Sessions

The adolescents argued that sexual education sessions are usually focused in the risks and diseases of sexual activity. One girl argued, *"For them sexual education is to talk about the risks of having sex, but it should not only be to talk about diseases and risks because there are also good things, it is not? And why not to talk about them..."*

Protective Factors

Protective School Environment and Connectedness to School

Some participants considered that going to school can work as protective factor for risk sexual behaviors. One male said, *"Going to school makes the person feel better on his own."*. One female affirmed, *"The school initiatives when they are good are very important because we spend a lot of time in school."*

Information And Sexual Education

It seems that for adolescents the main contribution of schools in healthy sexual behaviors promotion is in the area of information that can be made available to students, aspect referred in all of the interviewed groups. One girl said, *"Now that we are thinking about those things and we begun to have sexual relationships, it is very important that we can talk about sexual relationships and other things with somebody without consequences about what was said."*

Relationship with a Large Number of Peers and Other Adults

Schools allow a relationship with an enlarged group of peers and other adults which can be quite positive. One girl explained, *"Most of them don't speak to their parents and if they had support in school it would be easier. The youths acquire information mainly in school through their friends and talking with some teachers."*

Distribution Of Condoms

Many adolescents considered that condoms distribution in school is essential to obtained free condoms and that is a good strategy to increased access to condoms. One boy said, *"They should distribute condoms and give accurate information about the way it should be used. This is very important for us because sometimes we don't have good access to condoms."*

Community Factors

Risk Factors

Low-Income Neighborhoods

In the opinion of some adolescents, living in low-income neighborhoods, with poverty, high rate of crime and drugs users, can represent a risk factor. One boy said, *"The environment where they live is important... in more decaying neighborhoods there are many adolescents with inaccurate information, usually anyone take precautions so they will not also take it."*

Difficulty to Acquire Condoms

The majority of adolescents (some boys and most of the girls) stated that is constraining or difficult to buy condoms, despite their relatively good availability. There is a group of girls that admitted that they were unable of buying it, *"There are many places where to buy it, but they are very public, we feel embarrassed... everybody looking at me... I was not able to go and buy it."*

Social Norms Regarding Gender Role Differences

To male adolescents, heterosexual sex is an important defining element of masculinity, and a key component of the male sexual script. The script embodies elements of male dominance in sex, and an attitude of achievement when it comes to sex. From the discourses of participants, there is evidence that boys believe that sexually successful with girls is a way for a young male to prove to his peers that he has come of age, and he isn't a homosexual.

Girls participants expressed the view that they are more culturally restrained than boys, *"If a girl gets into a relationship with every boy that asks her, she gets a bad reputation. It is opposite for boys, if he goes with every girl that asks him, it's ok."* Females are expected to be more reserved, and are praised for sexual abstinence. Unlike boys, adolescent females who have sex with someone with whom they are not in a relationship are labeled as "dirty girl". *"If they know you slept with someone, they will talk badly of you."*

Social norms encroach on the extent to which young women are prepared to carry condoms with them. Participants mentioned that gossip is a constant source of conflict and that women carrying condoms risked being labeled a promiscuous. *"Girls think: they will see me buying it... they will think that I am a bad girl., "If girls have condoms with them they are misjudge... and they don't want that."*

Mass Media and Internet

In the opinion of some adolescents mass media and Internet can encourage sexual activity. One girl said, *"Television can stimulate people... everyone is always talking about that in TV and with that kind of films, I think it is common that sex happens more and more early."*

Protective Factors

Availability of Condoms

Although the majority said that it is easy to have access to condoms, just a minority affirms to feel comfortable when they are buying it. One boy affirmed, *"We should not feel embarrassment especially because we are protecting ourselves. Shame is who doesn't use."*

Some female participants said that they ignore social norms about carrying condoms and replace them with their own norms because they are aware that young women who are able to overcome social distrust of female condom carrying are protecting themselves in terms of pregnancy and disease.

Support of Pro-Social Institutions

Adolescents highlight positive roll of some institutions or associations in providing information and condoms distribution. One male described, *"I have a centre that is near my house that they give condoms for free. If I had problems I would speak with those psychologists of these institutions... people can go there..."*

Mass Media and Internet

Mass Media and Internet were seen by the majority of the groups as informative sources. Some adolescents indicated that they have talked with the parents about sexual issues because television programs. One boy said, *"Sometimes television pulls the subject, and then we talk about those subjects."* One female explained, *"People are informed because television is a good source of information sometimes is not very good... but informs."*

Health Services

A small minority noted that health services can be used, either to provide information or to distribute condoms and contraceptive methods. However, when questioned about their use, none of the adolescents that point the possibility to use health services affirms having done it. In the opinion of the majority, the adolescents don't feel comfortable in these services. One girl said, *"If we want information we can go to the health centers. I don't go there to ask for information, but you could go... "*

Conclusion

The data provided by this study suggest that majority of adolescents don't have sexual risk behaviors. However, adolescents identified as sexually active consisted largely of early initiators who by definition are seen to be at higher risk in relation to sexual behavior. In this study, 29.9% of the adolescents reported that they or their partner didn't use a condom last time they had engage in sexual intercourse. Societal discomfort with sexual issues (including parents and school), and fear that teaching about sexuality and protection will promote adolescent sexual activity, can contributed to youth not receiving the education necessary to make informed decisions about sexuality, and to expose adolescents to significant physical, emotional, and social risks (Kirby, 2002b; Schaalma et al., 2004).

There were gender differences emerging from this study. The gender gap was most evident when participants discussed social risks and benefits of sexual behavior. Girls were generally more concerned about impact that sex might have on their relationship, difficulty to negotiate sexual behaviors, and their social status, whereas boys were more concerned about social standing and having fun or pleasure (Hoppe et al., 2004). Our findings suggest that males and females may need different messages and a different set of skills to negotiate their sexuality.

Several themes related to condom used emerged and they included personal sense of powerlessness and male dominance, condom beliefs that may be barriers to use, and lack of skills in negotiating the use of condoms. In the field of condom use promotion it should take account of the range of factors that militate against condom use by young people, despite high levels of knowledge about sexual health-enhancing benefits of condoms (Eloundou-Enyegue, Meekers, and Calves, 2005; Rock, Ireland, Resnick, and McNeely, 2005).

Data indicated that non-Portuguese adolescents experience disproportionate rates of risk behaviors relative to Portuguese adolescents. The apparent influences of race/ethnicity may be confounded by a host of environmental factors (Fenton, et al., 2005; Ross, and Fernandez-Esquer, 2005). For example, poverty may be a risk factor where its direct association with race/ethnicity exerts an indirect influence on sexual behaviors (Forehand et al., 2005). Non-Portuguese adolescents' higher sexual risk behaviors can be traced to a greater proportion of these adolescents living in geographic clusters characterized by poverty, low educational attainment, compromised family structures and lower socio-economic status.

In general, adolescents have a good knowledge about the main HIV/AIDS transmission routes and how to protect them from becoming infected. However, in this study, like findings from other studies in this area, it was noticeable the existence of misconceptions and gaps in knowledge (Dias, Matos, Gonçalves, 2005; Potsonen, Kontula, 1999). Our findings provide some evidence for the influence of motivational mechanisms on risk judgments. Almost all adolescents admitted that any person having intercourse can get AIDS, but becoming infected seemed like a distant risk as far as the youth concerned. It appears that several participants may be underestimated their absolute or comparative risk of acquiring AIDS in the sense that their risk perception are not consistent with their reports of involvement in potentially risky behaviors, like other researches have suggested (Bettinger et al., 2004; Kershaw et al., 2003). In theirs discourses, adolescents classified new relationships as 'serious' so as to justify their sexual behavior and incorporate issues of trust that prevent them from using condoms in relationships in which they actually know very little about their partners. In addition, young men in particular rely on appearance and reputation to make decisions about certain women being 'safe' and therefore not requiring condoms for sexual intercourse. This has to be an area of consideration for policy makers and providers of sexual health intervention (Johnson, McCaul, and Klein, 2002).

Contrary to the theory that adolescents are unaware of the risks of sex, the majority of adolescents in this study identified salient health risks associated with having sex. The finding that the most frequently mentioned theme was the risk of pregnancy, more than STI/HIV, could be interpreted as suggestive of a heightened concern for pregnancy over STI/HIV. This could be due the fact that HIV/AIDS is not an immediate consequence to their lives. In light of current research further studies are needed to determine how these differences in level of concern for pregnancy and STI/AIDS influences sexual decision-making (Horowitz, 2003; Wulff, and Lalos, 2004).

These results clearly indicate that adolescents were able to identify a broad range of risky and beneficial outcomes of having sex and using or not using condoms. The results also suggest that decision-making involves consideration of not only risks, but also benefits. Indeed, not only health risks but also social risks and benefits play a key role in behavioral decision-making (Hoppe et al., 2004; Johnson, McCaul, and Klein, 2002).

Interventions often focus on educating adolescents about medically correct information about human reproduction, HIV/AIDS, other STI's, and risky outcomes, with particular emphasis on health outcomes. It is important, using methodology that can capture the adolescents' perspective, examine what adolescents identify as risky and beneficial outcomes related to sex, and understand and address the role that these outcomes might have in decision-making. Furthermore, intervention and educational programs with adolescents regarding safe sexual activity could benefit from widening communication from a focus on health risks to include discussion of psychosocial risks and benefits. Adolescents are likely to be best served by placing prevention interventions back within the framework of broader sexuality education. Interventions should also include develop communication within relationships, information, decision-making, negotiation and handling pressures skills (Hopkins, Tanner, and Raymond, 2004; who, 2003b). For example, providing students with concrete action plans or by a skills training component aimed at increasing perceived self-efficacy to adopt healthy behaviors.

In addition, our findings are consistent with previous research that has shown that risky sexual behaviors tend to co-occur with other types of risk behaviors (Carpenter, 2005; Guilamo-Ramos, Litardo, and Jaccard, 2005; Stueve and O'Donnell, 2005). The causality and links between adolescent risky behaviors is difficult to establish (Abbey, Saenz, and Buck, 2005). Greater understanding of this relationship will help shape future intervention and benefit health educators as they develop programs designed to reduce adolescent health-compromising behaviors. The challenge of "complexity" in adolescent health research is not new, yet exhaustive efforts are required to understand the linkages among healthy and unhealthy behaviors and health protective factors in the context of formative adolescent lifestyles (Goold, Bustard, Ferguson, Carlin, Neal, and Bowman,, 2006; Guilamo-Ramos, Litardo, and Jaccard, 2005).

Our findings also highlight that young people's sexuality is a complex process and adolescent decision-making around sexuality issues is an interaction of individual, social, family, peer, school, community and socio-cultural factors. Given this, interventions for adolescents should be planned at several levels based in a social-ecological perspective, incorporating the multi-dimensional context in which adolescent sexuality is constructed and negotiated (DiClemente, Salazar, Crosby, and Rosenthal, 2005; Henrich, Brookmeyer, Shrier, and Shahar, 2006; Kotchick, Shaffer, Forehand, and Miller, 2001).

Both singularly and in various combinations, the wide circle of influences present opportunities for the development and elaboration of protective and risk factors associated with sexual activity. In the light of our interest in factors shaping youth sexuality, our analysis results identify a core set of risk and protective factors for healthy sexual decision-making and consistent condom use among adolescents.

Risk factors included lack of skills for negotiate sexuality, social norms that support sexual risk behaviors, negative and unsupportive adult attitudes to youth sexuality, lack of parental support and monitoring, role models for risk behaviors, peer norms and pressures to engage in sexual risk behaviors, school disconnectedness, restricted availability of condoms, and broader social issues related to social construction of gender sexual role.

Protective factors that are amenable to intervention include high levels of self-efficacy related to refusing unwanted and unprotected sex, attitudes and beliefs that support consistent condom use, and avoidance of sexual risk behaviors, perceived norms of peers, families, and communities that encourage self-protective sexual behaviors, like peer and partners support for condom use, perceived parent support to sexual communication, strong sense of connection to family and schools, and high expectations for school achievement. The results highlight that interventions programs should capitalize on the power of protective of individual-level and environment factors to counteract risk, protect adolescents from involvement in risky sexual behaviors and promote healthy sexuality (Garwick et al., 2004; Ross, Godeau, Dias, 2004; Vesely et al., 2004).

The data provided by this study indicate that adolescents conduct their sexual lives through experiences and beliefs that have been generated through their membership of particular societies and communities. The results suggest that the perceptions of societal double standard in sex are still in teenage culture and may influence behavior. Sexuality and its expression take place in a larger context of structural gender power inequality that characterizes most societies. The social control of sexual behaviors and gender relations are complex phenomena that require sophisticated and varied methods of study. Employing focus group discussions have been shown to be very effective method in understanding young people's perspectives on many issues (Dias, Matos, Gonçalves, 2006; Hyde et al., 2005; Morgan, 2001).

Social constructions of masculinity that promote the idea men should engage in multiple sexual relationships combined with internalized negative attitudes towards condoms place their sexual health at risk. Social definitions of sexual relations with men needing sex further constrain women's to either refuse sex or negotiate safe sex. Therefore, girls, regarding preservation of reputation, often adhere to these norms limiting theirs opportunities for adopt healthy sexual behaviors. For example, young women often avoid carrying condoms and do not have condoms available due to the negative reputations and labels associated with women who look for sex. In addition, social pressures encourage young women not to engage in sex but those that do are expected to do so in the confines of 'serious' and 'trusting' relationships. This emphasis on 'serious' relationships encourages premature trust of partners and therefore the non-use of condoms. Research has been particularly concentrated on danger in which adolescents place their sexual health when adhering to traditional social norms (Foreman, 2003; Rosenthal et al., 2002; Wingood and DiClemente, 2000).

Our research findings indicate that a minority of adolescents challenge dominant social constructions of relationships defining their sexuality outside of these norms. The areas in which they challenged social norms included male domination over women, the idea that males 'need' sex and don't like using condoms and the idea that girl carrying condoms could be classified as sexually promiscuous. For this reason one key interest in research is to examine not only dominant representations of adolescent sexuality, but also the ways in which these representations might be deconstructed and reconstructed in ways that promote safe sex behavior. For intervention, young people who challenge stereotypical norms and adopt sexual healthy behaviors provide a fertile starting point for debates to developing new approaches to more effective interventions .

Much research has simplistically generalized adolescent sexuality in a stereotyped, homogenous and one-dimensional way with inadequate attention to views held by young people (Hopkins et al., 2004; Zwane et al., 2004). Several authors have argued that for failing to take account of wide of variations in adolescents' sexuality, such generalizations have played a key role in undermining the success of sexual health promotion among youth (Robin et al., 2004; Tanne, 2005). It is therefore vital that research focuses not only on the way in which dominant norms place young peoples' sexual health at risk, but also on the ways in which particular young people resist these norms, sometimes leading to alternative and less risky sexual behaviors and practices.

Our findings are consistent with research that suggests that parenting is related to adolescent sexuality outcomes via communication, values, monitoring, and a sense of connection with their teen (Huebner and Howell, 2003; Hutchinson, Jemmott, Jemmott, Braverman, and Fong, 2003; Rose, Koo, Bhaskar, Anderson, White, and Jenkins, 2005). Moreover, parents' influence can also buffer adolescents' against the influence of negative peer norms that encourage risky sexual behaviors (Li, Stanton et al., 2000). Emerging evidence suggests that several family-level interventions may be effective at reducing adolescents' sexual risk behaviors (Ahern and Kiehl, 2006; Shoveller et al., 2004). There have been attempts to strengthen parent-adolescent processes in hopes of promoting healthy adolescent sexual behavior. Parent education should stress the importance of parents being physically and psychologically available to their children, especially as they approach the teen years. These interventions may also attempt to increase parent-child communication and enhanced parental monitoring as well as foster a sense of increased family support.

Another important aspect is that adolescents are particularly influenced by their peers (Shoveller et al., 2004). The results indicate that in the majority of cases peer norms and behaviors encourage risk, as they pressure to engage in sexual intercourse, promote unsafe sexual behavior and encourage concern about sexual health to be viewed in a negative light. In contrast, a small group demonstrated that peer norms assist in the adoption of safe sexual behavior. As other researchers have found, perceived peer norms supportive of sexual protective behaviors can have a significant influence on the adoption and maintenance of preventive behaviors (Zimmer-Gembeck, 2004). It is essential that programs create ways of enhancing adolescents with risk-reduction skills by helping them to change peer norms and to develop negotiation and assertiveness skills to in order to resist peer pressure. Peer education provides context for renegotiation of dominant norms of behavior that might be placing young people's sexual health at risk, and for collective establishment of new healthy norms (Campbell, and MacPhail, 2002). Stems from the belief that well-liked and respected peers may be able to encourage others towards behaviors that promote sexual health rather than the high-risk behaviors usually associated with peer norms (Main, 2002). New norms and values negotiated by peer groups in this way provide health enhancing environments in which healthy sexual behavior is more likely to be maintained.

Schools offer an advantageous setting because they are the only venue where nearly all youth can be reached in a structured environment and because sexual health education can potentially be integrated into a broader (family, peers and community) context to reducing risks and creating opportunities for healthful adolescent development. An effort has to be made in order to improve the possibility of a sense of affiliation and agency of adolescents in schools settings, as a way to increase their perceived positive school "ethos" and thus their subjective perception of wellbeing, sense of belonging, perception of self-efficacy and worthfulness, and consequently their choices of healthier life style (Roche, Ellen, and Astone, 2005; McNeely, Nonnemaker, and Blum, 2002).

Bronfenbrenner argued that in addition to proximal environments, such as family, peers and school interactions, the larger environment also influences developmental outcomes (Bronfenbrenner, 1979). In addition to this influences, neighborhood or community issues have also been found to influence teen sexuality (Roche, Mekos, Alexander, Astone, Bandeen-roche, and Ensminger, 2005). Adolescents' affiliations with social organizations, adolescents who perceive that they have higher levels of social support, and positive school environments may serve as protective factors Indeed, recent research provides evidence that communities where the citizens and institutions focus on increasing both competencies of youth and external supports at all levels of the ecology are most likely to succeed in building strong and resourceful youth (Biglan, Mrazek, Carnine, and Flay, 2003; Shoveller et al., 2004). At community levels, meaningful involvement in extracurricular activities appears to serve an important function. These activities may provide positive peer influences, relationships with caring adults, skill building, hope and plans for the future, or other important protective factors that encourage adolescents to sexual healthy behaviors.

Other societal characteristic that plays a distinct role in sexual health of adolescents is the media. Whether they are seeking information (e.g. internet) or entertainment, the media plays a significant role in the socialization of adolescents shaping cultural norms and influencing behaviors (Eggermont, 2005; Ward, 2003). Unfortunately, little is known about the psychosocial mechanisms that might explain observed associations between the media and adolescents' sexual risk behavior (Brown, Halpern, and L'Engle, 2005).

In conclusion, the findings suggest that focus only at the individual level it will not make the substantial changes to families, institutions, communities or society that could promote adolescent sexual health. A comprehensive and coordinated integration of multiple levels of socio-ecological model is of critical importance to systematize new kinds of data, find out broader aspects regarding the range of influences of sexual behaviors, and, most important, create new and promising opportunities for effective sexual health promotion research and intervention (Ross, Godeau, Dias, Vignes, Gross, 2004).

Several authors argue that descriptive knowledge provided by quantitative methods is inadequate to sufficiently inform a comprehensive assessment of adolescent health and risk, consequently interventions to moderate these risks are imprecise in hitting the right targets for behavioral change (Crawford and Popp, 2003; Jackson and Cram, 2003; Power, 2002). Many of our research findings in quantitative and qualitative study about young people's sexual experiences are similar. However, focus groups highlighted areas of debate and differences in the views of our participants, which could provide space for depth understanding of this complex phenomenon that lead to the possibility of more effective behavior change interventions. Focus groups also underline the importance of find a model that recognizes the active role that adolescents can have in their choices within specific situation of opportunities and constrictions of their environmental context (Caskey and Rosenthal, 2005). Finally, although this results has been based on evidence from Portuguese adolescent populations it is important to note that similar commentaries have been provided based on adolescent sexual behavior research in diverse parts of the world.

Acknowledgements

The author thank the team "Aventura Social" for data collection and general analysis.

Thanks to Prof. Margarida G. Matos and Prof. Aldina Gonçalves for valuable insight during the research. The Portuguese study "Health Behaviour in School-Aged Children/2002-WHO", was partially supported by a grant of Fundação para a Ciência e Tecnologia FCT Project POCTI 37486/PSI/2001 and had technical and economic support of CNLCS (National Agency for AIDS study and prevention).

The author are grateful to all the participants for their cooperation.

References

Abbey, A., Saenz, C., and Buck, P. O. (2005). The cumulative effects of acute alcohol consumption, individual differences and situational perceptions on sexual decision making. *Journal of Studies on Alcohol, 66*(1), 82-90.

Ahern N., Kiehl E. (2006). Adolescent sexual health and practice--a review of the literature: implications for healthcare providers, educators, and policy makers. Family and Community Health, 29(4), 299-313.

Aggleton, P., Chase, E., and Rivers, K. (2004). *HIV/AIDS prevention and care among especially vulnerable young people: a framework for action.* London: WHO and DFID.

Barbour, R., and Kitzinger, J. (1999). *Developing focus group research: Politics, theory and practice.* London: Sage.

Bettinger, J. A., Adler, N. E., Curriero, F. C., and Ellen, J. M. (2004). Risk perceptions, condom use, and sexually transmitted diseases among adolescent females according to social network position. *Sexually Transmitted Diseases, 31*(9), 575-579.

Biglan, A., Mrazek, P. J., Carnine, D., and Flay, B. R. (2003). The integration of research and practice in the prevention of youth problem behaviors. The *American Psychologist, 58*(6-7), 433-440.

Bronfenbrenner, U. (1979). *Ecology of Human Development: Experiments by nature and by design.* Cambridge, MA: Harvard University Press.

Brown, J., Halpern, C. T., and L'Engle, K. L. (2005). Mass media as a sexual super peer for early maturing girls. *Journal of Adolescent Health, 36*(5), 420-427.

Campbell, C., and MacPhail, C. (2002). Peer education, gender and the development of critical consciousness: participatory HIV prevention by South African youth. *Social Science and Medicine, 55*(2), 331-345.

Carpenter, C. (2005). Youth alcohol use and risky sexual behavior: evidence from underage drunk driving laws. *Journal of Health Economics, 24*(3), 613-628.

Caskey, J. D., and Rosenthal, S. L. (2005). Conducting research on sensitive topics with adolescents: ethical and developmental considerations. *Journal of Developmental and Behavioral Pediatrics, 26*(1), 61-67.

Collins, J., Robin, L., Wooley, S., and al., e. (2002). Programs-that-work: CDC's guide to effective programs that reduce health-risk behavior of youth. *Journal of School Health, 72(3)*, 93-99.

Concoran, J. (2000). Ecological factors associated with sexual activity. *Social Work in Health Care, 30*(4), 93-111.

Crawford, M., and Popp, D. (2003). Sexual double standards: a review and methodological critique of two decades of research. *Journal of Sex Research, 40*(1), 13-26.

Currie, C., Roberts, C., Morgan, A., Smith, R., Settertobulte, W., Samdal, O., et al. (Eds.). (2004). *Young people's health in context. Health Behaviour in School-aged Children (HBSC) study: International report from the 2001/2002 survey.* Copenhagen: Who Regional Office for Europe (Health Policy for Children and Adolescents No. 4.

Deren, S., Oliver-Velez, D., Finlinson, A., Robles, R., Andia, J., Colon, H. M., et al. (2003). Integrating qualitative and quantitative methods: comparing HIV-related risk behaviors among Puerto Rican drug users in Puerto Rico and New York. *Substance Use Misuse, 38*(1), 1-24.

Dias, S., Matos, M.G., Gonçalves, A. (2005). Preventing HIV transmission in adolescents: an analysis of the Portuguese Data from health Behaviour School-aged Children Study and focus groups. *European Journal of Public Health,* 15 (3), 300-304.

Dias, S., Matos, M.G., Gonçalves, A. (2006). AIDS-related stigma and attitudes towards AIDS infected people among adolescents. *AIDS Care,* 18(3), 208-214.

DiCenso, A., Borthwick, V. W., Busca, C. A., Creatura, C., Holmes, J. A., Kalagian, W. F., et al. (2001). Completing the picture: adolescents talk about what's missing in sexual health services. *Canadian Journal of Public Health, 92*(1), 35-38.

DiClemente, R., Salazar, L. F., Crosby, R. A., and Rosenthal, S. L. (2005). Prevention and control of sexually transmitted infections among adolescents: the importance of a socio-ecological perspective--a commentary. *Public Health, 119*(9), 825-836.

DiIorio, C., Dudley, W. N., Soet, J. E., and McCarty, F. (2004). Sexual possibility situations and sexual behaviors among young adolescents: The moderating role of protective factors. *Journal of Adolescent Health, 35*(6), 528e11-528e20.

Eaton, D., Kann, L., Kinchen, S., Ross, J., Hawkins, J., Harris, W., Lowry, R., McManus, T., Chyen, D. Shanklin, S., Lim, C., Grunbaum, A., Wechsler, H. (2005). Youth Risk Behavior Surveillance - United States, 2005. *Morbity and Morality Weekly Report* 2006; 55(SS-5):1-108.

Eggermont, S. (2005). Young adolescents' perceptions of peer sexual behaviours: the role of television viewing. *Child: Care, Health and Development, 31*(4), 459-468.

Eloundou-Enyegue, P. M., Meekers, D., and Calves, A. E. (2005). From awareness to adoption: the effect of AIDS education and condom social marketing on condom use in Tanzania (1993-1996). *Journal of Biosocial Science, 37*(3), 257-268.

Fenton, K. A., Mercer, C. H., McManus, S., Erens, B., Wellings, K., Macdowall, W., et al. (2005). Ethnic variations in sexual behaviour in Great Britain and risk of sexually transmitted infections: a probability survey. *Lancet, 365*(9466), 1246-1255.

Fergus, S., and Zimmerman, M. A. (2005). Adolescent resilience: a framework for understanding healthy development in the face of risk. *Annual Review of Public Health, 26*, 399-419.

Forehand, R., Gound, M., Kotchick, B. A., Armistead, L., Long, N., and Miller, K. S. (2005). Sexual intentions of black preadolescents: associations with risk and adaptive behaviors. *Perspectives on Sexual and Reproductive Health, 37*(1), 13-18.

Foreman, 2003). Intimate risk: Sexual risk behavior among African American college women. *Journal of Black Studies, 33*(5), 637-653.

Frith, H. (2000). Focusing on sex: using focus groups in sex research. *Sexualities, 3*(3), 275-297.

Garriguet, D. (2005). Early sexual intercourse. *Health Reports, 16*(3), 9-18.

Garwick, A., Nerdahl, P., Banken, R., Muenzenberger-Bretl, L., and Sieving, R. (2004). Risk and protective factors for sexual risk taking among adolescents involved in Prime Time*1. *Journal of Pediatric Nursing, 19*(5), 340-350.

Goodwin, R., Kozlova, A., Nizharadze, G., and Polyakova, G. (2004). HIV/AIDS among adolescents in Eastern Europe: knowledge of HIV/AIDS, social representations of risk and sexual activity among school children and homeless adolescents in Russia, Georgia and the Ukraine. *Journal of Health Psychology, 9*(3), 381-396.

Goold, P. C., Bustard, S., Ferguson, E., Carlin, E. M., Neal, K., and Bowman, C. A. (2006). Pilot study in the development of an Interactive Multimedia Learning Environment for sexual health interventions: a focus group approach. *Health Education Research*, 21(1), 15-25.

Green, J., and Thorogood, N. (2004). *Qualitative methods for health research*. London: Sage.

Grzywacz, J. C., and Fuqua, J. (2000). The social ecology of health: leverage points and linkages. *Behavior Medicine, 26*(3), 101-115.

Guilamo-Ramos, V., Litardo, H., and Jaccard, J. (2005). Prevention programs for reducing adolescent problem behaviors: Implications of the co-occurrence of problem behaviors in adolescence. *Journal of Adolescent Health, 36*(1), 82-86.

Henrich, C. C., Brookmeyer, K. A., Shrier, L. A., and Shahar, G. (2006). Supportive relationships and sexual risk behavior in adolescence: An ecological-transactional approach. *Journal of Pediatric Psychology, 31*(3):286-97.

Hollander, J. (2004). The social context of focus groups. *Journal of Contemporary Ethnography, 33*(5), 602-637.

Hopkins, C. D., Tanner, J. F., Jr., and Raymond, M. A. (2004). Risk avoidance versus risk reduction: a framework and segmentation profile for understanding adolescent sexual activity. *Health Marketing Quarterly, 21*(3), 79-106.

Hoppe, M. J., Graham, L., Wilsdon, A., Wells, E. A., Nahom, D., and Morrison, D. M. (2004). Teens speak out about HIV/AIDS: Focus group discussions about risk and decision-making. *Journal of Adolescent Health, 35*(4), 345-346.

Horowitz, S. M. (2003). Applying the transtheoretical model to pregnancy and STD prevention: a review of the literature. *American Journal of Health Promotion, 17*(5), 304-328.

Huebner, A. J., and Howell, L. W. (2003). Examining the relationship between adolescent sexual risk-taking and perceptions of monitoring, communication, and parenting styles. *Journal of Adolescent Health, 33*(2), 71-78.

Hutchinson, M., Jemmott, J. B. I., Jemmott, L. S., Braverman, P., and Fong, G. T. (2003). The role of mother-daughter sexual risk communication in reducing sexual risk behaviors among urban adolescent females: A prospective study. *Journal of Adolescent Health*, 33(2), 98-107.

Hyde, A., Howlett, E., Brady, D., and Drennan, J. (2005). The focus group method: Insights from focus group interviews on sexual health with adolescents. Social Science and Medicine, 61(12):2588-99.

Jackson, S. M., and Cram, F. (2003). Disrupting the sexual double standard: young women's talk about heterosexuality. *The British Journal of Social Psychology, 42*(Pt1), 113-127.

Jacobson, K. C., and Crockett, L. J. (2000). Parental monitoring and adolescent adjustment: an ecological perspective. *Journal of Research on Adolescence, 10*(1), 65-97.

Johnson, R. J., McCaul, K. D., and Klein, W. M. P. (2002). Risk involvement and risk perception among adolescents and young adults. *Journal of Behavioral Medicine, 25*(1), 67-82.

Kershaw, T. S., Ethier, K. A., Niccolai, L. M., Lewis, J. B., and Ickovics, J. R. (2003). Misperceived risk among female adolescents: social and psychological factors associated with sexual risk accuracy. *Health Psychology, 22*(5), 523-532.

Kingon, Y., and Sullivan, A. (2001). The family as a protective asset in adolescent development. *Journal of Holistic Nursing, 19*(2), 102-121.

Kirby, D. (2002a). Antecedents of adolescent initiation of sex, contraceptive use, and pregnancy. *American Journal of Health Behavior, 26*(6), 473-485.

Kirby, D. (2002b). The impact of schools and school programs upon adolescent sexual behavior. *Journal of Sex Research, 39*(1), 27-33.

Kotchick, B. A., Shaffer, A., Forehand, R., and Miller, K. (2001). Adolescent sexual risk behavior: A multi-system perspective. *Clinical Psychology Review, 21*(4), 493-519.

Krueger, R. A., and Casey, M. A. (2000). *Focus groups: A practical guide for applied Research* (3rd Edition ed.). Thousand Oaks, CA: Sage Publications.

Li, X., Stanton, B., and Feigelman, S. (2000). Impact of perceived parental monitoring on adolescent risk behavior over 4 years. *Journal of Adolescent Health, 27*(1), 49-56.

Lipovsek, V., Karim, A., Gutiérrez, E., Magnani, R., and Gomez, M. (2002). Correlates of adolescent pregnancy in la Paz, Bolivia: findings from a quantitative-qualitative study. *Adolescence, 37*(146), 335-353.

Main, D. S. (2002). Commentary: Understanding the effects of peer education as a health promotion strategy. *Health Education and Behavior, 29*(4), 424-426.

Manlove, J., Ryan, S., and Franzetta, K. (2004). Contraceptive use and consistency in U.S. teenagers' most recent sexual relationships. *Perspectives on Sexual and Reproductive Health, 36*(6), 265-275.

McManus, R. (2002). Adolescent care: Reducing risk and promoting resilience. *Primary Care, 29*(3), 557-569.

McNeely, C., Nonnemaker, J., and Blum, R. (2002). Promoting school connectedness: evidence from the National Longitudinal Study of Adolescent Health. *Journal of School Health, 72*(4), 138-146.

Morgan, D. (1998). Practical strategies for combining qualitative and quantitative methods: applications to health research. *Qualitative Health Research, 8*(3), 362-376.

Morgan, D. (2001). Focus Group interviewing. In J. F. Gubrium and J. A. Holstein (Eds.), *handbook of interview research: context and method*. Thousand Oaks, CA: Sage.

Pantin, H., Schwartz, S. J., Sullivan, S., Prado, G., and Szapocznik, J. (2004). Ecodevelopmental HIV prevention programs for Hispanic adolescents. *The American Journal of Orthopsychiatry, 74*(4), 545-558.

Parker, R., Easton, D., and Klein, C. H. (2000). Structural barriers and facilitators in HIV prevention: a review of international research. *AIDS, 14*(Suppl 1), S22-32.

Peterson-Sweeney, K. (2005). The use of focus groups in pediatric and adolescent research. *Journal of Pediatric Health Care, 19*(2), 104-110.

Potsonen R, Kontula O. (1999).Adolescents' knowledge and attitudes concerning infection and HIV infected persons: how a survey and focus group discussions are suited for researching adolescents' HIV/AIDS knowledge and attitudes. Health Education Research, *14 (4)*: 473-484.

Power, R. (2002). The application of qualitative research methods to the study of sexually transmitted infections. *Sexually Transmitted Infections, 78*(2), 87-89.

Reininger, B. M., Evans, A. E., Griffin, S. F., Sanderson, M., Vincent, M. L., Valois, R. F., et al. (2005). Predicting adolescent risk behaviors based on an ecological framework and assets. *American Journal of Health Behavior, 29*(2), 150-161.

Robin, L., Dittus, P., Whitaker, D., Crosby, R., Ethier, K., Mezoff, J., et al. (2004). Behavioral interventions to reduce incidence of HIV, STD, and pregnancy among adolescents: a decade in review. *Journal of Adolescent Health, 34*(1), 3-26.

Roche, K. M., Ellen, J., and Astone, N. M. (2005). Effects of out-of-school care on sex initiation among young adolescents in low-income central city neighborhoods. *Archives of Pediatrics and Adolescent Medicine, 159*(1), 68-73.

Roche, K., Mekos, D., Alexander, C., Astone, N., Bandeen-roche, K., and Ensminger, M. (2005). Parenting influences on early sex initiation among adolescents: How neighborhood matters. *Journal of Family Issues, 26*(1), 32-54.

Rose, A., Koo, H. P., Bhaskar, B., Anderson, K., White, G., and Jenkins, R. R. (2005). The influence of primary caregivers on the sexual behavior of early adolescents. *Journal of Adolescent Health, 37*(2), 135-144.

Rosenthal, S., Stanberry, L. R., Griffith, J. O., Succop, P. A., Biro, F. M., Lewis, L. M., et al. (2002). The relationship between STD locus of control and STD acquisition among adolescents girls. *Adolescence, 37*(145), 83-92.

Ross, J., Godeau, E., and Dias, S. (2004). Sexual health. In C. Candace, R. Chris, M. Antony, S. Rebecca, S. Wolfgang, S. Oddrun and B. Vivian (Eds.), *Young people's health in context. Health Behaviour in School-aged Children (HBSC) study: international report from the 2001/2002 survey* (Vol. 4, pp. 153-160). Copenhagen: Who Regional Office for Europe (Health Policy for Children and Adolescents).

Ross, J., Godeau, E., Dias, S. (2004). Sexual health in young people: findings from HBSC study. Entre Nous: *The European Magazine for Sexual and Reproductive Health*, 58, 20-23.

Ross, J.,Godeau, E., Dias, S., Vignes, C., Gross, L. (2004). Setting politics aside to collect cross-national data on sexual health of adolescents. *SIECUS Report*, 32 (4),28-34.

Ross, M. W., and Fernandez-Esquer, M. E. (2005). Ethnicity in sexually transmitted infections and sexual behaviour research. *The Lancet, 365*(9466), 1209-1210.

Schaalma, H. P., Abraham, C., Gillmore, M. R., and Kok, G. (2004). Sex education as health promotion: what does it take? *Archives of Sexual Behavior, 33*(3), 259-269.

Shoveller, J. A., Johnson, J. L., Langille, D. B., and Mitchell, T. (2004). Socio-cultural influences on young people's sexual development. *Social Science and Medicine, 59*(3), 473-487.

Siqueira, L. M., and Diaz, A. (2004). Fostering resilience in adolescent females. *The Mount Sinai Journal of Medicine, 71*(3), 148-154.

Stueve, A., and O'Donnell, L. N. (2005). Early alcohol initiation and subsequent sexual and alcohol risk behaviors among urban youths. *American Journal of Public Health, 95*(5), 887-893.

Talashek, M. L., Norr, K. F., and Dancy, B. L. (2003). Building teen power for sexual health. *Journal of Transcultural Nursing, 14*(3), 207-216.

Tanne, J. H. (2005). Abstinence only programmes do not change sexual behaviour, Texas study shows. *British Medical Journal, 330*(7487), 326b.

UNESCO (2003). HIV/Aids and Education: a strategic approach. Retrieved July 20, 2005, from *http://portal.unesco.org/aids/iatt-education*

United Nations. (2005). Youth at the United Nations: World Youth Report. Retrieved July 20, 2005, from *http://www.un.org/esa/socdev/unyin/wyr05.htm*

Vesely, S. K., Wyatt, V. H., Oman, R. F., Aspy, C. B., Kegler, M. C., Rodine, S., et al. (2004). The potential protective effects of youth assets from adolescent sexual risk behaviors. *Journal of Adolescent Health, 34*(5), 356-365.

Ward, L. M. (2003). Understanding the role of entertainment media in the sexual socialization of American youth: A review of empirical research. *Developmental Review, 23*(3), 347-388.

Warr, D. (2005). "It was fun...but we don't usually talk about these things": Analyzing Sociable Interaction in Focus Groups. *Qualitative Inquiry, 11*(2), 200-226.

Weissberg, R., Kumpfer, K., and Seligman, M. (2003). Prevention that works with children and youth - an introduction. *American Psychologist, 58*(67), 425-432.

WHO (2003a). The World Health Report. Retrieved July 20, 2005, from *http://www.who. int/whr/2003/*

WHO (2003b). *Skills for Health: Skills-based health education including life skills: An important component of a Child-friendly/health-promoting school.* Geneva: The World Health Organization Information Series on School Health: Document 9.

WHO (2004a). *The World Health Report: Changing History.* Geneva: World Health Organization.

WHO (2004b). Guide to Monitoring and Evaluating National HIV/AIDS Prevention Programmes for young people. Retrieved July 20, 2005, from *http://www.who. int/hiv/pub/me/en/me_prev_intro.pdf*

Wingood, G., and DiClemente, R. (2000). Application of the theory of gender and power to examine HIV-related exposures, risk factors, and effective interventions for women. *Health Education and Behavior, 27*(5), 539-565.

Wulff, M., and Lalos, A. (2004). The condom in relation to prevention of sexually transmitted infections and as a contraceptive method in Sweden. The *European Journal of Contraception and Reproductive Health Care, 9*(2), 69-77.

Zimmer-Gembeck, M. J., Siebenbruner, J., and Collins, W. A. (2004). A Prospective Study of Intraindividial and Peer Influences on Adolescents' Heterosexual Romantic and Sexual Behavior. *Archives of Sexual Behavior, 33*(4), 381-394.

Zwane, I. T., Mngadi, P. T., and Nxumalo, M. P. (2004). Adolescents' views on decision-making regarding risky sexual behaviour. *International Nursing Review, 51*(1), 15-22.

In: Hygiene and Its Role in Health

Editors: P. L. Anderson and J. P. Lachan

ISBN 978-1-60456-195-1

© 2008 Nova Science Publishers, Inc.

Chapter 8

School Health Program: A New Perspective

Prakash Adhikari[*]

Healthy Human Society, Jorpati, Kathmandu, Nepal

Abstract

School Health Program (SHP) is defined with respect to environment, services, and education. It should be a plan with a good vision so that it will be fruitful. School Health Program is to be conducted to ensure a healthy environment in schools and to promote the health of the school children. It helps to prevent the different diseases and make the children conscious about their health. SHP makes easy for early diagnosis, treatment, follow-up, and check regularly to the diseased and non-diseased students. A new concept of SHP, which is an emerging need for developing countries, is also included in this study. It is one of the cost effective program if implemented at a national and international level and make aware all the nongovernmental organizations/international non-governmental organizations/donors to spend their money in this type of program.

Keywords: *School Health Program (SHP), problems, curriculum, new modality and students.*

Introduction

The school health program (SHP) is an important branch of community health [1], [2] and is responsible for looking after the health of school children. It is an economical and powerful means of raising the health of the community. Though it is carried out in many countries since eighty years, it has not been able to find its place in the majority of schools in

---

[*] Dr.Prakash Adhikari, President, Healthy Human Society, Jorpati, Kathmandu, Nepal. P.O. Box: 4972. E-mail: prakash_ooz@hotmail.com

developing countries like Nepal. It is a universal truth that a healthy child turns into a healthy adult in future and hence proper cares on the health of school children turns the foundation of a nation that consists of healthy people who can lead a healthy life and contribute to the development of a nation.

Today, many students have added agendas that influence their ability to learn. Some students are not adequately nourished, lack sleep, lack immunizations and are not properly clothed. Others are being reared in families in which there is domestic violence, chemical dependency, or some form of abuse. As we know that if the school children are not cared properly, they will suffer from many diseases. If the health education is not given to these school children, they will not know about the disease and they will not be more cautious about their health and hygiene of the surroundings.

Early detection and treatment of asymptomatic disease have emerged as a major strategy for secondary prevention of the chronic diseases. Screening is aimed at the presumptive identification of unrecognized disease or defect by the use of procedures that can be applied rapidly and economically to a population. Its purpose is to distinguish among apparently well persons those who probably have a disease from those who probably do not [3]. This article is related to the school health problems and mainly focuses on a new concept of school health program.

Health Problems

The centers for disease control and prevention has identified six categories of risk behavior in today's students [4].

1. Behaviours That Result in Unintentional and Intentional Injuries

A person's behaviour may be the main cause of health problem, but it can also be the main solution. By changing their behaviour these individuals can solve and prevent many of their own problems [5]. Relatively little is known about risk behaviours of elementary school children [6]. The prevalence of risk behaviours was higher in absent than present students [7]. Through health education, we help people understand their behaviour and how it affects their health. We encourage people to make their own choices for a healthy life. We do not force people to change.

Behaviours can result in intentional and unintentional injuries. Unintentional injuries are accidental. These include motor vehicle related accidents, burns and drowning Intentional injuries results from interpersonal violence (domestic violence, child abuse, bullying, fighting) and suicide. Urban area dwellers and especially inner-city residents, tend to experience much higher rates of interpersonal victimization and perpetration that do those who live in suburban and rural areas [8].

Educators are faced with the issues of assaults, rapes, suicide, gang membership and weapon carrying in their schools [9]. An increasing number of students and adolescents are not only becoming victims of violence but also are routinely witnessing violence in their communities [10]. It is a concern that is no longer limited to large urban areas, but extend to smaller cities and rural areas as well [11]. Seven of every ten inner city Chicago students report that they have witnessed a murder, shooting, stabbing or robbery- half of which involved friends , family members, class mates or neighbors [12]. Presences of violence in children contribute to a lack of motivation to achieve in school [13]. Once a gun is readily accessible, a youth can easily bring it to school [14]. Sexual harassment is unwanted and unwelcome. When school officials fail to respond appropriately, students may develop feelings that 'they are incapable of standing up to injustice or acting in associating with peers who are being harassed or buccied [15].

2. Tobacco Use

Most adults, who smoke / use tobacco, began it during childhood or early adolescence. The earlier they began, the less likely they will quit. Risky healthy practices, such as cigarette smoking, poor diet, physical inactivity and substance abuse are linked to poverty [16]. Children who grow up under these adverse environmental conditions show a higher risk of developing a pattern of processes in adolescence doing poorly in school, dropping out, becoming adolescent parents, becoming delinquent, and using a cycle of misery and hopelessness [17]. Passive smoking also causes thousands of children to develop asthma each year [18]. Research studies show that being exposed to high particulate levels increases the likelihood of having persistent causes, respiratory illness and severe asthmatic attacks [19].

3. Alcohol and Other Drugs Use

There is an increasing rate of using alcohol, marijuana, cocaine, anabolic steroids from school life. Drug free school zones show a united front of schools, students, parents and communities in working together to establish drug free school and communities by decreasing drug trafficking around school [20].

4. Sexual Behaviors That Result in HIV Infection, Other STDs and Unintended Pregnancy

The sexual behavior of today's students is alarming. By the age of 15, 25% of the students had sexual intercourse at least once. By the age of 17, 75% of both male and female students have had intercourse at least once. More than one third of the high school students reported having had more than two sexual partners. Human immunodeficiency viruses (HIV), sexually transmitted diseases (STDs), and unintended pregnancies are also one of the problems of school children. The number of 12-21 years old in the US who has become infected with HIV has increased by 77% since 1991.The significant proportion of young adults who currently have Acquired Immunodeficiency Syndrome (AIDS) were infected with HIV during adolescent years because of risk behaviors they practiced [21]. Commonly STDs reported in students include Chlamydia, Gonorrhea, Syphilis, Chancroids, Genital herpes and Genital Warts. One in six adolescents develops one or more of these STDs each year. This means that more than 3 million adolescents are infected each year with one or more STDs [22].

Students who chose to be sexually active often face the consequence of unintended pregnancy. Those becoming pregnant before the age of 15, 60% will have 3 children by the age of 19 [23].

5. Dietary Patterns That Contribute to Disease

The dietary guidelines should be strictly followed. Over 25% of high school students reported eating more than two servings of foods high in fat content [24].

6. Insufficient Physical Activities

There has been a significant decline in the percentage of adolescents who can satisfactorily perform a series of physical fitness tests when compared to adolescents of previous pregnancies.

The five major common health problems in the school children of developing countries like Nepal are:

1. Parasitic diseases
2. Infectious disease
3. Upper respiratory infections
4. Malnutrition
5. Disease related to skin, ear and dental problems

These conditions are the major causes of mortality and morbidity in children. Regular check up of children in their respective school together with emphasis on health education is believed to reduce the morbidity and mortality in children.

A child spends almost one third of daily time in the school. The school thus must be able to provide the child with a healthy environment to ensure best physical, social and emotional health of the children. A healthy environment can be created by keeping in mind the following points.

(a) Environment of the School

A safe and healthful school environment is an environment that attends to the physical and aesthetic surroundings and psychological climate and culture that maximizes the health and safety of students and staff. All students respond to their environment. Favorable environmental conditions stimulate healthful growth and development, unfavorable conditions impede well-being. The environment of the school makes a great difference in the health aspect of the children. The surrounding area including the environment must be safe and comfortable. Similarly, the school site, structure, classroom, furniture, lights both natural and artificial, colors, laboratories, canteens, ventilations, sanitation, water supply, prevention from accidents, ground for play and recreation must be good. There should be effective classroom management, emotional security positive nutritional environment as well as safe school transportation to protect students as they travel to and from school [25], [26].

(b) Health of the School Children and Staffs

Not only is the periodic medical examination of the school children but also the health of the staffs (teachers and other staffs) are important. At the initial time of examination, a thorough examination should be done. To be an effective teacher, a teacher must be aware of the health status of the students. A teacher must be committed to working with students to maintain and improve their health status. A totally awesome is a teacher who is committed to promoting health literacy, improving health, preventing diseases and reducing health related behaviors in the students, and to creating a dynamic and challenging classroom where students learn and practice life skills for health [27]. Today's teacher must be totally awesome [27]. Teachers should inform to the program coordinator about the health of the school children. They should be involved in early identification of visual and auditory impairment, attention deficit, learning disabilities, regarding the growth and development of children and others. Thus, teacher (especially the class teachers) should be more concerned to the health of the children of their class.

(c) Follow Up

Not only the initial examination is necessary, but also there should be a periodic health check up of both the children as well as the school staff.

(d) Prevention of Communicable Disease

There are many communicable diseases. So, to prevent from these, a thorough evaluation about the immunization is most emphasized in the school health program.

(e) First Aid Treatment

For the first aid and emergency care, the teachers should be trained on carrying out first aid measures in the school premises.

(f)Nutrition Aspects

Teachers of the school care hostel children. Therefore, they should be given adequate nutritious food. For the mid day school children, their tiffin should be observed. Well-facilitated filtered water and good canteen should be in the school. *"A carrot per day prevents the children from night blindness"*. Therefore, it is very important to realize that whatever the children eat in the school and hostel should be hygienic, nutritious and provide adequate carbohydrate, protein, fats, vitamins and minerals to take care for the overall development of a child and provide sufficient calorie. Childhood overweight is one of the most serious problems currently affecting individual and public health. Schools represent a logical site for prevention because children spend 6-8 hours a day there during most of the year [28].

(g) Health Education

Through health education, we help people understand their behaviour and how it affects their health [5]. We encourage people to make their own choices for a healthy life [5]. We do not force people to change [5]. Health education about the personal hygiene, food habits, exercise and physical fitness, about the diseases and environment health should be given to all the school children in simple understandable terms. A planned curriculum must be designed to school health education. It includes a variety of topics.

- Mental and emotional health
- Family livings
- Growth and development
- Nutrition
- Personal heath
- Alcohol, Tobacco and other drugs
- Com. And Chronic diseases
- Injury prevention and safety
- Consumer and community health
- Environmental health

(h) Counselling, Psychological and Social Services

These are services that provide broad bared individual and group assessments, interventions and referrals that attend to the mental, emotional and social health of students.

(i) Physical Education

Quality physical education should promote through a variety of planned physical activities, each students optimal physical, mental, emotional, and social development, should promote activities and sports that all students enjoy and can pressure throughout their lives. Almost half of young people from low-income families do not participate in any extra curricular activities [29]. By the time that young people reach high school, the spontaneous expression of physical activity has often been curtailed [30].

(j) Disaster and Emergency Preparedness

Emergency preparedness plans should be made a periodically revived, tested and updated [31].

School Health Curriculum

The health education imparted in the school should aim at bringing about desirable changes in health knowledge, attitude and practices related to health. It should go beyond just giving children. It should equip them to make decisions, explore attitudes and values and adopt healthy practices for leading a healthy life.

It is recommended that the concerned authority of that school be provided at least 4-6 classes per month about the health education to the school children. In addition, the health education impaired should emphasize on personal hygiene, environmental health, family life, nutrition, spread, and control of diseases.

Comprehensive School Health Program

The comprehensive School health program should focus on:

1. Providing health service given to school children and staffs.
2. Legislation of the environment of the school (inner and surrounding environment)
3. Informing through health education classes with 4-6 classes per month

A review of each of these national initiatives targets the need for comprehensive school health program (SHP) designed specially to meet the needs of today's students. Currently there is emphasis being placed on implanting a comprehensive SHP is every school district. A comprehensive SHP is an organized to protect and promote the health, safety, and wellbeing of students and staffs. The *eight* components of the comprehensive SHP are almost the same as described before in health problems [31].

These will change the lifestyle of the school children, teacher and their families. Thus, an achievement will be gained which leads to the healthy child.

The *three strands of thoughts* also have to be kept in mind while running the School Health Program:

1. School health program must be founded on organized and mutually reinforcing components.
2. Schools are dynamic organizations that can respond to changing needs and environments.
3. Successful health promoting program are built upon five areas: Policy, supportive environment, Community action, personal skills development, and a reorientation of health services.

Thus, school health program is defined with respect to environment, services and education.

Schools Role in Providing School Health Services

School services are services designed to appraise, protect, and promote the health of students. These health services are delivered through the cooperative efforts and activities of teachers, nurses, physicians, allied health personal, social workers and others to appraise, protect and promote the health of the students as well as school personals. Most schools do not have the money personnel to offer all of the services that could be included in a camp. Therefore, schools are increasingly relying upon community support and linkages. School can increase their capacity to offer a health need of students by community partnership with local clubs/ nongovernmental organizations/international nongovernmental organizations/donors.

Ignorance is the root of most of the health problems. Every school should more efficiently serve as an entry point for health promotion and a location for health intervention. Every school should enable children and adolescents at all levels to learn critical health and life skills. The community and the school should work together to support health and education. Policies, legislation and guidelines should be developed to ensure a comprehensive school health program at the local and national level. School health program should be a plan with a good vision so that it will be fruitful.

New Modality of School Health Program

The modality of running the School Health Program (SHP) proposed by author (Dr. Adhikari) includes 18 points. This is a new concept of SHP, which an emerging need for developing countries like Nepal. This new modality starts from essential criteria.

Essential Criteria

(A) If the program is run by the government itself or by an organization without taking fees from the school students; they can follow 1-15 points.

OR

(B) If the program is run by any private sector or by any organization taking school health fees from school students, then; they have to follow these 1-18 points.

Therefore, this essential criteria will follow the basis whether to run this program with which criteria. The program will be effective once this SHP is launched with one of the above essential criteria. Below are the *lists of points* of essential criteria i.e. *lists of points* of new modality of School Health Program.

1.   Health check up

There will be a school health camp six monthly. The school students, both diseased and nondiseased, can get benefit by doing health check up from the medical experts.

2.   Blood grouping

This test will be done at the time of admission. Blood grouping is much more useful in certain circumstances such as accidents, shock etc.

3. Stool examination

Several study done in developing countries revealed that the parasitic infestations are common in school students. Thus, stool examination will be done to all the school students for ova and cyst six monthly and medicines will be given according to the worm infestations.

4. School Health Curriculum

Health awareness class 4-6 classes per month by experts on Sanitation, tobacco use, smoking, alcohol, drug abuse, injury prevention and safety, environment and on different infectious and communicable diseases including Acquired immunodeficiency syndrome and sexually transmitted diseases.

5. School Health Environment

It includes:

(a) Improvement of physical, psychological and social environment
(b) Healthy organizational culture in the school
(c) Interaction between the School and the nearby community

6. Nutritional status

As already described that the child can study properly only when medical condition is is fit and fine. So, in this type of new school health program, assessment of the nutritional status of school children and recommendation will be done.

7. Establishing School Health Clinics and Referral system

There will be 4-5 Clinics in one district depending upon the number of students attending Schools. The clinic will remain open daily. Investigations done will be at the hospital rate in this clinic. Poor patient get medicine free of cost. There will be also a referral system to the well-equipped hospital where they get treatment in subsidized rate. This will be until the hospital for this program is not started. Long-term plan of this program is to establish at least 3-4 hospitals in one district/state so that these school children will great benefit.

8. Counseling Center

There will be counseling centers on every school health clinics. This center will be provided with three counselors. When students have their mental/psychological/social problems, they can meet the counselor and solve their problems. In certain conditions such as mass hysteria, counselor will also go to schools and solve their problems.

9. First aid box and service

All the teachers and students will be taught about the first aid measures. The first aid box will contain the most essential drugs and instruments.

10. Training to class teacher

Teachers (especially class teacher) are more responsible for their respective class. Therefore, these class teachers will be given the training for early identification of disease of school children such as hearing impairment, refractive error etc. There will be also training classes to class teachers about the first aid.

11. Health Insurance Scheme

There is also a provision of health insurance. This scheme will be very useful especially to the poorer students whose parents cannot afford money to treat their children. So, it can be an alternative for poor family.

12. One Call Service

Program Coordinator (who is a medical expert) and his team will try to solve students' health problems and queries if they give a call to the helpline number. It is like a telemedicine where parents can ask any problem, their children had and can get relief for the time being. Later on, they can go to the school health clinic.

13. School health management team

There will be a team including:

(a) Program coordinator (Medical expert)
(b) Principal
(c) Teacher (especially health teacher)
(d) Student representative
(e) Lower level staff (as they know more about sanitation/water/canteen/latrines)

This team will be in every School.

Mass casualty management team.

To manage a disaster problem in the school such as mass hysteria, diarrhea, cholera, accidents; there will be a mass casualty management team. The program coordinator of school health management team will coordinate in this type of disaster
This team includes:

(a) Program Coordinator of school health management team

(b) Principal

(c) 2 senior doctors

(d) 4 junior doctors

(e) 4 nurses

(f) 5 other staffs

(g) Ambulance contacts

(h) Hospital contact

This team will be also in every school.

14. School health records and Research

Personal file of the individual students should provide data about the health and disease of the school children, which should be useful in analyzing and evaluating School health program and providing a useful link between the home, School and the community. The SHP will also be research oriented. It can do knowledge, attitude and practices study / research on nutritional status, parisitic infestations/prevalence of different diseases such as ear disease, eye disease etc.

15. Internal Auditing of the School Health Program

The program will be successful only when it is audited properly. Registered auditors should audit every financial aspects of this program.

16. External Evaluation and Analysis Team and Recommendation from them

There will be the external evaluation of this school health program by the expert from nongovernmental organizations/international nongovernmental organizations/donors and give their expert opinion so that the program will attain a new height.

17. Annual Report

In every school, one of the auditors of SHP will present the audit in the anniversary day of every school so that every one can know the reality transactions and report of our program in that respected school. This can help to make a program more successful.

Conclusion

Therefore, I want to say, "Struggle for Health is Struggle for Justice". If we conduct such a program in a developing country like Nepal, then it is sure that we can reduce the mortality and morbidity of the children. So, I hope every health personnel will think it seriously about the concept of School Health Program. Initially it might be difficult in running but i hope this program will significantly reduce the health problem of school children Thus, SHP will definitely improve the health of large populations when implanted on a national scale.

Acknowledgements

I express my sincere gratitude to the following intellectuals of Nepal Medical College Teaching Hospital: Dr S.B.Rizyal, principal; Prof.G.P.Mathur, Professor and Head of Department of Pediatrics; Prof.S.K.Melhotra, Prof. and Head of department of Community Medicine. I would like to thank Er.Bipin Kadel and Dr. Binod Kadel for technical supports. Lastly, I am thankful to other members of Healthy Human Society, Katmandu.

References

[1]   K, Park. *Park's Textbook of Preventive and Social Medicine*. 15th Edition. India: Banarsidas Bhanot Publisher; 1997.

[2]   MC, G. Mahaja. *Textbook of Preventive and Social Medicine*. 3rd Edition. India: Jaypee Publishers; 2003.

[3]   Duncan, W. Clark and Brian, Mac Mohan. *Preventive and Community Medicine*. 2nd Edition. Boston: Little, Brown and Company; 1981.

[4]   Centers for disease control. (1993). Comprehensive School Health Education Programs: *Innovative Practices and issues in Setting Standards*. Atlanta, GA: Centers for Disease Control and Prevention.

[5]   Education for health. *A manual on health education in primary health care*. Geneva: *WHO publication*; 1988.

[6]   Jenifer Cartland, Holly S Ruch-Ross (2006). Health Behaviors of School-Age Children: Evidence from One Large City. *Journal of School Health* 76 (5), 175-180.

[7]   Pascal Bovet, Bharati Viswanathan, David Faeh, Wick Warren (2006). Comparison of Smoking, Drinking, and Marijuana Use Between Students Present or Absent on the Day of a School-Based Survey. *Journal of School Health* 76 (4), 133-137.

[8]   Ropp, L., Visintainer, P., Uman, J., and Trelor, D. (1992.) death in the City: An American Tragedy. *Journal of the American M. Association*, 267: 2905-2910.

[9]   Meeks, L., Heit, P; and Page, R. *Drugs, Alcohol, and Tobacco: Totally Awesome Teaching Strategies*. Columbus, OH; Meeks Heit Publishing Company: 1995.

[10]   Fitzpatrick, K. M. (1993). Exposure to violence and presence of depression among low-income, African- American youth. *Journal of Consulting and Clinical Psychology*, 61:528-531.

[11]   Morganthau, T. (1992). *It's not just New York...Big cities, small towns: More and more guns in younger hands*. Newsweek, March 9, 25-29.

[12]   Bell, C. (1991). Traumatic stress and children in danger. *Journal of Health Care for the Poor and Underserved*, 2:175-188.

[13]   Wallach, L.B. (1993). *Helping children cope with violence*. Young Children, May, 4-11.

[14] Harrington- Lueker, D. (1992). Blown away by scool violence. *American School Board Journal,* 179:20-26.

[15] Stein, N. *Stop sexual harassment in schools.* USA. USA Today; May 18,11A: 1993.

[16] Adler, N.E., Boyce, T., Chesney, M.AQ., Colens, S., Folkman, S., Kahn, R.L., and Syme, S.L. (1994). Socioeconomic status and health: The challenge of gradient. *Amercian Psychologist,* 49: 15-24.

[17] Kazdin A.E (1993). Adolescent mental health: Prevention and Treatment programs. *American Psychologist,* 48; 127-141.

[18] Environmental Protection Agency. (1993). *Secondhand Smoke: What you can do About Second hand Smoke as Parental, Decision makers, and Building Occupants.* Washington. DC. U.S.EPA.

[19] Schultz, D. (1994). *Lung Disease Data.* New York: American Lung Association.

[20] Thomas, C.F., English, J.L., and Bickel, A.S. (1993). *Moving Toward Integrated Services: A Literature Review for Prevention Specialists,* Portland, OR: Northwest Regional Education Laboratory.

[21] Kolbe, L.J. (1992). Statement. In select Committee on Children, Youth, and Family, U.S. House of Representatives, The risky business of adolescence: How to help teens stay safe- Part I. Hearing Before the select Committee on Children, Youth, and Families, 22-23. Washington, D.C.: U.S. Government Printing Office.

[22] American Medical Association. (1990). *America's Adolescents: How healthy are they?* Chicago. IL: American Medical Association.

[23] Attico, N.B; Hartner J. (1992). "Teenage pregnancy: Identifying the scope of the problem." *Family Practice Recertification,* Volume 14, No.6.

[24] Kann, L., Warren, W., Collins, J., Ross, J., Collins, B., and Kolbe, L.J. (1993). Results from the national school- based 1991 youth risk behavior survey and progress toward achieving related health objectives for the nation. *Public Health Reports,* 108 (Supplement 1), 47-67.

[25] Bever, D.L. (1992). *Safety: A Personal Focus.* St. Louis, MO: Mosby.

[26] Wilson, M.H., Baker, S.P., Teret, S.P., Shock, S., and Gatbarino, J. (1991) *Saving Children: A Guide to Injury Prevention.* New York: Oxford University Press.

[27] Linda Meeks, Philip Heit, Randy. *Comprehensive School Health Education*: 2nd Edition. Columbus OH; Meeks Heit Publishing Company: 1996.

[28] Brudkin, M. (1993). *Every kid counts. 31 ways to save our children.* New York: HarperCollins.

[29] Glover, B., and Shephard, J. (1983). *The Family Fitness Handbook.* New York: Penguin Books.

[30] New York State Disaster Preparedness Commission. (1990). *Planning Manual and Guidelines for School Emergency / Disaster Preparedness.* Albany, NY: New York State Department of Education.

[31] Allensworth, Diane. (1993). Research Base for Innovative Practices in School Health Education. In: *Centers for Disease Control. Comprehensive School Health Education Programs: Innovative Practices and Issues in Setting Standards.* Atlanta, GA: Centers for Disease Control and Prevention.

In: Hygiene and Its Role in Health
Editors: P. L. Anderson and J. P. Lachan

ISBN 978-1-60456-195-1
© 2008 Nova Science Publishers, Inc.

Chapter 9

Potential Hygiene Motivators and De-Motivators among Rural Communities in the Eastern Cape of South Africa

Nancy Phaswana-Mafuya[*]

Social Aspects of HIV/AIDS and Health,
Human Sciences Research Council,
Port Elizabeth, South Africa
and
University of the Western Cape

Abstract

This study describes potential personal, household and community hygiene motivators and de-motivators among 494 villagers in the Eastern Cape. Over 50% were 26-50 years, male, married, employed and had secondary education. Individual interviews were conducted using an interview schedule with open ended questions. More than 50% viewed access to regular water supply as a hygiene motivator and the lack thereof as a de-motivator. Personal hygiene (30%), refuse/solid waste disposal (14.2%), safe human excreta disposal (28.5%) and safe liquid waste disposal (12.0%) facilities were viewed as hygiene motivators and the lack of these as de-motivators. Hygiene education was identified as a motivator for personal (7.5%), household (7.6%) and community (7.8%) hygiene and the lack of it as a de-motivator. Protected household water storage facilities (10.2%), money to purchase both personal hygiene items (10.5%) and domestic hygiene detergents (8.4%) were seen as hygiene motivators and the lack of these as de-motivators.

Keywords: *Sanitation, rural communities, hygiene motivation, Eastern Cape, South Africa.*

[*] Correspondence Address: 10 Nederburgh Crescent, Tulbagh, Port Elizabeth, 6025, South Africa. Tel: +27 (41) 3602214; Fax: +27 (41) 3609791; Fax to Email: +27 (0) 865146608; Email: nphaswanamafuya@hsrc.ac.za

Introduction

Hygiene, sanitation and water supply are inextricably linked. Hygiene refers to practices, principles and conditions that help prevent diseases and maintain health at personal, household and community levels. Personal hygiene has to do with personal cleanliness within the setting where people live. It includes bathing, clothing and washing hands with soap (e.g. after going to the toilet or after changing the nappies of babies and before preparation of food, etc) as well as personal care (care of feet, nails, hair, teeth, spitting) (Department of Water Affairs and Forestry (DWAF), 2001). Household hygiene has to do with keeping the home and toilet clean, safe disposal of refuse and solid waste, cleanliness in areas where food is stored and prepared and ensuring that food and drinking water is kept covered and uncontaminated (DWAF, 2001). Community hygiene mainly has to do with safe excreta and sullage disposal, solid waste (refuse) as well as liquid waste and hygiene education (DWAF, 2001). Personal, household and community hygiene cannot be maintained without adequate sanitation and regular water supply.

Adequate sanitation is defined as the safe management of human excreta and includes both hardware (sanitation technologies such as toilets and hygienic latrines) and software (hygiene promotion such as hand-washing with soap) (Postnote, 2002). Global sanitation coverage rose from 49% in 1990 to 58% in 2002. Still, some 2.6 billion people live without improved sanitation as demonstrated in Figure 1 (The United Nations Children's Fund (UNICEF)/World Health Organisation (WHO) Joint Monitoring Program (JMP), 2004).

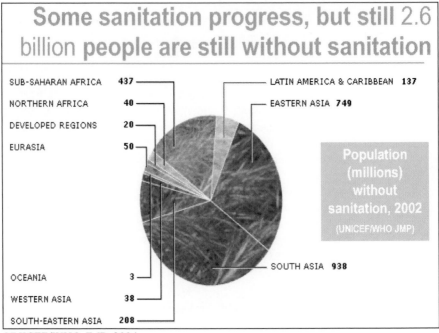

Source: UNICEF/WHO JMP, 2004.

Figure 1. Population without improved sanitation by region in 2002.

In Sub-Saharan Africa, coverage is a mere 36% as reflected in Figure 2 (UNICEF/WHO JMP, 2004).

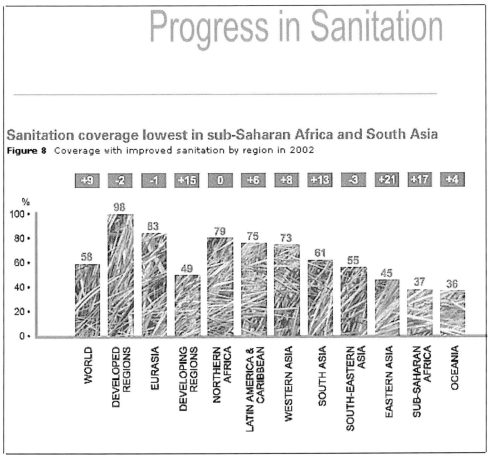

Source: UNICEF/WHO JMP, 2004.

Figure 2. Coverage with improved sanitation by region in 2002.

In South Africa, approximately 18 million people (38%) lacked access to adequate sanitation in 2001 (DWAF, 2001). Delivering the new sanitation target will require considerable political will together with significant financial, technical and human resources (Postnote, 2002).

Global water coverage progress looks good as reflected in Figure 3, but still 1.1 billion people are still without safe water (UNICEF/WHO JMP, 2004).

Figure 4 (UNICEF/WHO JMP 2004) shows that water coverage in Sub-Saharan Africa in 2002 was lower than that of other regions.

In South Africa, approximately 7 million (15%) people lacked access to adequate water supply in 2001 (DWAF, 2001). Figure 5 shows water supply and sanitation access by province in South Africa in 1996 (Development Bank of South Africa (DBSA), 2000).

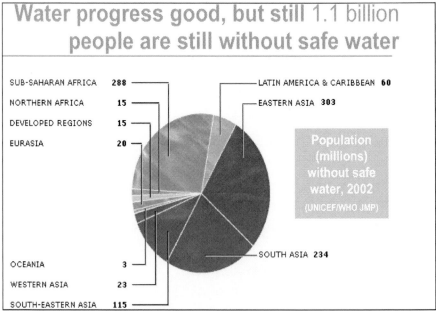

Source: UNICEF/WHO JMP, 2004.

Figure 3. Global water coverage by region in 2002.

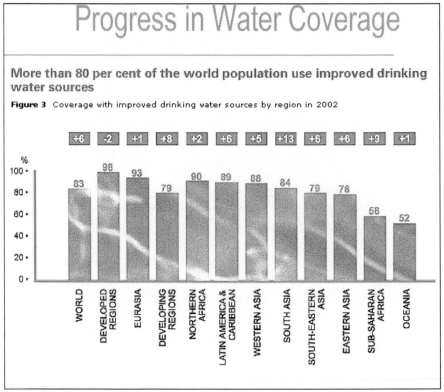

Source: UNICEF/WHO JMP, 2004.

Figure 4. Progress in Water Coverage.

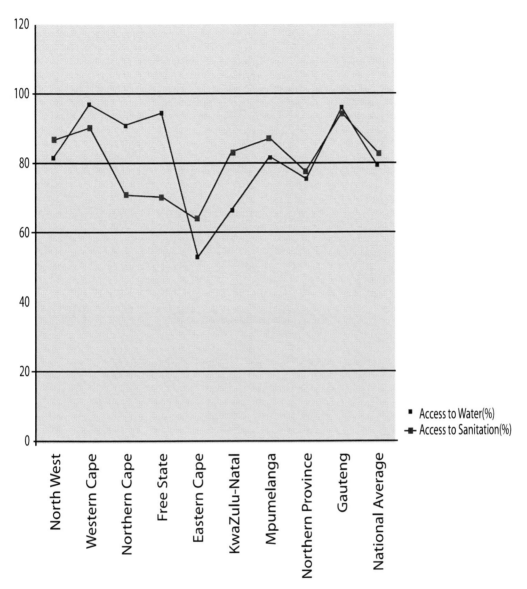

Source: DBSA, 2000.

Figure 5. Water Supply and Sanitation access by province in South Africa, 1996.

In the municipality where the current study was undertaken, it is estimated that 50% of the households have access to water supply from public stand pipes, 44% rely on natural resources and 38% on bore-holes especially in the rural villages (Political Information and Monitoring Service Centre (PIMS Centre), 2001). About 4% has access to water on-site and these are in the urban areas while only 14% have access to flush toilets. Most people use pit latrines (87%). However, some households (11%) have no toilet facility at all. About 98% of the population need proper sanitation (PIMS Centre, 2001). This is so in spite of the fact that the Constitution (1996) guarantees all South Africans the right to adequate sanitation.

Inadequate sanitation and irregular water supply may pose enormous challenges in as far as hygiene motivation is concerned be it at personal, household or community levels and may negatively impact on health as reflected in Figure 6.

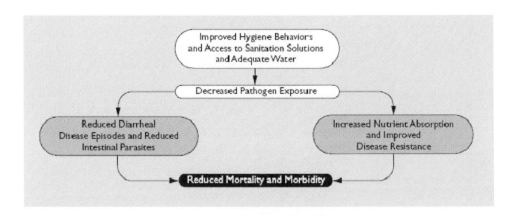

Source: Unknown

Figure 6. Impact of adequate water and sanitation on health.

Against this background, the current study was conducted to determine potential hygiene motivators and de-motivators among villagers in a rural municipality of the Eastern Cape, South Africa.

Materials and Methods

Design and Setting

A descriptive study was conducted in a rural municipality of the Eastern Cape, South Africa in 2003. The municipality has 112 villages spread across 14 wards. The total population is 93 997 people, made up of 20 757 households (PIMS Centre, 2001). The population is evenly spread across the 14 wards with the average number of people per ward being 6 714 (1 483) households. The average household size is 4.5% persons (PIMS Centre, 2001).

Sample and Procedure

Fourteen (14) villages were randomly selected from each of the 14 wards – one village per ward. In each village 50 villagers who were knowledgeable on hygiene issues were chosen; thus having a purposive sample of 700 villagers. From this sample, 494 villagers (70.6%) sample consented to participate in the study after being advised of their: a) their status as volunteers, (b) their right to refuse to answer any question, (c) the legal liabilities of their participation, (d) confidentiality, and (e) the limitations of anonymity due to the nature of the study. Only 29.4% did not participate in the study – 21.2% were not available at the time when the study was conducted and 8.2% declined to give consent to participate in the study. The distribution of respondents per each of the 14 villages in reflected in Table 1.

Table 1. Distribution of number of respondents across 14 villages

Villages	N
MC	45
BG	42
GS	42
QWK	41
MTT	41
DB	40
WR	40
GN	38
LX	33
NT	30
LQ	28
PE	28
MP	25
NB	19

The names of villages have not been provided for confidentiality and anonymity purposes. Over half of the sample was 26-50 years (64%), male (52.3%), married (54.1%), employed (64.8%) and possessed secondary education (63%).

Data Collection

Fourteen (14) trained field workers served as interviewers, one per each of the 14 villages. Before commencement of the interview, they gave respondents the definitions of personal, household and community hygiene, derived from DWAF (2001), as follows:

- Personal hygiene has to do with personal cleanliness (e.g. bathing and clothing) and washing hands (e.g. after going to the toilet or after changing the nappies of babies and before preparation of food, etc).

- Household hygiene has to do with keeping the home and toilet clean, safe disposal of refuse and solid waste, cleanliness in areas where food is stored and prepared and ensuring that food and drinking water is kept covered and uncontaminated.
- Community hygiene has to do with safe excreta and sullage disposal, solid waste (refuse), liquid waste, hygiene education for food vendors, keeping of animals and safe community storm water drainage.

Thereafter, they interviewed each responded using an interview schedule with the following open ended questions:

- Name one key motivator that would enable you to practice personal hygiene.
- Name one key motivator that would enable you to practice household hygiene.
- Name one key motivator that would enable you to practice community hygiene.
- Name one key de-motivator that would hinder you to practice personal hygiene.
- Name one key de-motivator that would hinder you to practice household hygiene.
- Name one key de-motivator that would hinder you to practice community hygiene.

The interviews were conducted in the local language (Xhosa). Each interview session lasted for about 30 minutes.

Data Analysis

Content analysis was conducted as described below. It must be stated that while the steps of analyzing data have been described as distinct activities, the process itself was recursive.

- The responses given for each question were phared differently. The researcher went through all responses in each interview schedule in order to develop a thorough and comprehensive description of hygiene motivators and de-motivators that the respondents provided at each hygiene level.
- The data was then classified or grouped and then coded according to the already existing categories that the researcher had i.e. hygiene motivators and hygiene de-motivators bearing in mind the research questions and put on Statistical Package for Social Services (SPSS) version 11 (Open coding).
- The researcher carefully examined data in each category and sub-categorised into already existing sub-categories, i.e. personal, household and community hygiene on SPSS.
- Responses given for each hygiene level were then compared for similarities and differences and the further sub-divided according to similarity (though expressed with different words) as reflected in the results section.
- The data was then captured on SPSS according to the identified categories and sub-categories which were continuously refined as the researcher came across new data.
- Frequency counts were then established and presented in the form of descriptive data on the tables as reflected in the results section.

The researcher adopted various strategies to ensure trustworthiness of the interpretation of the data espoused by Miles and Huberman (1994). These included:

- *Participant checking:* Periodic feedback sessions were held to present the results of the data collection to the participants to test whether they agree with them.
- *Data cross-checking:* this activity involved the researcher stepping back to consider what the analyzed data mean and to assess their implications for the questions at hand. This helped the researcher to ensure that the data are credible, defensible, warranted, and able to withstand alternative explanations.
- *Moderator reviews:* the interviewers had regular meetings to cross-check the quality of each other's data sets.
- *Ongoing reflection on data:* the researcher began the analysis almost in tandem with data collection. This helped the researcher to identify tentative interpretations or emerging hypotheses during the fieldwork process.
- *Peer reviews:* the researcher brought two peers who were knowledgeable on qualitative analysis as well as the substantive issues involved in the study, into the analytic process. Approximately 20% of the data were given to these peers to rate the initial codings. These peers served as a cross-check, sounding board, and source of new ideas and cross-fertilization. A 96% agreement rating was achieved.

Results

Potential Personal Hygiene Motivators and De-Motivators

Potential personal hygiene motivators were in descending order: access to regular supply of portable water (52%), availability of personal hygiene facilities (e.g. adequate means of hygienically washing and drying hands, including wash basins and a supply of hot and cold (or suitably temperature controlled) water; lavatories of appropriate hygienic design; and adequate changing facilities for personnel (30%), availability of money to purchase hygiene items such as toothpaste, toothbrush, soap, shampoo, deodorant, and comb (10.5%) and hygiene education (e.g. home visits by health workers, hygiene messages on TV and radio, hygiene training workshops) (7.5%).

Table 2. Potential personal hygiene motivators and de-motivators

Motivators: Availability of:	%	De-motivators: Lack of:	%
Regular portable water supply	52.0	Regular portable water supply	58.4
Personal hygiene facilities	30.0	Personal hygiene facilities	17.8
Money to purchase hygiene items	10.5	Money to purchase hygiene items	8.8
Hygiene Education	7.5	Hygiene Education	15.0

Potential personal hygiene de-motivators motivators were in descending order, lack of access to regular supply of portable water (58.4%), lack of personal hygiene facilities

(17.8%), lack of hygiene education (15.0%) and lack of money to buy personal hygiene items (8.8%).

Potential Household Hygiene Motivators and De-Motivators

Potential household hygiene motivators were in descending order: having regular portable water supply (52%), availability of refuse and solid waste disposal facilities (14.2%), availability of protected water storage facilities (10.2%), availability of money to purchase household detergents (8.4%), covered food storage (8%) and hygiene education (7.6%).

Potential household hygiene motivators were in descending order, lack of regular portable water supply (58.8%), lack of hygiene education (15.8%), lack of money to purchase household detergents (11.5%), lack of refuse and solid waste disposal facilities (10.9%), lack of protected water storage facilities (2%) and uncovered food storage (1%).

Table 3. Potential household hygiene motivators and de-motivators

Motivators: Availability of:	%	De-motivators: Lack of:	%
Regular portable water supply	52.0	Regular portable water supply	58.8
Refuse/solid waste disposal facilities	14.2	Refuse/solid waste disposal facilities	10.9
Protected water storage facilities	10.2	Protected water storage facilities	2.0
Covered food storage	8.0	Covered food storage	1.0
Sufficient income to buy detergents	8.4	Sufficient income to buy detergents	11.5
Hygiene Education	7.6	Hygiene Education	15.8

Potential Community Hygiene Motivators and De-Motivators

Potential community hygiene motivators were in descending order: access to regular portable water supply (51.6%), availability of facilities for safe disposal of human excreta (28.5%), availability of facilities for safe disposal of other solid and liquid wastes (12.0%) and hygiene education (7.8%).

Table 4. Potential community hygiene motivators and de-motivators

Motivators: Availability of:	%	De-motivators: Lack of:	%
Regular water supply	51.6	Regular water supply	50.3
Safe disposal of human excreta	28.5	Safe disposal of human excreta	27.7
Safe disposal of solid/liquid wastes	12.0	Safe disposal of solid/liquid wastes	6.8
Hygiene Education	7.8	Hygiene Education	15.2

Potential community hygiene motivators were in descending order, lack of access to regular portable water supply (50.3%), lack of facilities for safe disposal of human excreta

(27.7%), lack of hygiene education (15.2%) and lack of facilities for safe disposal of other solid and liquid wastes (6.8%).

Discussion

More than half of the respondents were of the opinion that access to regular portable water supply is a hygiene motivator for personal (52%), household (52%) and community (51.6%) hygiene and the lack thereof was perceived as a de-motivator for personal (58.4%), household (58.8%) and community (50.3%) hygiene. More worrying is the fact that most individuals, households and communities in rural areas do not have adequate portable water supply as alluded to in the introduction. Phaswana-Mafuya (2006a) found that water was generally perceived as "not enough" across the same communities studied here (92.9%) mainly due to rivers/dams being dry and taps closed/broken or not having water (71.4%). Tumwine, Thomson, Katui-Katua, Mujwahizi, Johnstone and Porras (2003), found in a review of 60 studies, that water availability (25%) was one of the largest benefits of hygiene improvements. Lack of sufficient quantities of clean water critically impairs the ability of most rural populations to engage in appropriate personal, household and community hygiene practices which would greatly assist in stemming the tide of infectious diseases (Phaswana-Mafuya, 2006b). Improving the quantity and quality of water available may enhance the adoption of better hygienic practices which interrupt the transmission of most faecal-oral diseases.

Hygiene education was also identified as a hygiene motivator for personal (7.5%), household (7.6%) and community hygiene (7.8%) and the lack thereof was perceived as a de-motivator for personal (15.0%), household (15.8) and community (15.2%) hygiene. The logical explanation to this is the fact that without knowledge of the importance of hygiene and the negative effects of hygiene on health, it is more unlikely that people would adopt safe hygienic practices. Phaswana-Mafuya and Shukla (2005) and Phswana-Mafuya (2006c) found that educational mechanisms such as training, advocacy; capacity building, social mobilisation, access to information and information exchange were critical in the adoption of safe hygiene practices. There was a consensus across all the stakeholders who participated in the study that, unhygienic practices, certain cultural beliefs in relation to hygiene, fears and perceptions of hygienic practices would have to be changed through raising awareness and education. Ineffective promotion and low public awareness, ignorance of people, lack of capacity building, lack of hygiene education and training, negligence of people were said to be de-motivating factors for adoption of safe hygienic practices. Further stakeholders expressed the need for more hygiene programmes. It was indicated that hygiene programmes should change long-held beliefs through mentioning the unmentionable; equally address the needs, preferences and behaviours of children, women and men; adopt approaches which recognise and allow optimal use of valuable community attributes such as participatory approaches; focuses on behaviour and facilities together (Phaswana-Mafuya and Shukla, 2005).

The results also show that availability of: personal hygiene facilities (30%), refuse and solid waste disposal facilities (14.2%), safe human excreta disposal facilities (28.5%), and safe liquid waste disposal facilities (12.0%) serve as hygiene motivators. The lack of: personal hygiene facilities (17.8%), refuse and solid waste disposal facilities (10.9%), safe human excreta disposal facilities (27.7%), and safe liquid waste disposal facilities (6.8%).

The concern however, is that, most rural communities overwhelmingly lack adequate arrangements for solid and liquid waste disposal. For example, Phaswana-Mafuya (2006a), found that 92.9% of the same communities studied here, had poor liquid waste disposal facilities. Alcock (1999) argues that most rural communities typically spill waste water from bathing and washing right outside houses, where it may soak into the ground or form stagnant pools in poorly drained areas. Where sewers exist, they are virtually always open drainage canals. The ground by the side of the shelters or in the alleyways serves as a frequent substitute for urinals. With regard to solid waste disposal, Phaswana-Mafuya (2006a) found that the same communities studied here generally adopted safe solid waste disposal practices as they mainly threw solid waste in the rubbish pit (78.6%) and when the rubbish pit is full they burned it (64.3%). However, other communities threw rubbish in the veld (21.4%), as that was the only means they had (7.1%). They neither had rubbish pits nor essential services for waste disposal (35.7%). Similar findings were reported by Tshibangu (1987). Unhygienic disposal of domestic waste (e.g. bottle tops, matches, brushes, small bottles, sanitary towels, toilet paper, newspaper, tampons, condoms, plastic/paper packets), has serious health and environmental implications (Alcock, 1999). The literature point out that safe disposal of solid waste is a major and necessary requirement for hygiene motivation (Tumwine *et.al.* 2003). Inadequate disposal of waste results in exposure and increased risks to personal safety. It is especially women and elderly who are the most inconvenienced (DWAF, 1996 and 2001). Further, inadequate disposal of waste leads to environmental pollution. Environmental pollution leads to poor health. Poor health keeps families in a cycle of poverty and lost income.

In as far as excreta disposal facilities are concerned the literature reveals that generally rural settlements, informal settlements and traditional villages have little or no basic safe human excreta disposal facilities compared to the large towns, even when they are located adjacent to the large towns (DWAF, 2002b). In Sub-Saharan Africa, sanitation coverage is a mere 36% and in South Africa, approximately 18 million people lacked access to adequate sanitation in 2001 as alluded to in the introduction. In general, villagers have improvised sanitation systems in rural areas to satisfy their perceived needs. Phaswana-Mafuya (2006c) found that in communities where there are no toilets, communities relief themselves in the veld (100%). Although it is difficult to quantify morbidity and mortality related to unsafe and inadequate sanitation because of lack of an effective monitoring and surveillance system and country-wide baseline survey, limited information on disease prevalence reported indicates that water-borne diseases are among the major causes of sickness and death (WHO, 2000/2003). The lack of sewerage systems threatens not only hygiene but also the health of the communities. A qualitative study conducted among 122 sanitation stakeholders in the Eastern Cape suggests that safe, acceptable and affordable sanitation technologies and flexible sanitation systems, incorporating respect for community values, perceptions and practices and appropriate to the resource base of the community and the physical environment in which it is located are critical for adoption of safe hygienic practices (Phaswana-Mafuya and Shukla (2005). Hemson (2004) points out that additional resources are needed not only to make sanitation services available to the rural poor but also to make access to services both reliable and really beneficial. Investing in sanitation can lead to reduced morbidity and mortality, increased life expectancy and savings in health care costs (DWAF, 2001). Adequate sanitation is an important way to minimise or manage the negative impact of human settlement on the environment.

Availability of protected water storage facilities (10.2%) was also cited as a hygiene motivator at household level and the lack thereof as hygiene de-motivator (2%). It is encouraging to note that Phaswana-Mafuya (2006a) found that the same communities studied here practiced safe water storage as they generally stored water in plastic containers (64.3%), outside (78.6%) and in direct sunlight (71.4%), being properly covered (35.7%) in order to prevent animals from drinking the water, germs, diseases. The communities used different containers for storing water and for rubbish collection (64.3%); washed their water containers once a day, twice a day and more than twice a day (64.3%) in order prevent germs, diseases and maintain hygiene. Similarly, Tshibangu (1987) found that the storage of water at household was safe in some communities. Unsafe water storage practices pose a threat to the health and hygiene of the communities as this may result in waterborne diseases such as diarrhoel diseases, intestinal infections, polio, typhoid and cholera (DWAF, 1996 and 2001). They may lead to disperse pollution of water sources (DWAF, 1996; DWAF, 2002b). This in turn increases the cost of downstream water treatment, as well as the risk of disease for communities who use untreated water.

Availability of money to purchase personal hygiene (10.5%) items and domestic hygiene detergents (8.4%) was also seen as a hygiene motivator and the lack thereof as hygiene de-motivators. In her study of the same communities, Phaswana-Mafuya (2006a) found that 7.1% of the communities did not treat their drinking water because they had no money to buy detergents (7.1%). Further, in a study of hygiene and sanitation stakeholders in the Eastern Cape, it was found that communities drank untreated water from unprotected streams, due to lack of money to buy disinfectants (Phaswana-Mafuya and Shukla, 2005). Availability of income was considered by all stakeholders to be one of the key motivating factors for adoption of safe hygienic practices. Unemployment, low incomes, poor living conditions, low literacy levels and lack of recreational facilities were perceived as de-motivating factors towards the adoption of safe hygienic practices. Similarly the high cost of water and sanitation to families of low income and the shortage of capital for investment were also cited as de-motivating factors. While even the lowest-income families can usually afford potable water as it is delivered, the provision of indoor connections close to the house can become unaffordable because of attendant costs that are not taken into account in project feasibility studies. People are always willing to pay for the type of service they want. It should be ensured that that the method of payment is the preferred one which best suit their circumstances. Special provision may have to be made for the poorest individuals and families.

Conclusions and Recommendations

The results of this study should be interpreted with caution because of the non randomness of the sample, the limited sample size and the qualitative nature of the study. Below, the preliminary conclusions and recommendations of the study are made. These preliminary conclusions and recommendations can be tested further with more representative samples and rigorous scientific methods. The following conclusions and recommendations are made:

- Availability of regular water supply is a key hygiene motivator and the lack therof a key hygiene de-motivator at personal, household and community hygiene levels. This is not surprising given the fact that water is not only necessary for consumption, but it is also necessary for cooking, personal and domestic hygiene requirements. Therefore, in order for communities to adopt safe hygiene practices, there should be sufficient, safe, acceptable, physically accessible, and affordable regular water supply. This is a challenge given the fact that 1.1 billion people lack access to an improved water source in developing countries as indicated in the introductory and discussion sections of this paper.
- Hygiene education is a critical hygiene motivator and the the lack thereof a hygiene de-motivator at personal, household and community hygiene levels. Therefore, hygiene education efforts need to be scaled up. Effective hygiene education may produce changes in knowledge and understanding; it may influence or clarify values; it may improve skills and eventually effect changes in behaviour.
- Availability of solid/liquid waste/human excreta disposal facilities serve as hygiene motivator and the lack therof as hygiene de-motivator at personal, household and community hygiene levels. It is imperative for these facilities to be made available in order to ensure safe hygienic practices. The safe disposal of waste is a prerequisite to protecting health. In the absence of basic sanitation facilities (for example), a number of major diseases can be transmitted through faecal pollution. These include diarrhoea, schitosomiasis, hepatitis A, cholera and typhoid. This is a challenge given the fact that 2.4 billion people in developing countries do not have access to improved sanitation facilities as indicated in the introductory and discussion sections of this paper.

A range of effective interventions can be implemented in the areas of policy, education, awareness raising, technology development and behavioural change. Such interventions can be extremely cost-effective and can be implemented by policy and decision makers, householders, communities, educators, government officials and many other stakeholders. Below a few indicative examples of actions that can be taken are given. The list is not exhaustive but illustrates a range of actions that can be considered. Of course, specific interventions that are implemented in any one setting will depend on the nature and the severity of the problem, the local context, the resources available and the priorities to be addressed.

- Extending access to improved water sources amongst the "unserved" in rural and urban areas
- Targeting hygiene education on key behaviours at both children and adults
- Ensuring availability of safe water storage facilities and treatment of water at home
- Improved access to safe sanitary facilities and availability of safe disposal of human excreta, solid and liquid wastes

Acknowledgements

The financing of the project by the Water Research Commission and the contribution of the members of the Steering Committee is acknowledged gratefully.

This study was successful with the co-operation of many individuals and institutions. Sincere thanks to:

The Limakhozu Development Agency team, for their dedication, team spirit and commitment to the study.

The Eastern Cape rural communities, for their wonderful co-operation in providing the information needed in such an honest and generous way. Without their commitment to the dissemination of information, this research would not have been successful.

The anonymous reviewers are thanked for their useful comments.

References

Alcock, P.G. 1999. *A water resources and sanitation systems source book with special reference to Kwa-Zulu Natal.* Part 6. WRC Report No 384/6/99.

DBSA. 2001. South Africa: Inter-Provincial Comparative Report. *DBSA*, Midrand, South Africa.

DWAF. 1996. *National Sanitation Policy*. National Sanitation Task Team. Republic of South Africa. Pretoria: Government Printers.

DWAF. 2001. *White Paper on Basic Household Sanitation*. Pretoria: Government Printers.

DWAF. 2002. *Draft White Paper on Water Services*, October 2002. Republic of South Africa.

Hemson, D. 2004 Beating the backlog: meeting targets and providing free basic services. Position Paper, January 2004. *Human Sciences Research Council: Integrated Rural and Regional Development.*

Phaswana-Mafuya, N. 2006a. Hygiene status of rural communities in the Eastern Cape of South Africa. *International Journal of Environmental Health Research*, 16 (4): 289-303.

Phaswana-Mafuya, N. 2006b. *Health aspects of sanitation among Eastern Cape (EC) rural communities*, South Africa. Curationis, 29 (2): 41-47.

Phaswana-Mafuya, N. 2006c. An investigation into the perceived Sanitation Challenges in EC rural communities. *Health SA/Gesondheid Accredited Interdisciplinary Research Journal,* 11 (1): 18-30.

Phaswana-Mafuya, N. and Shukla, N. 2005. Factors that could motivate people to adopt safe hygienic practices in the Eastern Cape, South Africa. *African Health Sciences*, 5 (1), 21-28.

PIMS Centre. 2001. *Integrated Development Planning of Ngqushwa District Municipality.* Eastern Cape, South Africa.

Postnote. 2002. *Access to sanitation in developing countries.* Postnote, December 2002 Number 190.

The Constitution of the Republic of South Africa, Act No.108 of 1996. Pretoria: Government Printers.

Tshibangu, N.N. 1987. Water Supplies and sanitary facilities in rural Transkei, *South African. Medical Journal*, 17 (6), 368-369.

Tumwine, J.K.; Thomson, J.; Katui-Katua, M.;Mujwahizi, M.; Johnstone, N. and Porras, I. 2003. Sanitation and hygiene in urban and rural households in East Africa. *Environmental Health Research* 13, 107-115.

WHO. 2000. *The World Health Report: Making a Difference.* Geneva: World Health Organisation.

WHO. 2003. *World Health Report 2003.* Shaping our future. World Health Organisation. ISBN 9241562439 (http://www.who.int/whr/en/).

WHO/UNICEF JMP. 2004. *Meeting the MGD Drinking Water and Sanitation: A Mid-Term Assessment of Progress.* Geneva: WHO/UNICEF. ISBN 9241562781.

WSSCC and WHO. 2005. *Sanitation and hygiene promotion: programming guidance.* Geneva: WHO Press.

In: Hygiene and Its Role in Health
Editors: P. L. Anderson and J. P. Lachan

ISBN 978-1-60456-195-1
© 2008 Nova Science Publishers, Inc.

Chapter 10

Assessment of the Impact of Activity on Health Status in the Elderly

A. Gebska-Kuczerowska, M. Miller and M. J. Wysocki

Department of Health Promotion in National Institute of Hygiene,
Warsaw, Poland

Abstract

Introduction: According to the opinion of gerontologists, it is possible to prevent or delay the negative influence of aging on mental and physical health status by healthy behaviors. "Active aging" people bring a lot for their societies and that's why activity is the value not only for the elderly but also for the societies.

Aim: The purpose of the research was to assess the impact of various forms of the activity (physical, pro-social and intellectual) on the health condition people who are 65 years old and older.

Material and Methods: The research was conducted by anonymous questionnaire forms. A nation-wide research had been preceded by a pilot study. After a preliminary qualification and selection of 2,072 questionnaires, a further analysis of 1,910 questionnaires (92.6%) have been finally classified. The condition of health has been evaluated on the basis of information: illness and health problems, self-evaluation of health condition, body weight, use of medical assistance, and other aids, hospitalization and reasons for it and presence of at least one group of disabled persons whose mobility is limited and reasons for these limitations. The extent of psycho-social health has been evaluated on the basis of moods such as sadness, depression, limited life enthusiasm, assessment of satisfaction resulting from contacts with relatives and other persons, and identification of problems connected with aging.

Results: Active persons determine their health condition more positively, they suffer from fewer CVDs and their health is more stable, they have a better psychological condition (loneliness, depression), and they are less often use medical services in hospitals.

Disability recognized in legal terms and formal disability, except 1st disability category (the hardest cases) and persons who are immobile does not constitute any barrier in becoming active. Similarly, diseases don't exclude activity, except pathologies that limit or prevent elderly people from partaking in any activities. Activity has a positive impact on keeping a proper body weight. Active persons stay independent, are satisfied with life more often, feel that they are needed, and their self-esteem is high. It seems that a barrier in the psychological sense in becoming active by elderly people is the fact that they are less willing to become active. The majority of respondents have admitted that their health condition has deteriorated drastically at the age of 63 to 64.

Conclusion: Analysis of results has confirmed the existence of a relation between activity and health condition. Activity (different kinds) is deciding about healthy aging and it is simultaneously a positive indicator.

Introduction

We have observed demographic aging of the Polish population like in most countries over the world. This is due to an increase in average life span and a decrease of the birthrate [1, 2, 3, 4].

The percentage of the population over 65 years old in Poland has increased in last decades as follows: 9.4% in 1985, 10.2% in 1990, 11.2% in 1995, 11.5% in 1996 and 11.7% in 1997. In the same period, the percentage of people aged 65-79 increased (from7.7 %) to 9.4%, and people above 90 years old from 1.8% to 2.0% [5].

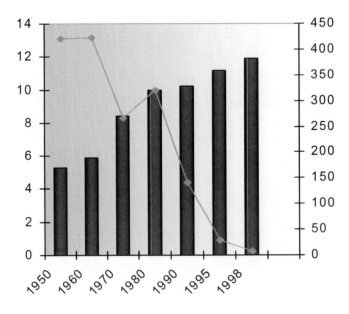

Figure 1. Population aging in Poland (left-percentage of 65+, right-actual increase of the population in thousand-red line).

The aging of the population causes many deontological, medical, social and economic consequences [5, 6, 7, 8]. The health promotion should be addressed also into the elderly population, despite better and more spectacular results of health promotion in younger age groups. According to the opinion of gerontologists it is possible to prevent or delay the negative influence of aging on mental and physical status. These influences change and improve adaptation mechanisms and modify environmental agents [9, 10, 11]. An active life style is one of the most important determinants of health status, due to its potential modification. It means that health status and also the aging process are dependent in the majority (50-60%) on modifiable factors [5, 12, 13, 14].

There is a strong implication that it is possible to minimize the negative results of the aging process by the creating or improving activities (and other healthy behaviors).

World Health Organization experts' opinion is that activities (different kinds of activities) play a special and important role for people over 65 years old. That's why WHO dedicated 1999 the year for seniors' activities ("Active aging makes differences")

"Active aging" people bring a lot for theirs societies and that's why activity is the value not only for the elderly but also for the societies [15]. The 2002 year for all generations was defined by WHO similarly as "Move for health" [16, 17].

The aim of the research made in 1999 was to analyze the health status, demographic structure and level of various kinds of activities of people 65 years old and over. Another goal was to assess the impact of activities (physical, pro-social and intellectual) on health condition in the study group.

Methods

Nationwide research was conducted by using anonymous questionnaire forms. Nationwide research has been preceded by a pilot research in 1998. After preliminary qualification and selection of 2,072 people aged 65 years old and older – 1,910 questionnaires (92.6%) have been finally classified. Students from the Third Age University have been included in that research due to low prevalence of activities (intellectual, physical and pro-social) in that age group [5]. In the questionnaire form were information on demographic data as follows: age, gender, education, legal status, accommodation. The health status was assessed on the basic information on illness and complaints, disability, inefficiency category, limitations of mobility and reasons for them, hospitalization and ambulatory visits – medical assistance, Body Mass Index, psychosocial problems as: sadness, depression, troubles with relationships, health status self-assessment and activities (kind and frequency of activity). The kind of activity has been assessed on the basis of responses to open questions. The information on activities has been grouped according to the adopted key (pro-social, intellectual and physical activities). The physical activity level was assessed by an equivalent of MET.

The database (health status, activity and demography) was created using the Epi-Info 6 program and the statistic analyzes by Chi2 test. The Stat-Graf and SAS programs were used for analyzing by logistic regression and Pearson's correlation.

Results

The Characteristic of the Study Group

In the research 1,910 respondents participated. There was 1,102 (57.7%) persons aged 65 to 74 years old (early period of senility), 755 (39.5%) aged 75 to 89 (advanced senility), 53 (2.8%) 90 years old and over (oldest old). Mean age was 74 years (+/- 6.9 years). Women constituted 65.9% of the group and they were in the majority of every age group (66% - 65 to 74 years old, 65% - 75 to 89 and 70% - 90 years old and over).

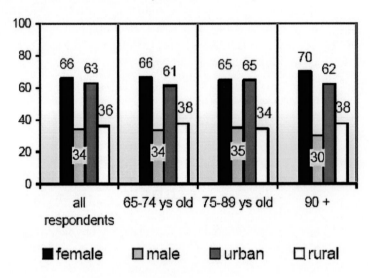

Figure 2. Study group by sex, age and dwelling-place (%).

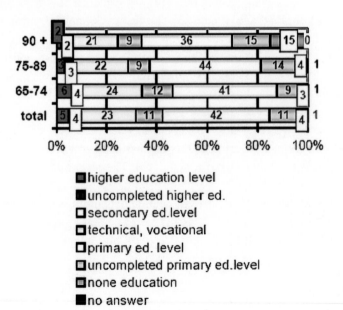

Figure 3. Education level of respondents.

Respondents with primary level education constituted 42.4% of the study population, 23.3% were with secondary level education (college, comprehensive or trade school), 11.3% with uncompleted primary level education and 10.7% finished trade schools. Subjects with a higher education level constituted 5% and respondents with uncompleted higher education – 3.7%. There were 3.7% persons without education at all. The lower education level was observed in older age groups. Women constituted 57% of the higher educated study group, but among women this percentage was lower than among men (4.1% v. 7%). There was two fold more men than women who finished trade schools (16% vs. 8%). Urban individuals constituted 62.7% (1,198). They were better educated than rural respondents were. Rural individuals finished only primary schools more frequently - 54%, 19% uncompleted primary schools and 5% were without education at all.

1/3 respondents aged 75-89 led a lonely life, ¼ in aged 65-74 and 1/5 in aged 90 years old and older. There were 21% individuals living temporarily or permanently in nursing homes. The number of respondents living in nursing houses increased with the aging. In the study group, 64% of women and 60% of men lived in urban areas. Approximately 1/3 of women and men led a lonely life; ½ of men and women lived with family and about 1/5 lived in nursing homes. The loneliness in the majority concerned older groups of respondents. In the study 51% of individuals were widowers and widows, 6% were single, 6% divorced or separated. Only 36% were in marriage and 0.4% in concubine. There were 26% of women who had a partner (at the time of research) and 74% led a lonely life. There were 42% of men who led a lonely life. In urban areas there were more subjects living alone (69%) than in rural areas (52%).

Individuals participating in the study most often suffered from cardiovascular diseases - CVD (87%), diseases of locomotor system (63%), respiratory system (25%), urinary system (22%) and other (less than 2% each). 4% of subjects were healthy (without any disease) and 16% of respondents were without any complaints. The number of respondents with complaints increased with age. There were two fold healthy men (6%) than women (3%) in the study. CVDs were the main health problem in every age group (86-89%). The prevalence of locomotor diseases, urinary system diseases and ophtalmological problems (cataract or glaucoma) increased with age. The prevalence of endocrine system diseases and neoplastic diseases and mood disorders decreased with age in the study group. Women suffered more frequently from CVDs, urinary system and locomotor system diseases, while men more frequently declared respiratory system diseases. Among CVDs were recognized most often: peripheral blood vessel diseases (veins and arteries – 67%) heart diseases (59%) and arterial hypertension (51%). In the large group of declared heart diseases most common were ischaemic heart diseases (29%) and dysrrhythmia (26%). Among locomotor system diseases more frequently degeneration diseases (78%) and osteoporosis with complications were found.

Respondents more frequently complained from: headaches and dizziness (answers for open questions - 26%), pain caused by osteoarticular system pathologies (21%), CVDs (15%), digestive system (10%), sense organs and other pain (10%). Women slightly more often (18%) reported ailments than men (15%). Women more often notified dizziness and headaches, locomotor system ailments caused by prosthesis or digestive system complains.

Men more often reported sense organs pathology, postoperative or postinjury complaints and pain.

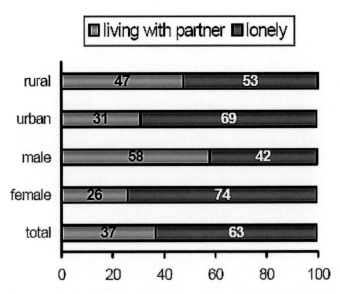

Figure 4. The status of household.

There was 47% of the study group who were disabled. It was noted that among disabled respondents, 1/5 was in the first degree of disability (the hardest cases, immobility – category I) and 1/10 was in the third degree. Slightly more frequently men (49%) than women (47%) and respondents from urban areas (48%) than from rural areas (45%) were disabled. The number of people without disability recognized in legal terms increased with age (but increased formal disability). There were 50% of disabled individuals in age 65-74, 44% in age 75-89 and 34% in 90+ groups. Among people aged over 75 years old, first disability category was found more frequently, whereas among younger respondents (aged 65-74 years old) second disability category was found more often. The number of people with third degree of disability category was lowest. Locomotor system diseases (38%) and CVDs (36%) were the most common reasons for movement confinements. These diseases caused more often (2-3 times) immobilization and serious movement confinements (movement difficulties) in comparison with other diseases. For both men and women locomotor system diseases were the first reason of movement confinements. In the understudied group, 36% of women and 26% of men declared locomotor system diseases as the reason of movement problems, and 25% of women and 30% of men - CVDs. The movement difficulties (different intensity) caused by these system diseases were declared more often by rural inhabitants. Locomotor system diseases and CVDs caused the biggest dynamic of increment of disabled persons with the aging process.

Ambulatory care was supplied by outpatients' clinics – GP (68%), specialist's clinics (25%), nursing houses (20%) and private clinics (15%). Only 5% of respondents did not use any medical assistance and 2% of individuals chose "non-conventional medical" help (paramedics, herbalist and bioenergotherapist). Medical supply by the specialists clinics and private medical care decreased with age and also the of nursing homes and private GPs visits and persons not using any medical help increased with age. There were more untreated (in medical meaning) men then women (7% v. 4%) and untreated rural individuals than urban residents (6% v. 4%). There was two fold women (2.5%) than men (1.2%) and rural inhabitants (2.7%) than urban residents (1.8%) used paramedic's help. Rural inhabitants (74%) more often used outpatient district clinics care and less often used specialist's clinics (town – 27%, country – 22%), private medical help, private clinics and nursing homes (town – 22%, country – 14%).

During the last five years, half of the respondents were hospitalized. The percentage of hospitalized men and women in rural and in urban areas were similar. The main reason for hospitalization was exacerbation of chronic diseases (61%). There were 31% hospitalized respondents because of a new disease or disorder, about 10% were due to diagnostic procedures or injury. Women were two times more frequently hospitalized due to planned diagnostic procedures or injury, whereas men were more often hospitalized because of decompensation of chronic diseases or a newly recognized disease or disorder. Urban residents were hospitalized slightly more often because of procedures or injury, whereas rural residents because of exacerbation of chronic disease and newly recognized disease or disorder. The hospitalization due to a new recognized disease or disorder and injury event was increased with age and hospitalization caused by planned diagnostics procedures decreased with the age of respondents. Hospitalization caused by decompensation of chronic disease was similar in the age group 65-89 years old (about 60%) and a little bit lower in the oldest age group (54%).

Individuals with normal Body Mass Index (BMI) constituted 47% of all respondents, overweight and obese respondents – 45% and underweight – 8%. The percentage of underweight persons was similar among men and women (7% v. 8%). There more overweight and obese women then men (49% v. 38%). The number of overweight and obese rural residents was higher than in urban areas residents (48% v. 44%) and also the number of underweight persons was lower (7% v. 9%). The prevalence of the underweight increased and the overweight and obesity decreased with age.

In the study group 84% of the respondents declared the progress or appearance of some new problems caused by growing old. More than half of respondents (despite of demographic determinants as gender, accommodation and age) declared lower energy (hypothymia) and unnecessity to be active. These were the main problems of senility pointed out by respondents. Individuals also declared financial (40%) and housekeeping (34%) problems. There were about 10% respondents with relationship problems, 12% with newly formed relationships, 11% contacts keeping with family and 10% of respondents declared problems with keeping contacts with acquaintances. Only 5% of respondents (the lowest percentage) declared problems with contact keeping with friends. There were 13% of women and about 20% of men who noted no problems at all. The financial problems (42% v. 35%), housekeeping problems (39% v. 25%) and necessity to be active (57% v. 53%) were more often pointed out by women than by men. Social problems (15% v. 11%) and contact keeping problems with friends were declared slightly often by men than by women. Urban residents more frequently than rural residents declared the contact keeping with friends as a problem. The housekeeping and house-organizing problems on the rural area were more often observed. The percentage of people with housekeeping and house-organizing problems, followed by relationship problems, family and friend contact keeping problems increased with age. Declared financial troubles decreased with age.

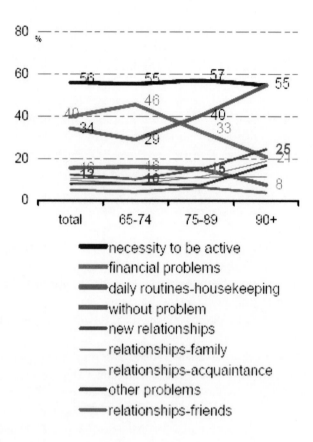

Figure 5. Declared problems by respondents (%).

Examined people assessed their family ties and relationships (life partner). The relationship with the life partner was evaluated as good and very good by 43% of respondents. Men defined their relations positively twice more frequently than women (61% v. 33%). Rural residents evaluated partner relationships better then urban residents (51% v. 38%). The percentage of positively assessed partners' relationships decreased with the age of respondents. Simultaneously the percentage of lack of response on this part of questionnaire increased with age.

The kind of help that was most required by respondents included daily-living routines (56%) and the sense of assurance (53%). A smaller number of individuals pointed out the necessity "to be useful for next of kin" (38%) and "to be loved by others" (29%) and some of them emphasized the role of any incidental help (20%). Women and urban residents were less frequently satisfied due to " be necessary and loved" and also these expectations were rarely fulfilled by family members in older groups. There were 52% of respondents who felt lonely; 20% of them permanently and 33% occasionally had this feeling. The percentage of feeling lonely increased with age (both permanent and incidental). Women felt lonely slightly more frequent than men. About 69% of respondents suffered from depression, several times a week

(16%) and also several times a month (16%). The percentage of depressed respondents increased with age. Generally lonely people, especially women, were more frequently depressed.

The health status was self-assessed as good and pretty good by 23% of respondents and as bad and very bad by 28% of individuals. Women self-assessed their health status more critically than men (the positive opinion on health status was more frequent among men than among women 28% v. 21% and also men evaluated less negatively their health).

The assessment of health status was well done similarly by rural and urban residents (23% v. 24%), but the negative opinion on health status (bad and very bad status) were given by rural residents (31% v. 26%). The number of positive opinions on health status was decreased with the age and simultaneously the number of negative opinions increased with the age of respondents.

In the study group the great number –1,679 of respondents were active in a different range (88%): 110 individuals (6%) took on only low intensity physical activities (as partly some housework, shopping, meals cooking, walks and other daily activities). There were 747 people (39%) took on medium intensity activities (independent housework, occasionally undertaken physical training, gardening) and 822 respondents (43%) took on high level intensity of activities (working out, regular physical training as gymnastics and others).

Intellectually active people constituted 10% of all respondents (differential aspects of intellectual activities) and civil active individuals constituted 36%. The majority of them (486 people - 25%) helped their family (take care of family members and others, housekeeping etc.) There were 198 respondents (10%) who declared more spectacular civil activity (help for non-family member, religious activities, political, NGOs and activities in other associations).

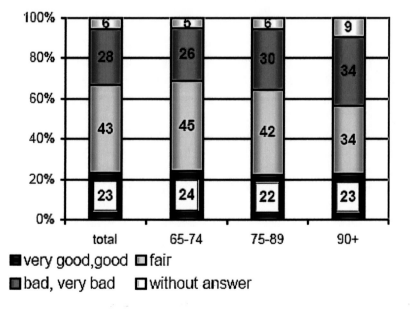

Figure 6a. Perceived health.

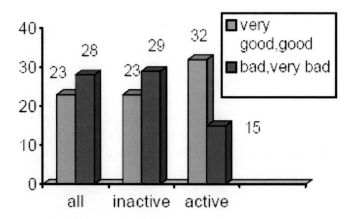

Figure 6b. Perceived health (extreme evaluation).

Impact of the Activity on Health Status

(1) *Active People Considered their Health Status More Positively*. Active respondents more frequently assessed their health status as good or pretty good (32%) than non active respondents (23%). Simultaneously active people evaluated their health status as bad and very bad more rarely then non active seniors (15% vs. 29%)

Worse self-assessment of health status was accompanied with the increasing of movement problems (r=0.34 p≤0.05) and also increasing number of CVDs (heart diseases r=0.25 p≤0.05 and peripheral vessel diseases r=0.2 p≤0.05). Less active respondents declared the lower level kind of efforts (r=0.2 p≤0.05) and they also declared depressive feelings more often (r=0.2 p≤0.05).

(2) *Majority of Respondents Declared that their Health Condition has Deteriorated Drastically at the Age of 63-64*.(See Figure 7)

(3) *Active Persons were Less Frequently Hospitalize*. Non-active respondents were admitted to the hospital more frequently than active respondents were in the period of last 5 years (p<0.05). The most common reason for hospitalization was chronic disease decompensation. The risk of hospitalization was 1.6 times greater for non-active people. Non-active people were significantly more often hospitalized because of chronic disease decompensation (p<0.05). The risk of hospitalization caused by this reason was two times bigger than the hospitalization event of active people. Active people were less frequently hospitalized due to injury or accidents and also more frequently because of planned diagnostics procedures or their new complains (p=NS).

(4) *The Prevalence of CVDs was Lower in the Group of Active Respondents or the Course of the Diseases as more Stabile*.

Non-active people suffered more frequently from peripheral vessels diseases (intermittent claudication p<0.005 OR=1.97). The heart diseases such as coronary heart disease, dysrhythmia and others were less frequently declared by active respondents (taking on different kinds of activities: physical, pro-social and intellectual) than non-active respondents (p=0.005 OR=0.6)

(5) *The Declared Physical Efficiency of Active Individuals* (Physical and Pro-Social Activities) was better than Non-active Respondents and also Non-active Individuals more Frequently Suffered from Mobility Problems (P<0.01).

The increasing problems of seniors' mobility limited their activity level.

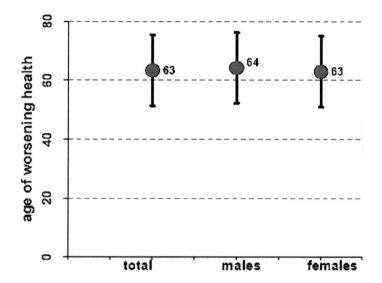

Figure 7.

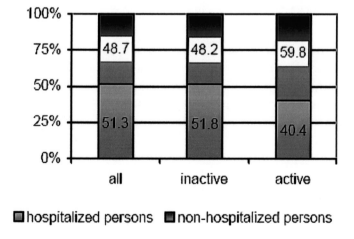

Figure 8. The hospitalization of respondents in 1994-1999 (p<0.05).

(6) *Active Seniors had Better Psychological Wellbeing.*

Non-active respondents emphasized more frequently that the senility process brings new difficulties of existing (p<0.01 OR=2.07). Active seniors declared less frequently the troubles caused by senility (physically active respondents – p=0.03

OR=0.5, intellectually active – p<0.01 OR=0.6, physically and pro-socially active – p=0.003 OR=0.6). Non-active individuals more frequently declared the feelings of loneliness (periodic loneliness p<0.05). Active persons significantly less frequently noted the feelings of loneliness (p<0.05). In the study group the correlation between depression and feelings of loneliness was revealed (p≤0.05 r=0.30). Non-active respondents (significantly) more frequently evaluated their relationship with partners positively (p<0.01 OR=6.9) but also active persons more often were satisfied by relationships with others. Feelings of their necessity (p <0.05) and satisfaction in private life (p <0.05) caused this satisfaction.

(7) *Biological and Legal Disability of Respondents (Except I Category of Disability and Immobilization) did not Limited the Activity Taking*

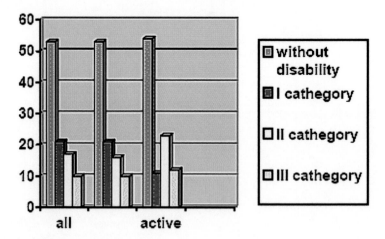

Figure 9. Disability In Study Group (%).

Approximately half of the study group (active and non-active persons) had no legal disability category. In the active group the most frequent II category of disability was predicated (medium kind of disability) – 23%, meanwhile in the none-active group the most frequent I category of disability was predicated (the hardest disability level) – 21%. Significant differences were noted among active and non-active groups in I disability category range (p<0.05).

(8) *Diseases did not Exclude the Activities, Except the Pathologies, which Restricted or Eliminated any Kind of Activities.*

In the group understudy the significant differences (the prevalence of diseases and complains) among active and non-active people were observed only in the frequency of peripherial vessels diseases (intermittent claudication p<0.005) and ophtalmological diseases such as cataracts (p<0.05). Moving problems concerned both groups. The differences, measured by frequency of events, were not significant in each level of movement's limitation except for complete immobilization.

(9) *The Barrier in Taking Activity were Lower Needs to become Active ("Smaller Motor")*

No active respondents were significantly less willing to become active (p<0.05 OR=1.7).

(10) *The Activities had a Positive Impact on Keeping a Proper Body Weight (Measured by BMI.*

Non-active people were overweight or obese more frequently (p<0.01), while among the active people no obese person was noted.

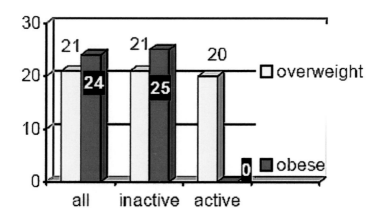

Figure 10. Overweight and obesity in study group.

Discussion

Analysis of the results has confirmed the presence of the relation between the taken activities and health status. The relation between activity and the lower prevalence of CVDs (heart and peripheral blood vessels diseases) was indicated. It confirms the fact of positive influence of the activity taking (or continuity) over the age of 65 on adequate efficiency maintenance and the smaller prevalence of the civilization-related diseases (like CVDs) [9, 11]. This dependence can be more complex due to multifactoral reasons. Also the activity may decide the lack of pathology, and the presence of the diseases can limit the activity. In this study we accepted that the elderly activities are caused by earlier active life style (behaviors).

Active seniors were hospitalized rarely, and the risk of hospitalization was 1.6 times higher for non-active people in the study group. Non-active people were admitted to the hospital more frequently because of chronic disease exacerbation. That is probably the consequence of a more labile clinical health status of non-active persons and the higher risk of the decompensation of their chronic diseases.

The moving problems (except complete immobilization) did not exclude the activities in the group's understudy. The main reason of moving restriction was caused by locomotive system diseases – 29.3% of active persons and 32.3% of no active persons. The next reasons for disability were CVDs, then the respiratory diseases and the others. According to the Central Statistical Office in Poland the main reasons for Polish elderly disability were caused by CVDs and locomotive diseases [5]. The most direct relation between limited mobility and activity was concerning the physical activity (OR=2.5 p<0.01) and pro-social activity (OR=1.6 p<0.01).

The prevalence of CVDs and the highest mortality in this group are connected with excessive body weight (measured by BMI). Also overweight conditions and obesity are the risk factors of many diseases as follows: respiratory system, osteoarticular and digestive systems diseases and its complications. In the active respondents group there were more underweight people than in the non-active respondents group (p<0.01). Also the active persons were rarely overweight (p<0.01). All obese people were recruited from the non-active group. This confirmed the profitable influence of activities on maintenance of appropriate body weight [11, 18].

The self-assessment of seniors' health status has prognostic meaning. It was assessed that health self-assessment corresponds to 60-70% to real biological health status. There are many other factors, which may influence the health assessment such as real health status (physical, functional), activity, age, gender, socio-economical status and education level [19].

The results of the research confirmed the relation between self-assessment of health status and the health status, measured by the presence of diseases and category and ethiology of disability. Worse self-assessment on health status was connected with the presence of circulatory system pathologies (diseases of heart and blood vessels) and mobile problems (mainly caused by diseases of locomotive and circulatory systems).

Analysis of the results confirmed that the retirement on pension is a negative factor of health status and its self-assessment [7]. The worsening of the health status of all respondents was indicated on the average age of 63-64 years (S.D. ± 12).

Among many determinants of satisfying and healthy aging are mentioned as follows: the health factors, psycho-social agents such as positive relationships, satisfied life occurrence and the presence of the goals [10, 19]. Emotional status of respondents (deteriorated by the depression) was correlated with the health status self-assessment. It can confirm the close relation between biological and emotional health status as well [20]. Simultaneously active people assessed their health status and also the level of their activity more positively.

One of the crucial problems for the people over 65 years old is caused by the inconvenience in daily routines (– activities daily living) [8]. That is why the majority of respondents (56%) needed help – offered by the relatives. Non-active respondents declared more frequently the presence of housekeeping problems and the risk of this event was 1.8 times lower among active respondents. The differences between active and non-active individuals were less willing to become active. Non-active respondents 1.7 times more frequently declared less energy and so less needs to become active than active respondents. It seems that the activity is caused by necessity (except extreme biological limits - disability). Therefore the motivation of this age group and also younger adults plays the fundamental and special role in health promotion for healthy aging.

Active respondents (physically, pro-socially and intellectually) rarely noticed problems and difficulties connected with aging. The risk of difficulties connected with the old age for physically active people was 0.5 times lower than for inactive, for intellectually active people is 0.6 times lower, and for physically and pro-socially (both activities) – 0.7 times lower. It means that the activity and its many forms (physical, pro-social and intellectual) has protective meaning in number of problems which is growing with age (efficiency, philosophy of life, attitude, coping).

Equally important are the elements of people's ability to function after 65 with other people, for example with life partner, friends and families [21, 22]. In the elderly group an understudy in the psycho-social health sphere found that there is a relation between depression and sense of loneliness. Sense of loneliness caused by legal status and hindered relations with relatives ("empty nest", disability, psychical barriers and other difficulties), causes the lonely people to be in the group of risk amounted to [19]. Lonely people constituted 65% of the active respondents and 63% of inactive people. In spite a of similar percentage of lonely people in both groups, inactive respondents more frequently confirmed the periodic sense of loneliness and the risk of this sense was 1.8 times greater (frequency) among non-active people. Analytically the people who suffered from depression had worse results (in their self-assessment of health condition).

Conclusion

Active people (intellectually, pro-socially and physically) after 65 are healthier and more able-bodied, and are less often hospitalized. Absence of physical, pro-social and intellectual activity is not always caused by pathology coexistence. Propagation of activity should concern every age group and should be continued during pensionable age. Activity deciding about healthy aging and is simultaneously an indicator of positive aging.

References

[1]   Golinowska, S; Holzer, J; Szwarc, H; Pędich, W. Starzenie się i starość; pojęcia, tendencje, cechy i struktury. Raport o rozwoju społecznym Polska 1999. *Warszawa: UNDP;* 1999; 7-13.

[2]   Jabłońska-Chmielewska A. Podstawowe wiadomości o demografii lekarskiej. Jabłoński, L, editor. *Epidemiologia.* Lublin: Folium; 1996; 39-51.

[3]   Jabłoński, L. Mierniki zdrowia. *Zdrowie w medycynie i naukach społecznych.* 2000: 39-55.

[4]   Magdzik, W; Naruszewicz-Lesiuk, D; Czarkowski, MP. Sytuacja demograficzna Polski w latach 1950-1998 i prognoza jej rozwoju do 2050 roku. *Przegląd Epidemiologiczny,* 2000 54, 201-225.

[5]   GUS. Seniorzy w polskim społeczeństwie 1999. Warszawa: *GUS;* 1999.

[6]   Indulski, J; Kowaleski, J. Proces starzenia się populacji jako determinanta sytuacji zdrowotnej oraz popytu na usługi w ochronie zdrowia. Sytuacja zdrowotna osób w starszym wieku w Polsce, *aspekt medyczny i społeczno-demograficzny.* 1998: 65-73.

[7]   Kopczyński, J. Choroby cywilizacyjne przyszłości. Aktualne problemy zdrowotne, zagrożenia i szanse. *Warszawa: Ignis;* 1999; 61-3.

[8]   WHO. The elderly in eleven countries. A sociomedical survey. Copenhagen: *WHO;* 1983.

[9]   Buchner, DM; Beresford, SA; Larson, EB; et al. Effects of physical activity on health status in older adults. II intervention studies. Annu. Rev. Public Health, 1992 13, 469-88.

[10] Szwarc, H. Profilaktyka starzenia. Analizy i opinie. Geriatria i gerontologia. *Warszawa;* 1975: 88-91.

[11] WHO. Cardiovascular care of the elderly. Geneva: *WHO;* 1987.

[12] Miller, M; Gębska-Kuczerowska, A. Ocena stanu zdrowia ludzi w starszym wieku w Polsce. *Gerontologia Polska*, 1998 VI (3-4), 18-23.

[13] Roszkowska, H; Goryński, P; Seroka, W. Stan zdrowia osób w wieku starszym w świetle danych o hospitalizacji. *Warszawa: PZH*; 1999.

[14] Wnuk-Lipiński, E; Golinowska, S; Topińska, I; Błędowski, P; Włodarczyk, C. Społeczeństwo i państwo wobec ludzi starszych. Opieka zdrowotna i usługi pielęgnacyjne dla ludzi starszych. Raport o rozwoju społecznym. Polska 1999. *Warszawa: UNDP;* 1999; 64-74.

[15] WHO. Ageing – exploding the myths. *WHO*; 1999.

[16] WHO. Agita Mundo, move for health. *WHO*; 2002.

[17] WHO. World Health Day 07.04.02. Move for health. *WHO*; 2002.

[18] Szałtynis, D; Kochańczyk, T. Sport dla wszystkich. Aktywność fizyczna w promocji zdrowego starzenia. *Warszawa: TKKF*; 1997.

[19] Tobiasz-Adamczyk, B. *Wybrane elementy socjologii zdrowia i choroby*. Kraków: UJ; 2000; 97-115.

[20] Beekman, AT; Deeg, DJ; Bramm, AW et al. Consequences of major and minor depression in later life: study of disability, wellbeing and service utilization. *Psychol. Med.* 1997 27(6) XI, 1397-409.

[21] Dyczewski, L; Adamczuk, L; Szatur-Jaworska, B et al. Potrzeby ludzi starszych uniwersalne i specyficzne. Raport o rozwoju społecznym Polska 1999. *Warszawa: UNDP*; 1999; 27-46.

[22] Golinowska, S; Wygnański, J; Żukowski, T. Ludzie starsi dla siebie oraz dla społeczeństw. Raport o rozwoju społecznym Polska 1999. *Warszawa: UNDP*; 1999; 75-96.

Index

D

E

incidence, viii, ix, 9, 15, 18, 19, 21, 24, 27, 30, 34, 38, 39, 40, 42, 47, 59, 63, 85, 130, 161, 166, 167, 173, 182, 183, 184, 185, 186, 187, 191, 195, 198, 199, 200, 201, 202, 203, 204, 208, 246

inclusion, 199

income(s), 152, 184, 234, 246, 254, 260, 272, 274, 275

increased access, 234

incubation, 96, 106, 108, 110, 159, 167

incubation period, 96, 106, 108, 110, 167

independent variable, vii, 2, 220

India, 183, 260

indication, 111

indicators, 127, 218

indigenous, 168

indirect effect, 22

individual characteristics, 217

individual differences, 242

individual students, 259

Indonesia, 149, 152, 183

induction, 67, 160

industrial, 142, 152

industrialized countries, 11

industry, 111, 142, 143, 171

inefficiency, 281

inequality, 210, 239

infancy, 201

infants, 98, 125, 132, 133, 201, 210

infarction, 13, 14

infectious disease(s), ix, x, 51, 85, 86, 89, 129, 181, 182, 183, 184, 189, 201, 202, 207, 208, 209, 210, 211, 212, 273

infestations, 257, 259

inflammation, 10, 18, 31, 33, 50, 51, 53, 55

inflammatory, 11, 12, 20, 21, 50

inflammatory disease, 50

inflammatory response, 12, 20

inflation, 205

influenza, 138, 142, 200, 211

information exchange, 273

ingestion, 17, 24, 25, 36, 45, 90, 132, 148, 167

inhibition, 17, 37, 159

inhibitor(s), 17, 43

initiation, 31, 107, 216, 218, 245, 246

injection(s), 14, 15, 46

injuries, 41, 78, 250

injury, 10, 12, 33, 142, 257, 285, 288

injustice, 251

innate immunity, 124

inoculation, 100, 179

insertion, vii, 1, 3, 4, 5, 6

insight, 241

inspections, 202

inspectors, 106

institutions, 90, 105, 111, 235, 240, 241, 277

instruction, ix, 18, 130, 183

instructors, 202

instruments, 18, 74, 258

insulin, 19, 20, 22, 23, 59, 61

insurance, 258

integration, 10, 23, 241, 242

integrin, 178

integrity, 32, 84

intensity, 37, 284, 287

intensive care unit, 212, 213

intentions, 243

interaction, vii, ix, 2, 3, 6, 11, 43, 130, 158, 159, 217, 238, 247, 257

interactions, vii, 1, 17, 57, 72, 91, 230, 240

interest, 223, 238, 239

interface, 92

interferon, 201

interleukins, 201

international, xi, 16, 58, 96, 124, 127, 171, 219, 245, 246, 249, 256, 259

internet, 235, 241

interpretation, 2, 5, 271

interstitial, 39

interval, 220

intervention, 15, 35, 50, 62, 64, 120, 138, 152, 183, 184, 185, 186, 187, 188, 189, 190, 191, 192, 193, 194, 195, 197, 198, 199, 200, 201, 202, 203, 204, 205, 206, 207, 208, 209, 210, 217, 218, 237, 238, 239, 241, 256, 294

intervention strategies, 152, 218

interview(s), xi, 184, 244, 245, 263, 269, 270

intestinal flora, 173

intestinal tract, 156

intestine, 131, 156, 157, 158, 160, 161, 165

intima, 55

intraoperative, 13

intravascular, 14

intravenous, 13, 18, 37, 98

intravenous fluids, 98

intravenously, 37

intrinsic, 16, 25

invading organisms, 14

invasive, 10, 12, 15, 16, 17, 21, 23, 26, 28, 33, 35, 44, 60, 61

investigations, 110, 137, 171, 257

S

T

U

V